120 Careers in the Health Care Field

2nd Edition

Stanley Alperin

Lisa A. Rose
Research Director

U.S. Directory Service, Publishers
655 N.W. 128 Street • Miami, Florida 33168

"A Trusted Source for Healthcare Information For Nearly A Quarter Century"

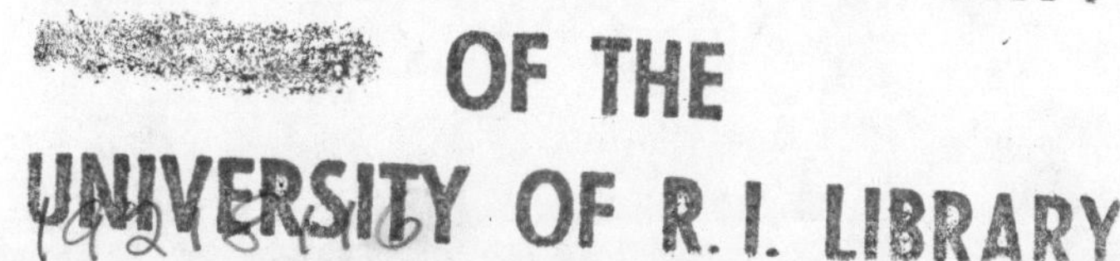

Printed in U.S.A.
Manufactured in U.S.A.

Federal ID Number 59-1387-264
Duns Number 07-600-0397

Published & Distributed Worldwide by

U.S. Directory Service
655 N.W. 128 Street
P.O. Box 1700
Miami, Florida 33168-2735 • U.S.A.
(305) 769-1700
Fax (305) 769-0548

International Standard Book Number: 0-916524-31-0
(First edition 0-88410-709-4)

Library of Congress Catalog Card Number: 79-53587

Stock Number: 102
120 Careers in the Health Care Field, 2nd edition

CONTENTS

PREFACE

This handbook is a concise, yet factual, reference source for careers in allied health. It is written primarily as a counseling guide for high school students but may also be used by community college students, by guidance counselors, healthcare recruiters, by persons who have been out of the work force for a period of time and wish to return, and for those who want to change careers. The discussion of each allied health career or occupational title in this handbook includes all or more of the following descriptions: job functions and responsibilities, work locations, training prerequisites and requirements, certification procedures, if applicable, recommended high school courses, financial aid information, potential salaries, and a list of community colleges, universities, vocational-technical schools, and other educational institutions that provide accredited training programs.

This is the second volume series of its kind to describe the range of careers in allied health and also to contain lists of schools in the United States that offer accredited training.

Compiled with reliable data obtained from medical and allied health associations and societies and from government publications, the information in this handbook is as current and as accurate as possible; however, because of the rapidly changing nature of scientific developments in medicine, the continued accreditation of new training programs, and the inflationary structure of wages, the publishers of the handbook cannot assume responsibility or liability for unintentional errors or omissions.

INTRODUCTION

This handbook describes the occupations and training of allied health personnel including administrators, assistants, auxiliary workers, technicians, technologists, and therapists. The handbook also includes- as its major feature- the listing of accredited training programs for most allied health occupations.

The student interested in a health-related career who finds it impossible or undesirable to meet the high costs and standards of education required by medical and dental schools should investigate a career in allied health. These careers represent excellent job opportunities in the ever-expanding fields of healthcare services and medical research and provide many of the same satisfactions, challenges, and benefits that are experienced by physicians, dentists, veterinarians, chiropractors, podiatrists, optometrists, pharmacists, and other professional medical practitioners- but with much less expensive, shorter, and less rigorous training requirements.

The reason for the present expansion in health services, which is causing a situation of demand exceeding supply in allied health personnel, is the increased demand for healthcare by the growing national population. People are living longer, and they have an increasing ability to pay for their healthcare, both because of higher personal incomes and because of the growth of public and private health insurance plans. Medical research is increasing the need for skilled allied health personnel, too, as it constantly develops new and specialized techniques and procedures for diagnosing, treating, and preventing diseases, illnesses, and injuries.

Though certain careers in allied health have been traditionally limited to either men or women in the past, the trend is now changing. Both men and women have equal opportunities for admittance into all training programs, for receiving financial aid, and for job placement.

There are certain personal qualifications all health workers must possess including good health, emotional stability, and an ability and desire to work with and help the sick and the injured. Healthcare personnel must also be accurate, thorough, responsible, sympathetic, versatile, and possess a willingness to keep abreast of new medical procedures and technical equipment. They must have an interest and aptitude for biological and physical sciences, and some, especially technologists and technicians, must be able to operate complicated electronic equipment and delicate instrumentation.

Many occupations in allied health, especially those of assistants or aides who work for physicians in their private practices, are excellent opportunities for persons who wish to work part-time in a health-related career.

According to the Bureau of Labor Statistics, more than eight million people work in health-related occupations in the United States, and projected employment in this industry is expected to reach over eleven million by the year 2000. The majority of healthcare workers are employed in hospitals while the remainder are employed by clinics, laboratories, nursing homes, research institutes, public health services, mental health facilities, private medical practices, and pharmaceutical companies. Health-related personnel are also employed by industry to administer basic healthcare and emergency first aid to workers, to inspect equipment and assure that safety measures are followed and to act as technical advisors and representatives in the manufacturing and marketing of medical equipment and supplies.

For the person planning a career in allied health, the education and training he or she receives is of extreme significance when applying for good, well-paying jobs. Educational requirements vary as much as the range of careers in allied health, and the selection of an appropriate training program is a major decision that will later influence job placement opportunities.

Educational requirements in allied health vary from one-to-two-months of on-the-job training to graduation from a master's degree program. This handbook has limited its selection of health-related careers to those that require a maximum of a bachelor's degree as their educational requirement; that is, with practically all of the careers described herein a student can be in the work force earning a reasonably good salary within one-to-four years after graduation from high school. However, a few careers listed require further education.

Most allied health occupations at the professional level, such as those of dietitian, physical therapist, and medical record administrator, require bachelor's degrees to obtain employment in all but supervising, teaching, and research positions where a master's degree is needed. In most paraprofessional occupations, that is, those carried out by technologists, technicians, and assistants, graduation with an associate degree or certificate awarded by a community (junior) college or vocational-technical school is required. Aides and auxiliary workers who occupy entry-level positions are usually trained on-the-job in hospitals and in other health services facilities. It should be noted that the U.S. Armed Forces offer training in many health career occupations, and persons interested in combining a career in the military and in healthcare should contact their local recruiting office.

The lists of educational programs contained in this handbook are comprised, for the most part, solely of programs that are accredited by their respective professional associations or societies or by the Committee on Allied Health Education and Accreditation of the American Medical Association. Graduates from accredited programs have much better chances of being hired for the jobs they desire, especially as some employers will not hire graduates of nonaccredited programs. Graduation from an accredited program is also often a major criterion for certification, or registration, with an occupation's respective professional health association.

In a few cases a school list will also include programs that are not accredited but have their accreditation pending. Where there are no accreditation procedures available for an occupation, all known schools offering programs are listed.

For some careers, such as for aides and auxiliary workers, there are training programs offered by hospitals, however the trend is for most allied health workers to obtain formal training in their respective occupation. It is beyond the scope of this handbook to list all hospital training programs. Employers often prefer graduates of universities, colleges, or vocational-technical schools because of their more well-rounded education that includes both classroom and clinical experience. Many hospital teaching programs are currently becoming associated with universities and colleges and thus providing their students with a more academic education. Hospital training programs, however, usually charge little or no tuition and in some cases even pay a minimal salary during training. For further information, persons interested in hospital training programs in a specific occupation, should contact their local hospital.

The reader is reminded that the listing of nonhospital educational programs are as current and accurate as possible. Omissions may occur, however, as new programs are constantly being accredited by their respective professional associations.

Persons interested in applying to a specific program should contact the school as early as possible. Considerable care should be taken in selecting a program, and information should be obtained on the following:

- entrance prerequisites
- length of program
- accreditation qualifications
- type of degree or certificate offered
- tuition and other costs
- types of employment obtained by recent graduates
- length of time the program has been operating
- types of scholarships and financial aid
- instructional facilities
- faculty qualifications

The potential student should apply to as many schools as reasonable to compare these data in different programs.

Where available, certification or registration by a professional health association is definitely beneficial to the allied health worker. Certification usually requires graduation from an accredited training program, successful completion of written or clinical examinations, and some work experience. The benefits of certification, however, include proof to future employers of the health worker's qualification, accessibility to a greater range of jobs, higher salaries, and greater potential for job advancement.

The data in the handbook on salaries are at best broad indicators of average incomes in recent years. The data are by no means completely accurate because salaries are affected by individual duties and responsibilities of each particular job, geographic location of employer, local hiring and salary policies, amount and quality of training and work experience, and fluctuating rates of inflation. In general, salaries are usually higher in industry than in government; they are usually higher in urban areas than in rural areas; and they are usually higher on the East and West coasts than in the rest of the country. Finally, although training and experience are probably the most important factors in determining individual salaries, the exact amount of any salary is often negotiable.

Most hospital employees work a 36-to-40 hour week that often includes working on Saturdays and Sundays. Overtime is also sometimes required. Fringe benefits for hospital employees usually include paid vacations, health insurance, and sick leave. Some hospitals even provide free education courses, pension programs, uniforms, and salaries for on-the-job training. Work surroundings in hospitals and in other healthcare facilities are usually bright, clean, and comfortable. But even though salaries, fringe benefits, and working conditions are favorable, the most satisfying reward for most healthcare workers is their own personal gratification of being able to provide humanitarian services to people and to relieve pain and suffering.

For the student interested in a career in allied health the handbook mentions recommended courses he or she should take while in high school. Good high school grades are important, especially in certain occupations where there is competition for the relatively few training facilities. In general, high school students should study biology, health, chemistry, physics, mathematics, and English. Being able to communicate effectively is also very important in health services, and the student should maximize his or her writing and speaking skills. A second language is often beneficial in applying for certain jobs in some areas of the country.

To develop an interest and prepare for a career in allied health, students should talk with their school guidance counselors and science teachers or with admissions counselors in schools of allied health. Students should also visit hospitals and other health facilities and talk with their respective personnel directors; or they should write to their state health departments to inquire about that state's particular healthcare needs and about career and training opportunities in their city or town. Students interested in locating hospitals in their area should refer to the *Hospital Phone Book,* published by U.S. Directory Service Publishers, 655 N.W. 128 Street, P.O. Box 68-1700, Miami, Florida 33168, a complete name and address book of hospitals in the United States. The health departments of all fifty states are listed in Appendix A. Students may also inquire about health careers, by writing to Career Information, American Hospital Association, 840 N. Lake Shore Drive, Chicago, Illinois 60611.

Volunteer programs are an excellent way for students to determine if they have the aptitude and interest to enter a career in the health field. Volunteers actively participate in and perform necessary functions in a variety of health facilities and many volunteer programs exist including those sponsored by the American Red Cross, the American Healthcare Association, and hospital teen volunteers or Candystripers. Students interested in becoming a volunteer should contact their local Red Cross office; the American Healthcare Association 1201 "L" Street, N.W., Washington, D.C. 20005; the American Society of Directors of Volunteer Services, 840 North Lake Shore Drive, Chicago, Illinois 60611; or the Director of Volunteer Services of their local healthcare facility. Sometimes preference for admission into training programs is given to those who have been volunteers while in high school.

Another source of acquiring experience in the health field while still in high school is by enrolling in cooperative health occupations, a work-study program offered by many high schools in which students receive part-time, on-the-job training and salaries in a health facility as part of their regular high school education.

A chapter on nursing is included in this handbook, but because of its scope, specific information on nursing careers is condensed. Those students interested in a career in nursing, should contact the American Nurses Association, 2420 Pershing Road, Kansas City, Missouri 64108, the National League for Nursing, 10 Columbus Circle, New York, New York 10019, or any of the above mentioned sources of health career information.

Membership in student healthcare organizations is also a valuable way to learn about health careers. One known organization, Health Occupations Students of America (HOSA), is a national vocational student organization for secondary, post-secondary, and adult students enrolled in a health occupations education course or instructional program. For information on this organization, write to: Health Occupations Students of America, 4108 Amon Carter Boulevard, Fort Worth, Texas 76155.

The author and the publisher wish to thank all the professional health associations and societies who have supplied the information used in compiling this handbook. A list of their addresses is included in the Acknowledgments as a reference source for additional information.

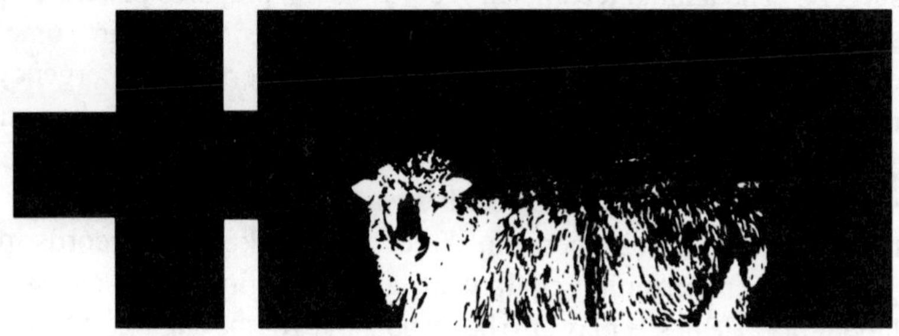

ANIMAL TECHNOLOGY

Animal technology is the allied health profession concerned with providing qualified technical support to the care, use, production, and husbandry of animals — both in animal health and in research. In animal health, the veterinarian, a doctor of veterinary medicine, treats sick and injured animals, and protects human health by preventing and controlling the spread of diseases transmissable from animals to humans. The assistance given by the animal technology team provides the veterinarian with more time to spend with his or her patients and clients. In research, conducted in clinical and research laboratories located in pharmaceutical companies, public health organizations, universities, hospitals, research institutions, and zoos, animals are essential for training surgeons and for testing the efficiency of drugs and numerous diagnostic, surgical and medical procedures. Scientists or senior technologists in the laboratory rely on the animal technology staff to assist them in the care and feeding of laboratory animals and in performing routine laboratory tests. Two careers in animal technology are those of the *animal technician* and *animal caretaker.*

Animal Technician

Also known as an *animal health technician* or as a *veterinary technician,* the animal technician is knowledgeable in animal care and handling and in routine laboratory and clinical procedures. The technician acts primarily as an assistant to veterinarians, biological research workers, and other scientists.

In veterinary practices the animal technician is supervised by the veterinarian and performs most of the same duties except those involving diagnosis, prescription, and surgery. The animal technician records cases; prepares patients, instruments, equipment and medication for surgery; collects specimens; assists in some medical procedures; dresses wounds; exposes and develops X-rays; performs emergency first aid; administers medication under the direction of the veterinarian; and consults with animal owners.

In clinical and research laboratories, the animal technician, often called a *laboratory animal technician*, is supervised by a scientist, or by a senior research or medical technologist, and may perform duties such as keeping records, performing laboratory procedures, maintaining equipment, and managing the business aspects of the animal laboratory. He or she may also be responsible for the caging, safety, basic health, sanitation and nutrition of the animals.

Most educational programs in animal technology are offered by community and junior colleges, are two years in length, and award associate degrees. There are a few four-year bachelor's degree programs also. Many veterinarians in private practice also conduct additional on-the-job training.

For animal technicians who are eligible and who have completed the academic and/or experience requirements, certification examinations are available from the Animal Technician Certification Board, sponsored by the American Association for Laboratory Animal Science. Nearly three-fourths (3/4) of the states presently require that practicing animal technicians be registered or certified. Certification requirements for animal technicians include successfully passing the certification examination, recommendation by supervisors and (1) high school diploma or equivalent, plus three years full time work as an animal technician in a laboratory animal facility with experience in animal care and use; or (2) graduation from an accredited two year program in animal technology, plus one year full time work in a laboratory animal facility.

Depending upon training and experience, average starting salaries for graduates of accredited animal technology programs equal $11,000 a year, while salaries for experienced graduates average $13,200, with some graduates earning salaries in the $20,000 range.

For more information on a career in animal technology write to the American Veterinary Medical Association, 930 North Meacham Road, Schaumburg, Illinois 60196. Certification information can be obtained through the American Association for Laboratory Animal Science, 70 Timber Creek Drive, Suite 5, Cordova, Tennessee 38019.

Following is a list of educational programs in animal technology, accredited by the American Veterinary Medical Association's Committee on Animal Technician Activities and Training. Two year programs are listed as well as a few that offer a four-year bachelor's degree. Four year programs are marked by an asterisk (*). Refer to the key below for each program's accreditation status.

KEY:

(1) Full accreditation

(2) Provisional or probational accreditation

SOURCES:
American Veterinary Medical Association
American Association for Laboratory Animal Science
Occupational Outlook Handbook

Animal Technician Programs

ALABAMA

Animal Hospital Technology Program (1)
Snead State Junior College
Boaz, Alabama 35957

CALIFORNIA

Animal Health Technology Program (1)
Cosumnes River College
8401 Center Parkway
Sacramento, California 95823

Animal Health Technician Program (1)
Hartnell College
156 Homestead Avenue
Salinas, California 93901

Animal Health Technology Program (2)
Los Angeles Pierce College
6201 Winnetka Avenue
Woodland Hills, California 91371

Animal Health Technology Program (1)
Mt. San Antonio College
1100 North Grand Avenue
Walnut, California 91789

Animal Health Technology Program (1)
San Diego Mesa College
7250 Mesa College Drive
San Diego, California 92111

Animal Health Technician Program (1)
Yuba College
2088 North Beale Road
Marysville, California 95901

COLORADO

Animal Health Technology Program (1)
Colorado Mountain College
Spring Valley Campus
3000 Colorado Road, 114
Glenwood Springs, Colorado 81601

Animal Technology Program (1)
Bel-Rea Institute of Animal Technology
1681 S. Dayton
Denver, Colorado 80231

CONNECTICUT

Laboratory Animal Technology Program (1,*)
Quinnipiac College
Mt. Carmel Avenue
Hamden, Connecticut 06518

FLORIDA

Veterinary Technology Program (1)
St. Petersburg Junior College
Box 13489
St. Petersburg, Florida 33733

GEORGIA

Veterinary Technology Program (1)
Abraham Baldwin Agricultural College
Box 8, ABAC Station
Tifton, Georgia 31793

Veterinary Technology Program (1)
Fort Valley State College
Fort Valley, Georgia 31030

ILLINOIS

Veterinary Technology Program (1)
Parkland College
2400 West Bradley Avenue
Champaign, Illinois 61821

INDIANA

Veterinary Technology Program (1)
Purdue University
School of Veterinary Medicine
West Lafayette, Indiana 47907

KANSAS

Animal Technology Program (1)
Colby Community College
1255 South Range
Colby, Kansas 67701

KENTUCKY

Veterinary Technology Program (1)
Morehead State University
Box 995
Morehead, Kentucky 40351

LOUISIANA

Veterinary Technology Program (1)
Northwestern State University of Louisiana
Dept. of Agricultural Sciences
Natchitoches, Louisiana 71457

MAINE

Animal Medical Technology Program (1)
University of Maine
Dept. of Animal & Veterinary Sciences
Orono, Maine 04473

MARYLAND

Animal Science Technology Program (1)
Essex Community College
7201 Rossville Blvd.
Baltimore, Maryland 21237

Animal Science Technology Program (2)
Essex Community College
Walter Reed Army Institute of Research
7201 Rossville Blvd.
Baltimore, Maryland 21237

MASSACHUSETTS

Veterinary Assistant Program (1)
Becker Junior College
1003 Old Main Street
Leicester, Massachusetts 01524

Veterinary Science Program (2,*)
Mount Ida College
777 Dedham Street
Newton Center, Massachusetts 02192

Animal Health Technician Program (1)
Newbury College
100 Summer Street
Holliston, Massachusetts 01746

MICHIGAN

Veterinary Technician Program (1)
Macomb Community College
Center Campus
44575 Garfield Road
Mt. Clemens, Michigan 48044

Veterinary Technology Program (1)
Michigan State University
College of Veterinary Medicine
East Lansing, Michigan 48823

Veterinary Technology Program (1)
Wayne Community College
c/o Wayne State University
540 East Canfield
Detroit, Michigan 48201

MINNESOTA

Veterinary Technician Program (1)
Medical Institute of Minnesota
2309 Nicollet Avenue
Minneapolis, Minnesota 55404

Animal Health Technology Program (2)
University of Minnesota
Waseca, Minnesota 56093

MISSOURI

Animal Health Technology Program (1)
Jefferson College
Hillsboro, Missouri 63050

Animal Health Technology Program (1)
Maple Woods Community College
2601 N.E. Barry Road
Kansas City, Missouri 64156

Animal Health Technology Program (1)
Northeast Missouri State University
Kirksville, Missouri 63501

NEBRASKA

Veterinary Technology Program (1)
University of Nebraska
School of Technical Agriculture
Curtis, Nebraska 69025

Animal Technician Program (2)
Omaha College of Health Careers
1052 Park Avenue
Omaha, Nebraska 68105

NEW JERSEY

Animal Science Technology Program (1)
Camden County College
P.O. Box 200
Blackwood, New Jersey 08012

NEW YORK

Animal Health Technology Program (2)
La Guardia Community College
The City University of New York
31-10 Thomson Avenue
Long Island City, New York 11101

Veterinary Science Technology Program (1)
State University of New York
Agricultural & Technical College
Agriculture & Life Sciences
Canton, New York 13617

Veterinary Science Technology Program (1)
State University of New York
Agricultural & Technical College
Delhi, New York 13753

Veterinary Science Technology Program (2)
State University of New York
Agricultural & Technical College
Farmingdale, New York 11735

NORTH CAROLINA

Veterinary Medical Technology Program (1)
Central Carolina Technical College
1105 Kelly Drive
Sanford, North Carolina 27330

NORTH DAKOTA

Animal Health Technician Program (1)
North Dakota State University
Dept. of Veterinary Science
Fargo, North Dakota 58102

OHIO

Animal Health Technology Program (1)
Columbus Technical Institute
550 East Spring Street
Columbus, Ohio 43215

Animal Health Technology Program (1)
Raymond Walters College
University of Cincinnati
Cincinnati, Ohio 45221

OKLAHOMA

Veterinary Technology Program (1)
Murray State College
Tishomingo, Oklahoma 73460

PENNSYLVANIA

Animal Health Technician Program (1)
Harcum Junior College
Bryn Mawr, Pennsylvania 19010

Veterinary Medical Technology Program (1)
Wilson College
Chambersburg, Pennsylvania 17201

SOUTH CAROLINA

Veterinary Technology Program (1)
Tri-County Technical College
P.O. Box 587
Pendleton, South Carolina 29670

SOUTH DAKOTA

National College (1)
Allied Health Division
321 Kansas City Street
P.O. Box 1780
Rapid City, South Dakota 57709

TENNESSEE

Animal Health Technology Program (1)
Columbia State Community College
Columbia, Tennessee 38401

TEXAS

Animal Medical Technology Program (1)
Cedar Valley College
3030 N. Dallas Avenue
Lancaster, Texas 75134

Animal Health Technology Program (1)
Sul Ross State University
Range Animal Science Dept.
Alpine, Texas 79830

Animal Technology Program (1)
Texas State Technical Institute
James Connally Campus
Waco, Texas 76705

UTAH

Animal Health Technology Program (2,*)
Brigham Young University
Provo, Utah 84602

VIRGINIA

Animal Technology Program (1)
Blue Ridge Community College
Box 80
Weyers Cave, Virginia 24486

Animal Science Technology Program (1)
Northern Virginia Community College
Loudoun Campus
1000 Harry Flood Byrd Highway
Sterling, Virginia 22170

WASHINGTON

Animal Technology Program (1)
Pierce College at Fort Steilacoom
9401 Farwest Drive, S.W.
Tacoma, Washington 98498

WEST VIRGINIA

Veterinary Technology Program (1)
Fairmont State College
Fairmont, West Virginia 26554

WISCONSIN

Animal Technician Program (1)
Madison Area Technical College
3550 Anderson
Madison, Wisconsin 53704

WYOMING

Animal Health Technology Program (1)
Eastern Wyoming College
3200 West C. Street
Torrington, Wyoming 82240

Animal Caretaker

Also known as an *animal health assistant, animal attendant* or *animal hospital attendant,* the animal caretaker works in a clinical or research laboratory, kennel, pound, or animal hospital, in an entry-level position. The caretaker cleans and sterilizes the animal's cages, pens, and the surrounding areas, prepares their meals and feeds them according to schedules and diet restrictions. The animal caretaker also keeps records on laboratory procedures, maintains prescribed temperature and humidity levels in the rooms, orders feed and supplies, and reports on any abnormal behavior in the animals. In general, the animal caretaker is responsible for the general health and well-being of animals.

A high school education, with courses in biology and chemistry, is the usual entrance prerequisite for admittance into a one-to-three-month on-the-job training program, usually offered by laboratories and animal hospitals. Training may also be available in secondary schools, or in college level programs that are less than two years.

For career opportunities as an animal caretaker, contact area animal hospitals, clinics or research laboratories, or refer to the classified employment section in local newspapers.

SOURCES:

American Veterinary Medical Association
Dictionary of Occupational Titles

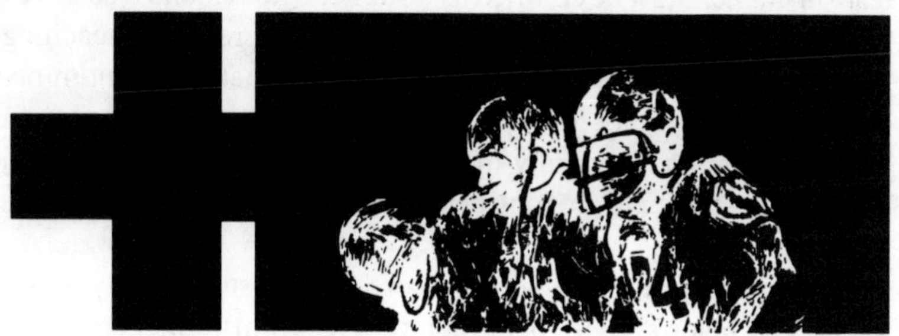

ATHLETIC TRAINING

Athletic training is that part of the medical aspect of an athletic program that is concerned with the prevention and treatment of athletic injuries.

Athletic Trainer

The *athletic trainer* is a trained professional who implements prevention-of-injury programs and who, under the direction of the team physician, supervises the treatment and rehabilitation of the injured athlete. Working closely with the team physician, the coaches, and the administration, the athletic trainer is concerned with the athlete's fitness, performance, and overall physical and emotional well being. The athletic trainer must be a skilled individual with a thorough knowledge of anatomy, physiology, psychology, kinesiology (the study of human muscular movements), hygiene, nutrition, conditioning, prevention-of-injury methodology, taping, and protective equipment.

Responsibilities of an athletic trainer may include treating an injured athlete with ice and heat, supervising strength and conditioning programs, inspecting athletic equipment to insure that it is working properly, taping knees and ankles to prevent or lessen injury, designing special equipment such as pads or braces and educating athletes on the prevention of injuries.

Athletic trainers are employed by high schools, school districts, colleges, universities, and by professional sports teams. According to the National Athletic Trainers Association the area of greatest employment potential-and often better salaries-is the high school level, where the trainer is also a teaching faculty member.

Since few high schools can afford a full time athletic trainer, many offer a position as a teacher-trainer, who's day is divided between the classroom and the training room. The teacher-trainer must be certified as an athletic trainer and also have a teaching license. The National Athletic Trainers Association does not require a teaching license specifically in health or physical education but recommends that a student minor in one of these areas. Athletic training is not restricted to males. The number of women participating in athletic training programs is rapidly increasing and according to the National Athletic Trainers Association, there is a growing demand for female athletic trainers, especially at the college level.

To become a certified athletic trainer (ATC), a student may follow one of two routes: (1) obtain a bachelor's degree or master's degree from a college, sponsoring an athletic training education program, and accredited by the National Athletic Trainers Association, or (2) obtain a bachelor's or master's degree in a related health field plus complete an 1800 hour internship under the direct supervision of an athletic trainer certified by the National Athletic Trainers Association. In both cases, certification requirements also include (a) current certification in first aid, and (b) current certification in CPR (cardiopulmonary resuscitation) and (c) successful completion of the National Athletic Trainers Association certification examination. Certification in first aid must be obtained through the American National Red Cross. For information on first aid certification contact the American National Red Cross, 431 18th Street, N.W., Washington, DC 20006 or your local Red Cross branch office. Certification in CPR can be obtained from either the American National Red Cross or the American Heart Association. The American Heart Association has information on certification in CPR at either their local branch offices or at the national headquarters, American Heart Association, 7320 Greenville Avenue, Dallas, Texas 75231.

Recommended high school courses included health, biology, physiology, chemistry, physics, general science, and first aid. It is suggested that high school students interested in a career of athletic training should work as a student trainer or manager at the high school or college level.

Salaries vary with location and experience, but athletic trainers could earn starting annual salaries of $16,000 working at the college level and may earn $25,000 in professional athletics. At the high school level, a newly hired teacher-trainer would normally earn an entry level teacher's salary plus an additional supplement for duties as an athletic trainer.

Athletic trainers may be a part of a facility's sports department, physical education department or as a member of a team's staff. An athletic trainer may be required to attend team activities, practices and games and may be expected to travel.

The following is a list of institutions that offer academic programs approved by the National Athletic Trainers Association. Most of the schools listed offer bachelor's degrees in athletic training, however, some graduate degree programs are also included.

For more information on internships, certification requirements or athletic training education programs, contact either the individual schools or the National Athletic Trainers Association, P.O. Drawer 1865, Greenville, North Carolina 27834.

KEY:

(1) Undergraduate Athletic Training Education Programs

(2) Graduate Athletic Training Education Programs

SOURCE:

National Athletic Trainers Association
Occupational Outlook Quarterly

Athletic Trainer Programs

ARIZONA

Department of Exercise & Sport Science (2)
University of Arizona
Tucson, Arizona 85721

CALIFORNIA

Department of Physical Education
& Recreation (1)
California State University, Fresno
Fresno, California 93740

Department of Health, Physical Education
& Recreation (1)
California State University, Fullerton
Fullerton, California 92634

Department of Physical Education (1)
California State University, Long Beach
Long Beach, California 90840

Department of Physical Education (1)
California State University, Northridge
Northridge, California 91330

Department of Physical Education (1)
California State University, Sacramento
Sacramento, California 95819

DELAWARE

College of Physical Education, Athletics
& Recreation (1)
University of Delaware
Newark, Delaware 19716

IDAHO

Department of Physical Education (1)
Boise State University
Boise, Idaho 83725

ILLINOIS

Department of Physical Education (1)
Eastern Illinois University
Charleston, Illinois 61920

Department of Health, Physical Education,
Recreation & Dance (2)
Illinois State University
Normal, Illinois 61761

Department of Physical Education (1)
Southern Illinois University
Carbondale, Illinois 62901

Department of Physical Education (1)
University of Illinois
Urbana, Illinois 61801

College of Health, Physical Education
& Recreation (1)
Western Illinois University
Macomb, Illinois 61455

INDIANA

Department of Men's Physical Education (1)
Ball State University
Muncie, Indiana 47306

Department of Physical Education (1,2)
Indiana University
Bloomington, Indiana 47405

Department of Physical Education (1,2)
Indiana State University
Terre Haute, Indiana 47809

Department of Physical Education, Health
& Recreation Studies (1)
Purdue University
West Lafayette, Indiana 47907

IOWA

Department of Exercise Science & Physical Education (1)
University of Iowa
Iowa City, Iowa 52242

KENTUCKY

College of Health, Physical Education, Recreation & Athletics (1)
Eastern Kentucky University
Richmond, Kentucky 40475-0933

MASSACHUSETTS

Department of Health, Physical Education & Recreation (1)
Bridgewater State College
Bridgewater, Massachusetts 02324

Department of Health, Sport & Leisure Studies (1)
Northeastern University
Boston, Massachusetts 02115

Department of Health, Physical Education & Recreation (1)
Springfield College
Springfield, Massachusetts 01109

MICHIGAN

Department of Physical Education (1)
Central Michigan University
Mount Pleasant, Michigan 48859

Department of Physical Education & Athletics (1)
Grand Valley State College
Allendale, Michigan 49401

Department of Health, Physical Education & Recreation (2)
Western Michigan University
Kalamazoo, Michigan 49008

MINNESOTA

Department of Health, Physical Education & Athletics (1)
Gustavus Adolphus College
St. Peters, Minnesota 56082

Department of Physical Education (1)
Mankato State University
Mankato, Minnesota 56001

MISSISSIPPI

Department of Athletic Administration & Coaching (1)
University of Southern Mississippi
Hattiesburg, Mississippi 39406-5105

MISSOURI

Department of Physical Education (1)
Southwest Missouri State University
Springfield, Missouri 65804

MONTANA

Department of Health & Physical Education (1)
University of Montana
Missoula, Montana 59812

NEBRASKA

Department of Health, Physical Education & Recreation (1)
University of Nebraska
Lincoln, Nebraska 68588-0618

NEVADA

School of Health, Physical Education, Recreation & Dance (1)
University of Nevada - Las Vegas
Las Vegas, Nevada 89154

NEW JERSEY

Department of Physical Education, Health & Recreation (1)
Kean College of New Jersey
Union, New Jersey 07083

Department of Movement Sciences and Leisure Studies (1)
William Patterson College of New Jersey
Wayne, New Jersey 07470

NEW MEXICO

Department of Health, Physical Education & Recreation (1)
University of New Mexico
Albuquerque, New Mexico 87131

NEW YORK

Department of Physical Education (1)
Canisius College
Buffalo, New York 14208

Department of Health, Physical Education & Recreation (1)
Ithaca College
Ithaca, New York 14850

Department of Physical Education & Exercise Science (2)
State University of New York at Buffalo
Buffalo, New York 14214

Department of Physical Education (1)
State University of New York at Cortland
Cortland, New York 13045

NORTH CAROLINA

Department of Health, Physical Education & Recreation (1)
Appalachian State University
Boone, North Carolina 28608

Department of Health, Physical Education, Recreation & Safety (1)
East Carolina University
Greenville, North Carolina 27834

Department of Physical Education (2)
University of North Carolina
Chapel Hill, North Carolina 27514

NORTH DAKOTA

Department of Health, Physical Education, Recreation & Athletics (1)
North Dakota State University
Fargo, North Dakota 58105

Department of Health, Physical Education & Recreation (1)
University of North Dakota
Grand Forks, North Dakota 58202

OHIO

Department of Health, Physical Education & Recreation (1)
Bowling Green State University
Bowling Green, Ohio 43403

Department of Sports Medicine (1)
Marietta College
Marietta, Ohio 45750

Department of Health, Physical Education & Recreation (1)
Miami University of Ohio
Oxford, Ohio 45056

Department of Health & Sport Sciences (1)
Ohio University
Athens, Ohio 45701

Department of Physical Education & Exercise Science (1)
University of Toledo
Toledo, Ohio 43606

OREGON

Department of Physical Education (1)
Oregon State University
Corvallis, Oregon 97331

Department of Physical Education (1)
University of Oregon
Eugene, Oregon 97403

PENNSYLVANIA

College of Education (1)
California University of Pennsylvania
California, Pennsylvania 15419

Department of Professional Physical Education (1)
East Stroudsburg University
East Stroudsburg, Pennsylvania 18301

Department of Health & Science (1)
Lock Haven University
Lock Haven, Pennsylvania 17745

Department of Health, Physical Education & Recreation (1)
Pennsylvania State University
University Park, Pennsylvania 16802

Department of Health, Physical & Recreational Education (1)
University of Pittsburgh
Pittsburgh, Pennsylvania 15261

Department of Health Sciences (1)
Slippery Rock University
Slippery Rock, Pennsylvania 16057

Department of Physical Education (1)
West Chester University
West Chester, Pennsylvania 19383

SOUTH DAKOTA

Department of Health, Physical Education & Recreation (1)
South Dakota State University
Brookings, South Dakota 57007

TENNESSEE

Department of Physical Education & Recreation (1)
East Tennessee State University
Johnson City, Tennessee 37614-0002

TEXAS

Department of Physical Education & Recreation (1)
Southwest Texas State University
San Marcos, Texas 78666

Department of Kinesiological Studies (1)
Texas Christian University
Fort Worth, Texas 76129

UTAH

College of Physical Education Sports (1)
Brigham Young University
Provo, Utah 84601

VERMONT

Department of Human Development Studies (1)
University of Vermont
Burlington, Vermont 05405

VIRGINIA

Department of Health & Physical Education (1)
James Madison University
Harrisonburg, Virginia 22807

Department of Health, Physical Education,
Recreation & Athletics (2)
Old Dominion University
Norfolk, Virginia 23508

Department of Health & Physical Education (2)
University of Virginia
Charlottesville, Virginia 22903

WASHINGTON

Department of Physical Education, Sport
& Leisure Studies (1)
Washington State University
Pullman, Washington 99164

WEST VIRGINIA

Department of Health, Physical Education
& Recreation (1)
Marshall University
Huntington, West Virginia 25701

Department of Professional Physical Education (1)
West Virginia University
Morgantown, West Virginia 26506-6116

WISCONSIN

Department of Health, Physical Education
& Recreation (1)
University of Wisconsin - La Crosse
La Crosse, Wisconsin 54601

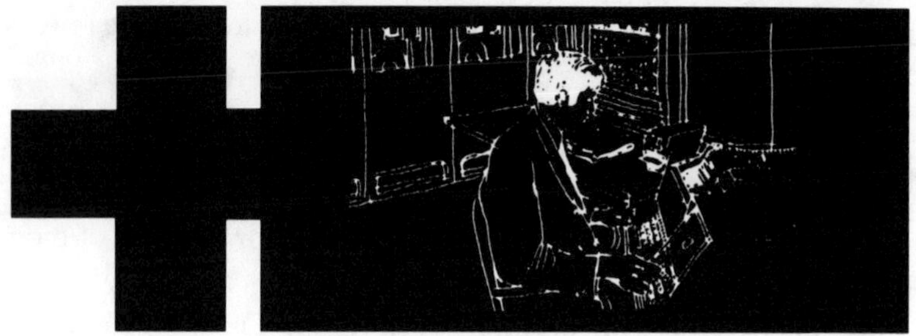

BIOMEDICAL ENGINEERING

Biomedical engineering is the application of engineering principles and methods to biomedical research and healthcare. In this field of allied health, aspects of engineering, physics, and technology are combined to understand and solve problems in life science research, medical diagnosis, medical therapy, and prevention of human disease. It is a very diverse health field and involves career specializations in the following areas: healthcare delivery; hospital safety; rehabilitation; public health; data processing and systems analysis; biomechanics; artificial organs and assist devices; chemical and nuclear energy sources; and performance evaluation of drugs, surgery, and instrumentation. In these specializations there are two career occupations: the *biomedical engineer* and the *biomedical equipment technician.*

Biomedical Engineer

The *biomedical engineer* is primarily an engineer who has had specific training in various aspects of biology or medicine. There are three main specializations in which the biomedical engineer may work: bioengineering, medical engineering and clinical engineering.

In one area of bioengineering the biomedical engineer researches the engineering aspects of biological (often nonmedical) systems, including the structure, function, and pathology of man and animals. In another, he or she is engaged in what is known as *bioenvironmental engineering* in which research is conducted to improve environmental quality and protect human, animal, and plant life from pollutants and toxicants. The bioenvironmental engineer may also apply engineering principles to the study of animal migrations and other ecological events or to the study of biological systems in the processing and production of food and fibers.

In *medical engineering* the biomedical engineer uses engineering concepts and technology to design and develop medical instrumentation, diagnostic and therapeutic devices, artificial organs, and other equipment including lasers for surgery and cardiac pacemakers. As a member of the healthcare team this type of biomedical engineer works closely with physicians in surgical and intensive care units.

In *clinical engineering* the biomedical engineer adapts computers to medical science and designs and builds healthcare delivery systems to modernize laboratory, hospital and clinical facilities and procedures.

Career opportunities are varied and plentiful in this field with biomedical engineers working in universities, colleges, research institutions, and hospitals. They are also employed as researchers in the automotive, aerospace, pharmaceutical, electronic, computer, and medical and hospital supply industries; in the National Aeronautics and Space Administration, Food and Drug Administration, Veterans Administration, Department of Defense, Department of Transportation, Department of Health and Human Services; and in state and local agencies.

The minimum educational requirement for a biomedical engineer is a four-year bachelor's degree from a biomedical engineering program or from an established program in electrical, mechanical, chemical, civil, aerospace, or industrial engineering with courses in biology, anatomy and behavioral sciences. Established engineering programs are available throughout the country at university and college schools of engineering. Many offer special courses in biomedical engineering as a minor, or option, for those students who are majoring in one of the more traditional engineering disciplines. The list below is comprised only of those schools that have specific departments and bachelor's degree programs in biomedical engineering.

The bachelor's degree should not generally be regarded as a terminal degree, as many graduates go on to graduate or medical school. For students interested in research and university teaching, a doctorate is the prerequisite.

Courses in high school for interested students in biomedical engineering should emphasize mathematics, science, and communication skills.

Information on certification can be obtained through the Association for the Advancement of Medical Instrumentation at the address listed below.

For further career information in biomedical engineering, contact the Biomedical Engineering Society, P.O. Box 2399, Culver City, California 90231 or the Association for the Advancement of Medical Instrumentation, 3330 Washington Blvd., Arlington, Virginia 22201.

Below is a list supplied by the Biomedical Engineering Society of programs in biomedical engineering accredited by the Accreditation Board for Engineering and Technology.

SOURCES:

Association for the Advancement of Medical Instrumentation
Biomedical Engineering Society
Accreditation Board for Engineering and Technology
Occupational Outlook Handbook

Biomedical Engineering Programs

ILLINOIS

Biomedical Engineering Program
Northwestern University
Evanston, Illinois 60201

IOWA

Biomedical Engineering Program
University of Iowa
Iowa City, Iowa 52242

LOUISIANA

Biomedical Engineering Program
Louisiana Technical University
Ruston, Louisiana 71272

Biomedical Engineering Program
Tulane University
New Orleans, Louisiana 70118

MASSACHUSETTS

Biomedical Engineering Program
Boston University
Boston, Massachusetts 02215

MARYLAND

Biomedical Engineering Program
John Hopkins University
Baltimore, Maryland 21218

NEW YORK

Biomedical Engineering Program
Rensselaer Polytechnic Institute
Troy, New York 12180

NORTH CAROLINA

Biomedical Engineering Program
Duke University
Durham, North Carolina 27706

OHIO

Biomedical Engineering Program
Case Western Reserve University
Cleveland, Ohio 44106

RHODE ISLAND

Biomedical Engineering Program
Brown University
Providence, Rhode Island 02912

WISCONSIN

Biomedical Engineering Program
Marquette University
Milwaukee, Wisconsin 53233

Biomedical Equipment Technician

Also known as a *biomedical engineering technician*, the biomedical equipment technician is involved with all phases of biomedical engineering. They install, calibrate, inspect, maintain, and repair general biomedical and related technical equipment that is used to help diagnose and treat disease. Able to understand medical and biological terminology, the technician both assists physicians, nurses, and researchers in carrying out clinical procedures, and experiments, and also instructs the medical staff in proper use and safety of the biomedical equipment. The technician repairs equipment such as electrocardiograph and dialysis machines, which must be safe and accurate in their operation and which must experience minimum down time when they are being repaired.

Entry-level biomedical equipment technicians are supervised by biomedical engineers, but with experience they may advance to intermediate or senior levels where they work on a variety of medical instruments, or to supervisory positions where they may train other biomedical equipment technicians.

The educational requirement for a biomedical equipment technician is an associate degree from a college or university in biomedical equipment technology, electronics, or a related engineering field.

Certification as a (CBET) certified biomedical equipment technician is granted by the International Certification Commission for Clinical Engineers and Biomedical Technicians after successfully passing a national examination and meeting the education and experience requirements.

Recommended high school courses for students interested in a career in this field include electronics, mechanics, algebra, biology and physiology.

For further information on certification or a career as a biomedical equipment technician write to the Society of Biomedical Equipment Technicians, 3330 Washington Blvd., Arlington, Virginia 22201.

Following is a list of educational programs in biomedical equipment technology.

Sources:

Association for the Advancement of Medical Instrumentation
Society of Biomedical Equipment Technicians
Occupational Outlook Handbook

Biomedical Equipment Technician Programs

ALABAMA

Biomedical Equipment Technician Program
Regional Technical Institute
University of Alabama
University Station
Birmington, Alabama 35294

ARKANSAS

Biomedical Instrumentation Technician Program
University of Arkansas
North Little Rock Division
VA Medical Center, 10A-4A
N. Little Rock, Arkansas 72114

CALIFORNIA

Biomedical Equipment Technician Program
Los Angeles Valley College
5800 Fulton Avenue
Van Nuys, California 91401

COLORADO

Biomedical Engineering Technician Program
Colorado Technical College
4435 N. Chestnut
Colorado Springs, Colorado 80907

FLORIDA

Biomedical Equipment Technician Program
Brevard Community College
1519 Clear Lake Road
Cocoa, Florida 32922

MASSACHUSETTS

Biomedical Equipment Technician Program
Franklin Institute of Boston
41 Berkeley Street
Boston, Massachusetts 02116

Biomedical Equipment Technician Program
Springfield Technical Community College
1 Armory Square
Springfield, Massachusetts 01105

MICHIGAN

Biomedical Equipment Technician Program
Schoolcraft College
18600 Haggerty Road
Livonia, Michigan 48152

NEW YORK

Biomedical Engineering Technician Program
Monroe Community College
1000 E. Henrietta Road
Rochester, New York 14623

OHIO

Biomedical Equipment Technician Program
Kettering College of Medical Arts
3737 Southern Boulevard
Kettering, Ohio 45429

Biomedical Equipment Technician Program
Owens Technical College
Caller No. 10,000-Oregon Road
Toledo, Ohio 43699

OKLAHOMA

Biomedical Equipment Technician Program
Tulsa Junior College
Tenth & Boston
Tulsa, Oklahoma 74119

TENNESSEE

Biomedical Equipment Technician Program
State Technical Institute at Memphis
5983 Macon Cove
Memphis, Tennessee 38134

TEXAS

Biomedical Equipment Technician Program
Amarillo College
P.O. Box 447
Amarillo, Texas 79178

Biomedical Equipment Technician Program
Texas State Technical Institute
Waco, Texas 76705

WISCONSIN

Biomedical Electronic Technician Program
Western Wisconsin Technical Institute
304 N. Sixth St.
LaCrosse, Wisconsin 54602

Biomedical Electronic Technician Program
Milwaukee Area Technical College
700 W. State Street
Milwaukee, Wisconsin 53233

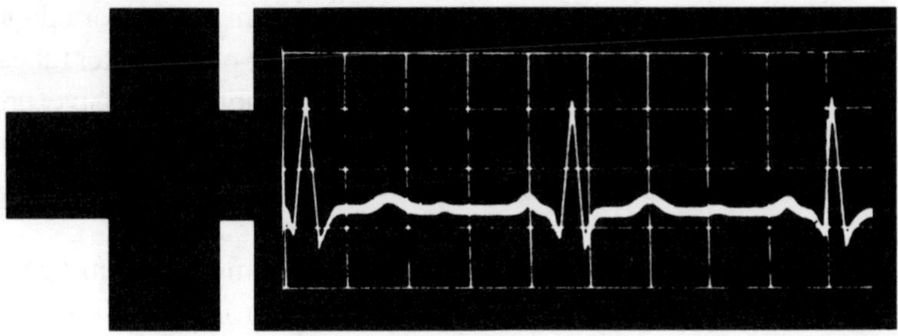

CARDIOVASCULAR TECHNOLOGY

Cardiovascular technology, also referred to as cardiology technology, is the allied health field that records and analyzes the functioning of the heart and blood vessels. Cardiovascular technology utilizes sophisticated testing procedures which assists the cardiologist (a physician who specializes in heart conditions) in the diagnosis and treatment of heart and circulatory problems.

Cardiovascular technology is one of the fastest growing career areas. Cardiovascular disease is a leading cause of death and disability in the United States and with the development of procedures to diagnose coronary disease, cardiovascular testing is not only being performed for patients who suffer or are suspected of having heart problems, it is also being used before most kinds of major surgery and as a more standard diagnostic test for routine physical examinations. As a result, cardiovascular technologists with specialized education and training should be in demand.

There are two career occupations in cardiovascular technology; the *cardiovascular technologist* and the *cardiographic (EKG) technician.*

Cardiovasular Technologist

The *cardiovascular technologist* provides supportive services to the cardiologist in the use of sophisticated diagnostic procedures in the diagnosis and treatment of diseases of the heart and blood vessels.

Cardiovascular technologists perform a variety of tasks but generally specialize in either invasive cardiovascular technology or non-invasive cardiovascular technology. In invasive procedures, a foreign substance or instrument is inserted into the body. One such procedure, cardiac catheterization involves the use of a catheter tube inserted into the blood vessels in the heart. Coronary angiography, another invasive procedure, involves the injection of radiopaque dyes to enhance x-ray images. Non-invasive tests involve the placing of electrodes on specific parts of the patient's body to obtain diagnostic information, such as with an E.K.G.

In addition to being fully capable of, and sometimes performing all the duties of an EKG technician (described in detail in the next section), the cardiovascular technologist may perform more complex tests including echocardiography (recording of heart ailments with the use of high frequency sound waves), vectorcardiography (recording of three-dimensional tracings), telemetry (monitoring heart rhythm patterns to detect abnormal pattern variances), cardiac catheterization, and coronary angiography.

Cardiovascular technologists are employed in hospitals, clinics, home health organizations, comprehensive healthcare centers, and outpatient care facilities.

Recommended high school courses included health, biology, anatomy, physiology, typing, and computer science.

Training for the cardiovascular technologist involves a 12-24 month training program to master and understand complex cardiology equipment. Training programs are offered at community and junior colleges, vocational-technical institutes and in some hospitals. Some two-year associate degrees are available, which include classroom and clinical experience to prepare the technologist to assist with complex catheterization and angiographies.

Credentials are available with the Cardiovascular Credentialing International (CCI). Applicants who meet the educational and/or experience requirements plus pass CCI's credentialing examination are eligible to apply for the status of Registered Cardiovascular Technologist (RCVT). For more information on registration, write to Cardiovascular Credentialing International, 2801 Farhills, Dayton, Ohio 45419.

Career information in cardiovascular technology can be obtained from the American Cardiology Technologists Association, 1980 Isaac Newton Square South, Reston, Virginia 22090.

Only a few formal training programs for cardiovascular technologists have received approval by the American Cardiology Technologists Association and a list can be obtained by writing to them at the above address. For other educational programs contact the Personnel Director in area healthcare facilities or contact local community colleges, junior colleges, and vocational-technical institutes.

SOURCES:

American Cardiology Technologists Association
Cardiovascular Credentialing International
Dictionary of Occupational Titles
Occupational Outlook Handbook

Cardiographic Technician (EKG Technician)

The *cardiographic technician,* also referred to as an *EKG technician,* is trained in the operation of electrocardiograph (EKG) equipment. EKG equipment monitors variations in the electrical potential produced by the heart. Electrical changes that occur during a heartbeat are recorded as tracings on an electrocardiogram. The record is used by the cardiologist to diagnose irregularities in heart action.

In operating EKG equipment, the cardiographic technician records pulse rates by attaching electrodes to specified areas of the patient's body. The technician also moves chest electrodes in a specific pattern across the patient's chest to record variations in electrical potential in different parts of the heart. The technician is able to detect abnormalities or false readings in the electrocardiograms and to correct technical errors in the machine.

Most cardiographic technicians are employed in EKG departments of large hospitals, while others are employed in small hospitals, clinics, and physicians' offices.

Cardiographic technicians, in addition to performing electrocardiograms, may perform other diagnostic tests including Holter monitoring and cardiac stress testing.

Training for the cardiographic technician is usually performed on-the-job and generally lasts from four-to-six weeks. With additional training, the cardiographic technician may perform more complex cardiovascular procedures (see section on cardiovascular technologist). Some community and junior colleges, hospitals, and vocational-technical institutes offer formal training programs, lasting from 12-24 months, but to date only a few programs have received approval from the American Cardiology Technologists Association.

The credentials of CCT (Certified Cardiographic Technician) are awarded to individuals who meet specific training and experience requirements and pass a credentialing examination. Write to the Cardiovascular Credentialing International (CCI), 2801 Farhills, Dayton, Ohio 45419, for more information on certification of cardiographic technicians.

Recent starting annual salaries for the cardiographic technician averaged $12,800, while those with additional experience earned $16,300. Cardiographic technicians who perform more sophisticated tests usually earn higher salaries.

Persons interested in a career as a cardiographic technician should contact the American Cardiology Technologists Association, 1980 Isaac Newton Square, Reston, Virginia 22090.

SOURCES:

American Cardiology Technologists Association
Cardiovascular Credentialing International
Occupational Outlook Handbook

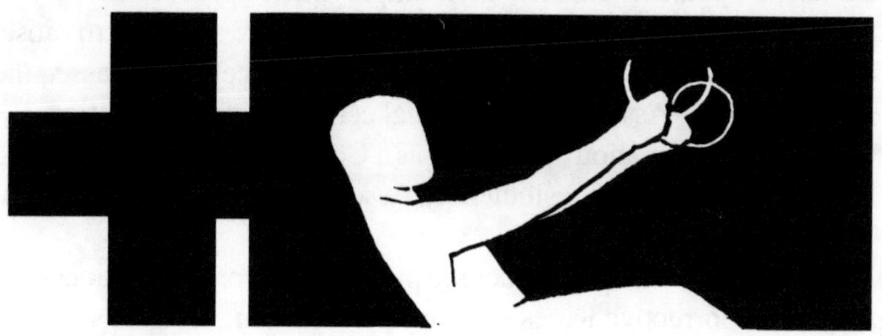

CORRECTIVE KINESIOTHERAPY

Corrective kinesiotherapy, formerly called *corrective therapy,* uses exercise and movement in the prevention of muscular deterioration resulting from disease, injury, congenital defects or other disabilities that may limit mobility. Through medically prescribed exercise programs corrective kinesiotherapy strives to improve movement, increase self-confidence and independence, and promote social interaction.

Corrective Kinesiotherapist

Under the supervision of a physician, the certified corrective kinesiotherapist develops and executes therapeutic exercises, education and other physical activities adapted to each individual's needs.

Corrective kinesiotherapists work for Veterans Administration hospitals, in rehabilitation facilities, hospitals, clinics, nursing homes, schools for the handicapped and home healthcare programs. Corrective kinesiotherapists may work with a variety of individuals or may specialize in geriatric healthcare, psychiatric healthcare, long term care, care of physically handicapped children, developmentally disabled or in the rehabilitation of cardiac patients or amputees.

A bachelor's degree in physical education, with a specialization in corrective kinesiotherapy, plus clinical training experience, is the requirement for students pursuing a career in corrective kinesiotherapy. The Corrective Kinesiotherapy Association suggests that graduates of corrective kinesiotherapy programs, who have also achieved a teaching license, may further enhance their employment opportunities.

The credentials of certified kinesiotherapist are awarded to those individuals who meet academic and clinical requirements and have successfully passed the American Corrective Kinesiotherapy Association's national certification examination.

For more information on a career as a Corrective Kinesiotherapist, write to the Executive Director, American Kinesiotherapy Association, Inc., 259-08 148th Road, Rosedale, New York 11422.

Below is a list of bachelor degree programs in corrective kinesiotherapy, provided by the American Corrective Kinesiotherapy Association.

SOURCE

American Corrective Kinesiotherapy Association

CALIFORNIA

Corrective Kinesiotherapy Program
California State University-Long Beach
Long Beach, California 90840

ILLINOIS

Corrective Kinesiotherapy Program
University of Illinois at Chicago
Chicago, Illinois 60680

MISSISSIPPI

Corrective Kinesiotherapy Program
University of Southern Mississippi
Hattiesburg, Mississippi 39406

NEW YORK

Corrective Kinesiotherapy Program
Adelphi University
Garden City, New York 11530

OHIO

Corrective Kinesiotherapy Program
The University of Toledo, Ohio
Toledo, Ohio 43600

OREGON

Corrective Kinesiotherapy Program
Portland State University, Oregon
Portland, Oregon 97207

Corrective Kinesiotherapy Program
San Jose State University
San Jose, California 95192

PENNSYLVANIA

Corrective Kinesiotherapy Program
Slippery Rock University, Pennsylvania
Slippery Rock, Pennsylvania 16057

VIRGINIA

Corrective Kinesiotherapy Program
Norfolk State University, Virginia
Norfolk, Virginia 23504

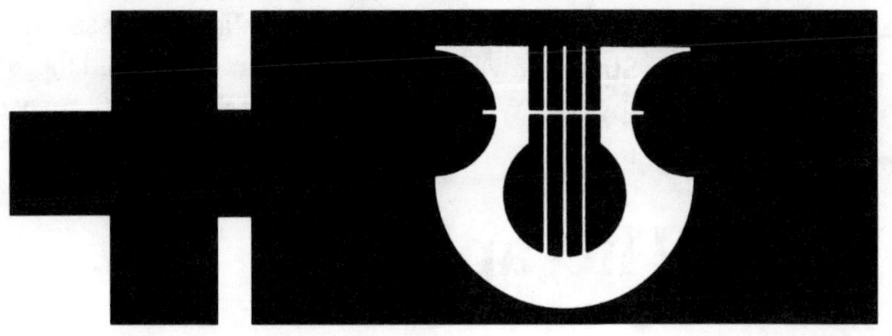

CREATIVE ARTS THERAPY: MUSIC THERAPY, DANCE THERAPY, ART THERAPY

Music, dance, and art therapies involve the respective application of the principles and techniques of each art form in a prescribed and scientific manner to accomplish therapeutic rehabilitation; that is, the restoration, maintenance, and improvement of physical and mental health. By employing motivational and creative programs each of these therapies attempts to bring about positive changes in patients' behavior, such as extended attention span, improved coordination, increased verbalization, and increased socialization.

Emotionally disturbed, handicapped, mentally retarded, and physically or learning disabled patients are the primary concerns of the creative arts therapies, but normal school children and adults, such as geriatric patients, also benefit from the programs.

Music, dance, and art goals play a secondary role to the social, communicational, and behavioral betterment goals of the therapies, which help the patient acquire self-confidence, self-awareness, and personal satisfaction and thereby adjust to an illness or disability. The therapy may serve as one integral part of a larger treatment program or actually act in some cases as the primary method of therapy.

As members of the therapeutic team, which may include physicians, psychiatrists, psychologists, teachers, nurses, families of patients, and others; music, dance, and art therapists help plan and perform treatment plans and analyze their effectiveness.

The careers of *music therapist, dance therapist* and *art therapist* are discussed in this chapter. Persons interested in career opportunities and training in *drama* and *poetry therapy* as well should contact the National Association for Drama Therapy, 19 Edwards Street, New Haven, Connecticut 06511 and the National Association for Poetry Therapy, 225 Williams St., Huron, Ohio 44839, respectively.

Music Therapist

Able to sight-read music, play by ear, improvise, and accompany other performers, the *music therapist* organizes and conducts medically prescribed musical programs to assist in the rehabilitation of patients who suffer from mental or physical illness or disability. Music therapy programs involve vocal, rhythmic, instrumental, and listening activities and include individual and group sessions with orchestras, bands, and choruses; instrument instruction; music appreciation and theory; composition instruction; general music; and folk ensembles.

The music therapist arranges concerts, sometimes performed by members of the hospital staff or by talented and capable patients, for the other patients and also accompanies and conducts group singing and folk and square dancing, with the emphasis always on therapy and rehabilitation. The music therapist may use music along with other activities, including exercise, games, art and relaxation training, as a means of achieving therapeutic goals.

Music therapists may be employed in hospitals, clinics, nursing homes, day care facilities, public and private school systems, community mental health agencies, special service agencies and in private practice.

The minimum educational requirement for a music therapist is a bachelor's degree with major emphasis on music including music theory, history, conducting, arranging, instrumental and vocal studies and group performance. Other college courses must be in biological sciences, humanities, sociology, anthropology, English composition and psychology. A six months' clinical training internship is to be completed after university or college course work and generally must be completed before a degree is granted. Teaching credentials must also be obtained if the music therapist wants to teach in a state public school system. Master's degrees are available for individuals interested in advanced education.

A student who completes specific academic and clinical requirements may obtain credentials from one of two professional music therapy associations.

Registration as a Registered Music Therapist (RMT) is available with the National Association for Music Therapy, after graduating from an approved bachelor's degree program and completing a clinical internship. Information on educational and registration requirements is available from the National Association for Music Therapy, Inc., 505 Eleventh Street, S.E., Washington, D.C. 20003.

Certification as a Certified Music Therapist (CMT) is available with the American Association for Music Therapy, 66 Morris Avenue, P.O. Box 359, Springfield, New Jersey 07081. Certification is available after completing an approved bachelor's degree program and internship requirement.

In addition to registration or certification, a music therapist may apply for the status of Music Therapist - Board Certified (MT-BC) which recognizes professional competence in the field of music therapy. Board certification is granted after successfully completing academic and clinical training requirements and successfully passing a written job-related independent examination. Information on the board certification requirements can be obtained through the Certification Board for Music Therapists, c/o ASI Processing Center, 718 Arch Street, Philadelphia, Pennsylvania 19106.

For persons interested in entering this career as much music as possible should be studied and performed while in high school. It is also recommended that volunteer work or summer employment in a rehabilitation setting would give a student experience in the music therapy field.

Currently, music therapy students with bachelor's degrees entering the field of music therapy can expect to earn $18,000 to $22,000 annually while students with advanced degrees generally earn more. Salaries may vary based on experience, amount of education and geographic location.

Below is a list of bachelor's degree programs in music therapy that are recognized by the National Association for Music Therapy, Inc. as having received approval of the National Association of Schools of Music. Those marked with an asterisk (*) offer master's degrees. Also listed are approved schools of the American Association of Music Therapy. For specific information on programs contact the Director of Music Therapy at the individual schools.

KEY:

(1) Programs recognized by the National Association for Music Therapy, Inc. as having received approval of the National Association of Schools of Music.

(2) Programs approved by the American Association of Music Therapy.

SOURCES:

American Association for Music Therapy
National Association for Music Therapy, Inc.
Certification Board for Music Therapists

Music Therapist Programs

ALABAMA

Music Therapy Program (1)
University of Alabama
University, Alabama 35486

ARIZONA

Music Therapy Program (1)
Arizona State University
Tempe, Arizona 85281

CALIFORNIA

Music Therapy Program (1)
California State University
Long Beach, California 90840

Music Therapy Program (1)
California State University
North Ridge, California 91330

Music Therapy Program (1*)
University of the Pacific
Stockton, California 95211

COLORADO

Music Therapy Program (1*)
Colorado State University
Fort Collins, Colorado 80523

DISTRICT OF COLUMBIA

Music Therapy Program (1)
Howard University
Washington, DC 20056

FLORIDA

Music Therapy Program (1*)
Florida State University
Tallahassee, Florida 32306

Music Therapy Program (1*)
University of Miami
Coral Gables, Florida 33124

GEORGIA

Music Therapy Program (1)
Georgia College
Milledgeville, Georgia 31061

Music Therapy Program (1*)
University of Georgia
Athens, Georgia 30602

ILLINOIS

Music Therapy Program (1)
Illinois State University
Normal, Illinois 61761

Music Therapy Program (1)
Western Illinois University
Macomb, Illinois 61455

INDIANA

Music Therapy Program (1)
Indiana University-Fort Wayne
Fort Wayne, Indiana 46815

Music Therapy Program (1)
University of Evansville
Evansville, Indiana 47702

Music Therapy Program (2)
St. Mary-Of-The-Woods College
Department of Music Therapy
St. Mary-of-the-Woods, Indiana 47876

IOWA

Music Therapy Program (1)
University of Iowa
Iowa City, Iowa 52242

Music Therapy Program (1)
Wartburg College
Waverly, Iowa 50677

KANSAS

Music Therapy Program (1*)
University of Kansas
Lawrence, Kansas 66045

LOUISIANA

Music Therapy Program (1*)
Loyola University
New Orleans, Louisiana 70118

MASSACHUSETTS

Music Therapy Program (1)
Anna Maria College
Paxton, Massachusetts 01612

Music Therapy Program (2)
Emmanuel College
Department of Music
400 Fenway
Boston, Massachusetts 02115

MICHIGAN

Music Therapy Program (1)
Eastern Michigan University
Ypsilanti, Michigan 48197

Music Therapy Program (1*)
Michigan State University
East Lansing, Michigan 48824

Music Therapy Program (1)
Wayne State University
Detroit, Michigan 48202

Music Therapy Program (1*)
Western Michigan University
Kalamazoo, Michigan 49008

MINNESOTA

Music Therapy Program (1)
Augusburg College
Minneapolis, Minnesota 55454

Music Therapy Program (1)
College of Saint Teresa
Winona, Minnesota 55987

Music Therapy Program (1*)
University of Minnesota
Minneapolis, Minnesota 55455

MISSISSIPPI

Music Therapy Program (1)
William Carey College
Hattiesburg, Mississippi 39401

MISSOURI

Music Therapy Program (1)
Maryville College
St. Louis, Missouri 63141

Music Therapy Program (1*)
University of Missouri-Kansas City
Kansas City, Missouri 64111

MONTANA

Music Therapy Program (1)
Eastern Montana College
Billings, Montana 59101

NEW JERSEY

Music Therapy Program (1)
Montclair State College
Upper Montclair, New Jersey 07043

NEW MEXICO

Music Therapy Program (1)
Eastern New Mexico University
Portales, New Mexico 88130

NEW YORK

Music Therapy Program (1)
Nazareth College of Rochester
Rochester, New York 14610

Music Therapy Program (1)
State University College-Fredonia
Fredonia, New York 14063

Music Therapy Program (1)
State University College-New Paltz
New Paltz, New York 12561

Music Therapy Program (2)
New York University
Department of Music Education and Therapy
777 Education Bldg. 35 W. 4th Street
New York, New York 10003

NORTH CAROLINA

Music Therapy Program (1)
East Carolina University
Greenville, North Carolina 27834

Music Therapy Program (1)
Queens College
Charlotte, North Carolina 28274

OHIO

Music Therapy Program (1)
Baldwin-Wallace College
Berea, Ohio 44017

Music Therapy Program (1)
Case Western Reserve University
Cleveland, Ohio 44106

Music Therapy Program (1)
Cleveland State University
Cleveland, Ohio 44114

Music Therapy Program (1)
College of Wooster
Wooster, Ohio 44691

Music Therapy Program (1)
Oberlin College
Oberlin, Ohio 44074

Music Therapy Program (1)
College of Mt. St. Joseph on the Ohio
Mt. St. Joseph, Ohio 45051

Music Therapy Program (1*)
Ohio University
Athens, Ohio 45701

Music Therapy Program (1)
University of Dayton
Dayton, Ohio 45469

OKLAHOMA

Music Therapy Program (1)
Phillips University
Enid, Oklahoma 73701

Music Therapy Program (1)
Southwestern Oklahoma State University
Weatherford, Oklahoma 73096

OREGON

Music Therapy Program (1)
Willamette University
Salem, Oregon 97301

PENNSYLVANIA

Music Therapy Program (1)
Combs College of Music
Bryn Mawr, Pennsylvania 19010

Music Therapy Program (1)
College Misericordia
Dallas, Pennsylvania 18612

Music Therapy Program (2)
Immaculata College
Department of Music
Immaculata, Pennsylvania 19345

Music Therapy Program (1*)
Duquesne University
Pittsburgh, Pennsylvania 15282

Music Therapy Program (1)
Elizabethtown College
Elizabethtown, Pennsylvania 17022

Music Therapy Program (1,2*)
Hahnemann University
Department of Music
230 North Broad Street, MS 424
Philadelphia, Pennsylvania 19102

Music Therapy Program (1)
Mansfield University
Mansfield, Pennsylvania 16933

Music Therapy Program (1)
Marywood College
Scranton, Pennsylvania 18509

Music Therapy Program (1)
Slippery Rock University
Slippery Rock, Pennsylvania 16057

Music Therapy Program (1,2)
Temple University
Department of Music Education and Therapy
1938 Park Mall, TV 298-00
Philadelphia, Pennsylvania 19122

SOUTH CAROLINA

Music Therapy Program (1)
Baptist College at Charleston
Charleston, South Carolina 29411

TENNESSEE

Music Therapy Program (1)
Tennessee Technological University
Cookeville, Tennessee 38501

TEXAS

Music Therapy Program (1)
Sam Houston State University
Huntsville, Texas 77341

Music Therapy Program (1*)
Southern Methodist University
Dallas, Texas 75275

Music Therapy Program (1*)
Texas Woman's University
Denton, Texas 76204

Music Therapy Program (1)
West Texas State University
Canyon, Texas 79016

UTAH

Music Therapy Program (1)
Utah State University
Logan, Utah 84322

VIRGINIA

Music Therapy Program (1*)
Radford University
Radford, Virginia 24142

Music Therapy Program (1)
Shenandoah College and Conservatory of Music
Winchester, Virginia 22601

WISCONSIN

Music Therapy Program (1)
Alverno College
Milwaukee, Wisconsin 53215

Music Therapy Program (1)
University of Wisconsin-Eau Claire
Eau Claire, Wisconsin 54701

Music Therapy Program (1*)
University of Wisconsin-Milwaukee
Milwaukee, Wisconsin 53201

Music Therapy Program (1)
University of Wisconsin-Oshkosh
Oshkosh, Wisconsin 54901

Dance Therapist

With an extensive level of training and education in dance, dance theory, improvisation, choreography and kinesiology (study of movement), the *dance therapist* also referred to as a *movement therapist,* incorporates dance and movement in the rehabilitation and treatment of physical, behavioral, and mental disorders.

Through the use of movement and dance, the dance therapist encourages patients to express themselves non-verbally. With therapeutic goals in mind, the dance therapist helps the patient improve coordination, acquire self-confidence and increase socialization skills.

Dance therapists may be employed in hospitals, community mental health centers, nursing homes, correctional and rehabilitation facilities and in some cases, private practice.

The minimum educational requirement for a dance therapist is a master's degree in dance therapy. A bachelor's degree, with emphasis in psychology, liberal arts, dance and dance therapy is required for preparedness for graduate study. Master degree curricula include courses in dance and movement therapy, theory and practice, psychotherapy, psychology and human development.

Registration as a Registered Dance Therapist (D.T.R.) is available from the American Dance Therapy Association after meeting specific academic and clinical requirements. Advance credential status, as a member of the Academy of Dance Therapists Registered (A.D.T.R.), is granted to those individuals who have met additional requirements.

Salaries for dance therapists vary by location, level of experience and type of facility. Generally, starting salaries range from the mid-teens to the low-twenties annually.

Below is a list of master's degree programs in dance therapy provided by the American Dance Therapy Association. The American Dance Therapy Association does not endorse any of these programs, but does provide them as a service to interested students. For a list of other graduate degree programs, write to the American Dance Therapy Association at the address below.

For further information on registration and careers in dance therapy, write to the American Dance Therapy Association, 2000 Century Plaza, Suite 108, Columbia, Maryland 21044.

SOURCE:

American Dance Therapy Association

Dance Therapy Programs

CALIFORNIA

Graduate Dance Movement Therapy Program
U.C.L.A.
405 Hilgard Avenue
Los Angeles, California 90024

MARYLAND

Dance Therapy Program
Goucher College
Dulaney Valley Road
Baltimore, Maryland 21204

NEW HAMPSHIRE

Dance Therapy Program
Antioch/New England Graduate School
103 Roxbury Street
Keene, New Hampshire 03431

NEW YORK

Dance Therapy Program
Hunter College
425 E. 25th Street
New York, New York 10010

Graduate Dance Movement Therapy Program
New York University
35 W. 4th Street
New York, New York 10003

PENNSYLVANIA

Dance Therapy Program
Hahnemann University
230 North Broad Street
Philadelphia, Pennsylvania 19102

Art Therapist

Using drawings and other art forms, the *art therapist* works with patients, generally on a one-to-one basis, in the treatment and rehabilitation of mental and emotional disorders. Art therapy may also be incorporated in the rehabilitation of substance abuse, sexual and physical abuse and in marriage and family counseling.

Art therapy provides a means of non-verbal expression and communication. Often a patient can express feelings or thoughts through the creative process of art. The art therapist works with the patient towards reconciling emotional conflicts and acquiring self-confidence and self-awareness.

Art therapists are employed in hospitals, clinics, community mental health agencies, day care facilities, public and private school systems, special service agencies, and in some cases, in private practice.

The minimum educational requirement for the art therapist is a master's degree in art therapy. Preparation for the master's degree program is a bachelor's degree from an accredited university with a major in studio art and/or psychology.

Master's degree course curricula include courses in psychology, psychotherapy, counseling, plus the history, theory, and practice of art therapy.

Graduates of approved master's degree programs are eligible to apply for registration status of Registered Art Therapist (A.T.R.).

Students interested in a career in art therapy should develop a strong background in the fine arts through education and training. Volunteer work or summer employment in a rehabilitation setting would give a student experience in the art therapy field.

Starting salaries for art therapy graduates generally range from $18,000 to $22,000 annually, although those with administrative capacities earn considerably more. Salaries can vary by experience level, geographic location, type of facility and education.

Following is a list of master's degree programs approved by the American Art Therapy Association, Inc.

For more information on a career as an art therapist plus a list of other known (although not approved) educational art therapy programs, write to the American Art Therapy Association, Inc., 505 East Hawley Street, Mundelein, Illinois 60060.

SOURCE:

American Art Therapy Association

Art Therapist Programs

CALIFORNIA

Art Therapist Program
College of Notre Dame
Belmont, California 94002

Art Therapist Program
Loyola Marymount University
Loyola Boulevard at West 80th Street
Los Angeles, California 90045

DISTRICT OF COLUMBIA

Art Therapist Program
George Washington University
Department of Art Therapy
2129 G Street, N.W.
Washington, DC 20052

ILLINOIS

Art Therapist Program
University of Illinois at Chicago
Art Therapy Department
School of Art and Design, Box 4348
Chicago, Illinois 60608

KENTUCKY

Art Therapist Program
University of Louisville
Department of Expressive Therapies
Belknap Campus
Louisville, Kentucky 40292

MASSACHUSETTS

Art Therapist Program
Lesley College
Institute for the Arts and Human Development
29 Everett Street
Cambridge, Massachusetts 02238

NEW YORK

Art Therapist Program
College of New Rochelle
New Rochelle, New York 10805

Art Therapist Program
Hofstra University
Department of Counseling, Psychology and Research in Education
Hempstead, New York 11550

Art Therapist Program
New York University
735 East Building
239 Greene Street
New York, New York 10003

Art Therapist Program
Pratt Institute
Creative Arts Therapy Department
East Building, Third Floor
Brooklyn, New York 11205

Art Therapist Program
State University College at Buffalo
1300 Elmwood Avenue
Buffalo, New York 14222

OHIO

Art Therapist Program
Wright State University
228 Creative Arts Center
Dayton, Ohio 45435

PENNSYLVANIA

Art Therapist Program
Hahnemann University of Health Sciences
Broad and Vine Streets, M.S. 424
Philadelphia, Pennsylvania 19102

Art Therapist Program
Marywood College
Scraton, Pennsylvania 18509

VERMONT

Art Therapist Program
Vermont College of Norwich University
Montpelier, Vermont 05602

VIRGINIA

Art Therapist Program
Eastern Virginia Medical School
P.O. Box 1980
Norfolk, Virginia 23501

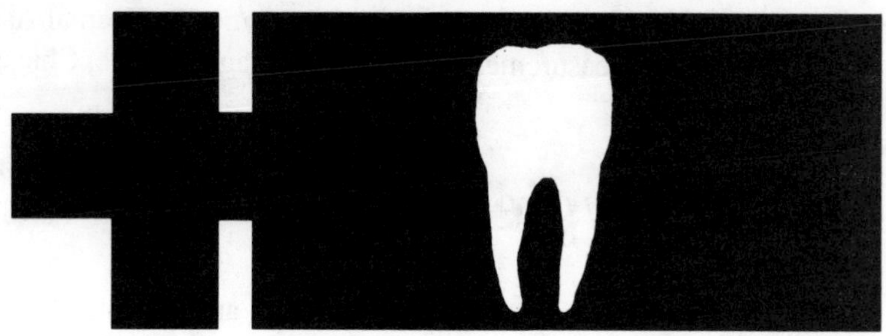

DENTAL SERVICES

Dentistry is the health profession that maintains, improves, and corrects the health of the teeth and the supporting oral structures. Dentists are the major practitioners of dental care and have final responsibility for all dental services. Dentists are highly educated and often are very specialized professionals. Dental school curricula are generally four years in length, and admission to dental school requires a minimum of two-to-four years of undergraduate college. Dental students interested in going into a dental specialty will require at least two to three years of additional schooling.

There are eight dental specialties recognized by the American Dental Association: orthodontics (dentistry concerned with straightening teeth), periodontics (dentistry that treats diseases of the gums), prosthodontics (dentistry to make artificial teeth and dentures), pedodontics (dentistry of children), endodontics (dentistry dedicated to treating diseases of the dental pulp usually with root canal therapy), oral pathology (dentistry that involves performing tests to diagnose disease), public health dentistry (dentistry in community clinics or with the federal government) and dental surgery.

The future for graduates entering the dental field looks bright. Employment of dentists and other dental auxiliary personnel should continue to grow well into the mid-1990's. Many factors, including changes in population size, increased public knowledge of dental health, rising incomes and the availability of dental insurance, may account for the increase.

Persons employed in allied dental health are known as dental auxiliaries, and there are three kinds of dental auxiliary careers: *dental hygienist, dental assistant* and *dental laboratory technician.* Each of the three undertakes specific functions that allow the dentist to devote more time to the specialized activities of the chairside operative and restorative dentistry they are trained and qualified to perform.

For more information on a career in dentistry, contact either the auxiliary dental associations listed in this chapter or the American Dental Association, Division of Educational Measurements, 211 East Chicago Avenue, Chicago, Illinois 60611.

Dental Hygienist

The *dental hygienist* is an oral health clinician and educator, whose goal is to improve the dental health of their patients. Under the dentist's supervision the dental hygienist may examine, clean and polish teeth, give fluoride treatments, take and process X-rays, educate the dental patient about proper oral hygiene, provide dietary recommendations for healthy teeth, take medical and dental histories and work within the community to educate on dental health. In some states the dental hygienist may also give local anesthetics. Duties of the dental hygienist are governed by state law and may vary from state to state.

Most dental hygienists work in private dental offices while the remainder work in schools, clinics, and hospitals, health maintenance organizations, and in private industry.

Training in dental hygiene can be obtained in a two year certificate or associate program offered at a community college or a vocational-technical school, or the prospective dental hygienist may complete a four year bachelor's degree program at a college or university. A high school degree is the minimum educational requirement for admission to dental hygiene schools. A two year degree would prepare a student for private practice office work, however, a student wishing to do research, teach or work in school health programs would require at a minimum, a bachelor's degree.

All states require the dental hygienist, like the dentist, to obtain a license to practice. A license can be obtained from the state's Board of Dental Examiners after graduating from an accredited dental hygiene program, and successfully passing both the national board examination (given by the American Dental Hygienists' Association) and the state or regional examination.

Recent starting salaries for dental hygienists with no experience working for the federal government ranged from $12,900 to $14,400 a year, while those with experience working for the federal government earned average annual salaries of $17,000. Dental hygienists working in private dental offices earned salaries between $12,000-$16,000 a year.

Below is a list of schools that offer dental hygiene programs accredited by the Commission on Dental Accreditation as part of the American Dental Association. The American Dental Hygienists' Association strongly recommends that students request an admission application from schools of interest at least a full year prior to desired admission date.

The ADHA (American Dental Hygienists' Association) Institute for Oral Health offers several scholarships to needy dental hygiene students enrolled in their second year of an accredited training program. For eligibility requirements and an application form write to ADHA Institute for Oral Health, 444 North Michigan Avenue, Suite 3400, Chicago, Illinois 60611.

For other information on accredited programs and educational requirements, contact the American Dental Hygienists' Association, 444 North Michigan Avenue, Suite 3400, Chicago, Illinois 60611.

For information on licensing requirements, contact the State Board of Dental Examiners (located in the *state capital*) or the American Association of Dental Examiners, 211 East Chicago Avenue, Chicago, Illinois 60611.

SOURCES:

American Dental Hygienists' Association
American Dental Association
Occupational Outlook Handbook

Dental Hygienist Programs

ALABAMA

Dental Hygiene Program
University of Alabama
School of Dentistry
University Station
Birmingham, Alabama 35294

ALASKA

Dental Hygiene Program
Anchorage Community College
University of Alaska
2533 Providence Drive
Anchorage, Alaska 99508-4670

ARIZONA

Dental Hygiene Program
Northern Arizona University
Box 15065
Flagstaff, Arizona 86011

Dental Hygiene Program
Phoenix College
1202 W. Thomas Road
Phoenix, Arizona 85013

ARKANSAS

Dental Hygiene Program
University of Arkansas for Medical Sciences
4301 West Markham Street
Little Rock, Arkansas 72205

CALIFORNIA

Dental Hygiene Program
Cabrillo College
6500 Soquel Drive
Aptos, California 95003

Dental Hygiene Program
Cerritos College
11110 East Alondra Boulevard
Norwalk, California 90650

Dental Hygiene Program
Chabot College
25555 Hesperian Boulevard
Hayward, California 94545

Dental Hygiene Program
Cypress College
9200 Valley View
Cypress, California 90630

Dental Hygiene Program
Diablo Valley College
321 Golf Club Road
Pleasant Hill, California 94523

Dental Hygiene Program
Foothill College
12345 El Monte Road
Los Altos Hills, California 94022

Dental Hygiene Program
Fresno City College
1101 East University
Fresno, California 93741

Dental Hygiene Program
Loma Linda University
School of Dentistry
Loma Linda, California 92350

Dental Hygiene Program
Pasadena City College
1570 East Colorado Blvd.
Pasadena, California 91106

Dental Hygiene Program
Sacramento City College
3835 Freeport Boulevard
Sacramento, California 95822

Dental Hygiene Program
University of California
School of Dentistry
San Francisco Medical Center
San Francisco, California 94143

Dental Hygiene Program
University of South California
School of Dentistry
University Park-MC0641
Los Angeles, California 90007

Dental Hygiene Program
West Los Angeles College
4800 Freshman Drive
Culver City, California 90230

COLORADO

Dental Hygiene Program
Colorado Northwestern Community College
Kennedy Drive
Rangely, Colorado 81648

Dental Hygiene Program
University of Colorado
School of Dentistry
4200 East Ninth Ave., Med. Ctr.
Denver, Colorado 80262

Dental Hygiene Program
Pueblo Vocational Community College
415 Harrison Avenue
Pueblo, Colorado 81004

CONNECTICUT

Dental Hygiene Program
Tunxis Community College
Routes 6 & 177
Farmington, Connecticut 06032

Dental Hygiene Program
University of Bridgeport
Fones School-Dental Hygiene
30 Hazel Street
Bridgeport, Connecticut 06601

DELAWARE

Dental Hygiene Program
Delaware Technical & Community College
Wilmington Campus
333 Shipley
Wilmington, Delaware 19801

DISTRICT OF COLUMBIA

Dental Hygiene Program
Howard University
College of Dentistry
600 "W" Street N.W.
Washington, DC 20059

FLORIDA

Dental Hygiene Program
Florida Junior College
4501 Capper Road
Jacksonville, Florida 32218

Dental Hygiene Program
Miami-Dade Community College
Medical Center Campus
950 N.W. 20th Street
Miami, Florida 33127

Dental Hygiene Program
Palm Beach Junior College
4200 S. Congress Avenue
Lake Worth, Florida 33461

Dental Hygiene Program
Pensacola Junior College
5555 Highway 98
Pensacola, Florida 32507

Dental Hygiene Program
St. Petersburg Junior College
P.O. Box 13489
St. Petersburg, Florida 33733

Dental Hygiene Program
Santa Fe Community College
Box 1530
Gainesville, Florida 32602

Dental Hygiene Program
Tallahassee Community College
444 Appleyard Drive
Tallahassee, Florida 32304

Dental Hygiene Program
Valencia Community College
1800 South Kirkman Road
Orlando, Florida 32811

GEORGIA

Dental Hygiene Program
Albany Junior College
2400 Gillionville Road
Albany, Georgia 31707

Dental Hygiene Program
Armstrong State College
11935 Abercorn
Savannah, Georgia 31406-7197

Dental Hygiene Program
Clayton Junior College
5900 Lee Street
Morrow, Georgia 30260

Dental Hygiene Program
Columbus College
Algonquin Drive
Columbus, Georgia 31993-2399

Dental Hygiene Program
Dekalb Community College
2101 Womack Road
Dunwoody, Georgia 30338

Dental Hygiene Program
Macon Junior College
5357 Raley Road
Macon, Georgia 31297

Dental Hygiene Program
Medical College of Georgia
School of Allied Health Science
1120 15th Street
Augusta, Georgia 30912

HAWAII

Dental Hygiene Program
University of Hawaii
2528 The Mall
Honolulu, Hawaii 96822

IDAHO

Dental Hygiene Program
Idaho State University
741 South 8th Street
Pocatello, Idaho 83209

ILLINOIS

Dental Hygiene Program
Illinois Central College
East Peoria, Illinois 61635

Dental Hygiene Program
Lake Land College
South Route 45
Mattoon, Illinois 69138

Dental Hygiene Program
Loyola University
School of Dentistry
2160 South First Avenue
Maywood, Illinois 60153

Dental Hygiene Program
Northwestern University
School of Dentistry
240 East Huron Avenue
Chicago, Illinois 60611

Dental Hygiene Program
Parkland College
2400 West Bradley
Champaign, Illinois 61820

Dental Hygiene Program
Prairie State College
202 South Halsted Street
Chicago Heights, Illinois 60411

Dental Hygiene Program
Southern Illinois University
School of Technical Careers
Carbondale, Illinois 62901

Dental Hygiene Program
William Rainey Harper College
Algonquin & Roselle Roads
Palatine, Illinois 60067

INDIANA

Dental Hygiene Program
Indiana University Northwest
Dental Auxiliary Education
3400 Broadway
Gary, Indiana 46409

Dental Hygiene Program
Indiana University-Purdue University at Fort Wayne
2101 Coliseum Boulevard East
Fort Wayne, Indiana 46805

Dental Hygiene Program
Indiana University-Purdue University at Indianapolis
1121 West Michigan Street
Indianapolis, Indiana 46202

Dental Hygiene Program
Indiana University at South Bend
Riverside Hall
1700 Mishawaka Avenue
South Bend, Indiana 46615

Dental Hygiene Program
University of Southern Indiana
8600 University Boulevard
Evansville, Indiana 47712

IOWA

Dental Hygiene Program
Des Moines Area Community College
2006 Ankeny Boulevard
Ankeny, Iowa 50021

Dental Hygiene Program
Hawkeye Institute of Technology
1501 E. Orange Rd.-Grundy Hall
Waterloo, Iowa 50701

Dental Hygiene Program
University of Iowa
College of Dentistry
Iowa City, Iowa 52242

KANSAS

Dental Hygiene Program
Johnson County Community College
College Blvd. & Quivira Rd.
Overland Park, Kansas 66210

Dental Hygiene Program
Wichita State University
College of Health Professions-Box 144
1854 Fairmount
Wichita, Kansas 67208

KENTUCKY

Dental Hygiene Program
Ashland Community College
1400 College Drive
Ashland, Kentucky 41101

Dental Hygiene Program
Lexington Community College
Cooper Driver-Oswald Building
Lexington, Kentucky 40506

Dental Hygiene Program
Southeast Community College
Cumberland, Kentucky 40823

Dental Hygiene Program
University of Louisville
School of Dentistry
Louisville, Kentucky 40292

Dental Hygiene Program
Western Kentucky University
Academic Complex
Bowling Green, Kentucky 42101

LOUISIANA

Dental Hygiene Program
Louisiana State University
School of Dentistry
1100 Florida Avenue
New Orleans, Louisiana 70199

Dental Hygiene Program
Northeast Louisiana University
700 University Avenue
Monroe, Louisiana 71209

MAINE

Dental Hygiene Program
University of Maine-Orono
University College
Lincoln Hall
Bangor, Maine 04401

Dental Hygiene Program
Westbrook College
716 Stevens Avenue
Portland, Maine 04103

MARYLAND

Dental Hygiene Program
Allegany Community College
P.O. Box 870
Willowbrook Road
Cumberland, Maryland 21502

Dental Hygiene Program
Community College of Baltimore
2901 Liberty Heights Avenue
Baltimore, Maryland 21215

Dental Hygiene Program
University of Maryland
School of Dentistry
666 West Baltimore Street
Baltimore, Maryland 21201

MASSACHUSETTS

Dental Hygiene Program
Bristol Community College
777 Elsbree Street
Fall River, Massachusetts 02720

Dental Hygiene Program
Cape Cod Community College
Route 132
West Barnstable, Massachusetts 02668

Dental Hygiene Program
Forsyth School of Dental Hygiene
140 The Fenway
Boston, Massachusetts 02115

Dental Hygiene Program
Middlesex Community College
Springs Road
Bedford, Massachusetts 01730

Dental Hygiene Program
Quinsigamond Community College
670 West Boylston Street
Worcester, Massachusetts 01606

Dental Hygiene Program
Springfield Technical Community College
1 Armory Square
Springfield, Massachusetts 01105

MICHIGAN

Dental Hygiene Program
C S Mott Community College
1401 East Court Street
Flint, Michigan 48503

Dental Hygiene Program
Delta College
University Center, Michigan 48710

Dental Hygiene Program
Ferris State College
School of Allied Health
901 South State Street
Big Rapids, Michigan 49307

Dental Hygiene Program
Grand Rapids Junior College
143 Bostwick, N.E.
Grand Rapids, Michigan 49502

Dental Hygiene Program
Kalamazoo Valley Community College
6767 West 'O' Avenue
Kalamazoo, Michigan 49009

Dental Hygiene Program
Kellogg Community College
450 North Avenue
Battle Creek, Michigan 49016

Dental Hygiene Program
Lansing Community College
419 North Capital Avenue
Lansing, Michigan 48901

Dental Hygiene Program
Oakland Community College
Highland Lakes Campus
7350 Cooley Lake Road
Union Lake, Michigan 48085

Dental Hygiene Program
University of Detroit
School of Dentistry
2985 East Jefferson Avenue
Detroit, Michigan 48207

Dental Hygiene Program
University of Michigan
School of Dentistry
1101 North University
Ann Arbor, Michigan 48109

Dental Hygiene Program
Wayne County Community College
Greenfield Center
8551 Greenfield
Detroit, Michigan 48228

MINNESOTA

Dental Hygiene Program
Mankato State University
Box 81
Mankato, Minnesota 56001

Dental Hygiene Program
Normandale Community College
9700 France Avenue
South Bloomington, Minnesota 55431

Dental Hygiene Program
University of Minnesota
School of Dentistry
515 Delaware, S.E.
Minneapolis, Minnesota 55455

Dental Hygiene Program
University of Minnesota-Duluth
10 University Drive
Duluth, Minnesota 55812

MISSISSIPPI

Dental Hygiene Program
Meridian Junior College
5500 Highway 19 North
Meridian, Mississippi 39301

Dental Hygiene Program
Northeast Mississippi Junior College
Booneville, Mississippi 38829

Dental Hygiene Program
University of Mississippi
Medical Center
2500 North State Street
Jackson, Mississippi 39216

MISSOURI

Dental Hygiene Program
Missouri Southern State College
Newman & Duquesne Roads
Joplin, Missouri 64801

Dental Hygiene Program
St. Louis Community College-Forest Park
5600 Oakland Avenue
St. Louis, Missouri 63110

Dental Hygiene Program
University of Missouri-Kansas City
School of Dentistry
650 East 25th Street
Kansas City, Missouri 64108

MONTANA

Dental Hygiene Program
Carroll College
Guadalupe Hall
Helena, Montana 59625

NEBRASKA

Dental Hygiene Program
Central Technical Community College
P.O. Box 1024
Hastings, Nebraska 68901

Dental Hygiene Program
University of Nebraska
College of Dentistry
40th & Holdrege Streets
Lincoln, Nebraska 68583-0740

NEVEDA

Dental Hygiene Program
Clark County Community College
3200 E. Cheyenne Avenue
North Las Vegas, Nevada 89030

NEW HAMPSHIRE

Dental Hygiene Program
New Hampshire Technical Institute
Institute Drive
Concord, New Hampshire 03301

NEW JERSEY

Dental Hygiene Program
Bergen Community College
400 Paramus Road
Paramus, New Jersey 07652

Dental Hygiene Program
Camden County College
P.O. Box 200
Blackwood, New Jersey 08012

Dental Hygiene Program
Fairleigh Dickinson University
School of Dentistry
110 Fuller Place
Hackensack, New Jersey 07601

Dental Hygiene Program
Middlesex County College
153 Mill Road
Box 3050
Edison, New Jersey 08818

Dental Hygiene Program
Union County College
1033 Springfield Avenue
Cranford, New Jersey 07016

Dental Hygiene Program
University of Med-Dent of New Jersey
School of Health Professions
100 Bergen Street
Newark, New Jersey 07103

NEW MEXICO

Dental Hygiene Program
University of New Mexico
Novitski Hall
Albuquerque, New Mexico 87131

NEW YORK

Dental Hygiene Program
Broome Community College
Upper Front Street
Binghamton, New York 13902

Dental Hygiene Program
Columbia University
School of Dental & Oral Surgery
630 West 168th Street
New York, New York 10032

Dental Hygiene Program
Erie Community College-North Campus
Main St. & Youngs Road
Buffalo, New York 14221

Dental Hygiene Program
Eugenio Maria De Hostos College
475 Grand Concourse
Bronx, New York 10451

Dental Hygiene Program
Hudson Valley Community College
80 Vanderburgh Avenue
Troy, New York 12180

Dental Hygiene Program
Monroe Community College
1000 East Henrietta Road
Rochester, New York 14623

Dental Hygiene Program
New York City Technical College
300 Jay Street
Brooklyn, New York 11201

Dental Hygiene Program
Onondaga Community College
Route 173
Syracuse, New York 13215

Dental Hygiene Program
Orange County Community College
115 South Street
Middletown, New York 10940

Dental Hygiene Program
State University of New York
Farmingdale Campus
Melville Road
Farmingdale, New York 11735

NORTH CAROLINA

Dental Hygiene Program
Ashville-Buncombe Technical College
340 Victoria Road
Asheville, North Carolina 28801

Dental Hygiene Program
Central Piedmont Community College
1141 Elizabeth
P.O. Box 35009
Charlotte, North Carolina 28235

Dental Hygiene Program
Coastal Carolina Community College
444 Western Boulevard
Jacksonville, North Carolina 28540

Dental Hygiene Program
Fayetteville Technical Institute
2201 Hull Road
P.O. Bos 35236
Fayetteville, North Carolina 28303

Dental Hygiene Program
Guilford Technical Community College
P.O. Box 309
Jamestown, North Carolina 27282

Dental Hygiene Program
University of North Carolina
School of Dentistry
405 Brauer Hall
Chapel Hill, North Carolina 27514

Dental Hygiene Program
Wayne Community College
Dental Auxiliary Department
P.O. Box 8002
Goldsboro, North Carolina 27530

NORTH DAKOTA

Dental Hygiene Program
North Dakota State
School of Science
Wahpeton, North Dakota 58075

OHIO

Dental Hygiene Program
Cuyahoga College
Metropolitan Campus
2900 Community College Ave.
Cleveland, Ohio 44115

Dental Hygiene Program
Lakeland Community College
Route 306 & 90
Mentor, Ohio 44060

Dental Hygiene Program
Lima Technical College
4240 Campus Drive
Lima, Ohio 45804

Dental Hygiene Program
Ohio State University
College of Dentistry
305 West 12th Avenue
Columbus, Ohio 43210

Dental Hygiene Program
Owens Technical College
Caller No. 10,000 Oregon Rd.
Toledo, Ohio 43699

Dental Hygiene Program
Shawnee State College
940 Second Street
Portsmouth, Ohio 45662

Dental Hygiene Program
Sinclair Community College
444 West Third Street
Dayton, Ohio 45402

Dental Hygiene Program
University of Cincinnati
Raymond Walters College
9555 Plainfield Road
Cincinnati, Ohio 45236

Dental Hygiene Program
Youngstown State University
Technical & Community College
410 Wick Avenue
Youngstown, Ohio 44555

OKLAHOMA

Dental Hygiene Program
Rose State College
6420 Southeast 15th Street
Midwest City, Oklahoma 73110

Dental Hygiene Program
Oklahoma Univ-Health Science Ctr.
College of Dentistry
P.O. Box 26901
Oklahoma City, Oklahoma 73190

OREGON

Dental Hygiene Program
Lane Community College
4000 East 30th Avenue
Eugene, Oregon 97405

Dental Hygiene Program
Mt. Hood Community College
26000 S.E. Stark Street
Gresham, Oregon 97030

Dental Hygiene Program
Oregon Institute of Technology
Campus Drive
Klamath Falls, Oregon 97601

Dental Hygiene Program
Oregon Univ-Health Science Ctr.
School of Dentistry
611 S.W. Campus Drive
Portland, Oregon 97201

Dental Hygiene Program
Portland Community College
12000 S.W. 49th Avenue
Portland, Oregon 97219

PENNSYLVANIA

Dental Hygiene Program
Community College of Philadelphia
1600 Spring Garden Street
Philadelphia, Pennsylvania 19130

Dental Hygiene Program
Luzerne County Community College
Prospect St. & Middle Rd.
Nanticoke, Pennsylvania 18634

Dental Hygiene Program
Montgomery County Community College
340 Dekalb Pike
Blue Bell, Pennsylvania 19422

Dental Hygiene Program
Northampton County Community College
3835 Green Pond Road
Bethlehem, Pennsylvania 18017

Dental Hygiene Program
Temple University
School of Dentistry
3223 North Broad Street
Philadephia, Pennsylvania 19140

Dental Hygiene Program
Thomas Jefferson University
College of Allied Health Science
Health Sciences Center
Philadelphia, Pennsylvania 19107

Dental Hygiene Program
University of Pittsburgh
School of Dental Medicine
337 Salk Hall
Pittsburgh, Pennsylvania 15261

Dental Hygiene Program
Williamsport Area Community College
1005 West Third Street
Williamsport, Pennsylvania 17701

PUERTO RICO

Dental Hygiene Program
University of Puerto Rico
School of Dentistry
G.P.O. Box 5067
San Juan, Puerto Rico 00936

RHODE ISLAND

Dental Hygiene Program
University of Rhode Island
8 Washburn Hall
Kingston, Rhode Island 02881

SOUTH CAROLI NA

Dental Hygiene Program
Florence-Darlington Technical College
P.O. Drawer F-8000
Florence, South Carolina 29501

Dental Hygiene Program
Greenville Technical College
P.O. Box 5616, Station B
Greenville, South Carolina 29606

Dental Hygiene Program
Medical University of South Carolina
College of Allied Health Science
171 Ashley Avenue
Charleston, South Carolina 29425

Dental Hygiene Program
Midlands Technical College
P.O. Box 2408
Columbia, South Carolina 29202

SOUTH DAKOTA

Dental Hygiene Program
University of South Dakota
East Hall
Vermillion, South Dakota 57069

TENNESSEE

Dental Hygiene Program
Chattanooga State Tech. Community College
4501 Amnicola Highway
Chattanooga, Tennessee 37406

Dental Hygiene Program
East Tennessee State University
College of Public & Allied Health
Johnson City, Tennessee 37614-0002

Dental Hygiene Program
Meharry Medical Coll.-Tennessee State Univ.
School of Allied Health Professions
3500 Centennial Boulevard
Nashville, Tennessee 37203

Dental Hygiene Program
University of Tennessee
Center for Health Sciences
7777 Court Ave.
Memphis, Tennessee 38163

TEXAS

Dental Hygiene Program
Amarillo College
School of Biomedical Arts
P.O. Box 447
Amarillo, Texas 79178

Dental Hygiene Program
Baylor College of Dentistry
Caruth School of Dental Hygiene
3302 Gaston Avenue
Dallas, Texas 75246

Dental Hygiene Program
Bee County College
Dental Hygiene Department
3800 Charco Road
Beeville, Texas 78102

Dental Hygiene Program
Del Mar College
Baldwin at Ayers Streets
Corpus Christi, Texas 78404

Dental Hygiene Program
El Paso Community College
P.O. Box 20500
El Paso, Texas 79998

Dental Hygiene Program
Howard County Junior College
1001 Birdwell Lane
Big Spring, Texas 79720

Dental Hygiene Program
Lamar University
Lamar University Station
Box 10096
Beaumont, Texas 77710

Dental Hygiene Program
Midwestern State University
3400 Taft
Wichita Falls, Texas 76308

Dental Hygiene Program
Tarrant County Junior College
Northeast Campus
828 Harwood Road
Hurst, Texas 76011

Dental Hygiene Program
Texas Women's University
Institute of Health Sciences
Box 22665-TWU Station
Denton, Texas 76204

Dental Hygiene Program
Tyler Junior College
Henderson Highway
Tyler, Texas 75711

Dental Hygiene Program
Univ. of Texas-Dental Branch
P.O. Box 20068
Houston, Texas 77030

Dental Hygiene Program
Univ. of Texas-Health Sciences
Center at San Antonio
7703 Floyd Curl Drive
San Antonio, Texas 78284

Dental Hygiene Program
Wharton County Junior College
911 Boling Highway
Wharton, Texas 77488

UTAH

Dental Hygiene Program
Weber State College
3750 Marrison Boulevard
Ogden, Utah 84408

VERMONT

Dental Hygiene Program
University of Vermont
School of Allied Health Science
Rowell Building
Burlington, Vermont 05405

VIRGINIA

Dental Hygiene Program
Northern Virginia Community College
8333 Little River Turnpike
Annandale, Virginia 22003

Dental Hygiene Program
Old Dominion University
Technology Building
Norfolk, Virginia 23508-8512

Dental Hygiene Program
Virginia Commonwealth University
School of Dentistry
Health Science Division
Richmond, Virginia 23298

Dental Hygiene Program
Virginia Western Community College
3095 Colonial Avenue, S.W.
Roanoke, Virginia 24015

WASHINGTON

Dental Hygiene Program
Clark College
1800 E. McLoughlin Boulevard
Vancouver, Washington 98663

Dental Hygiene Program
Eastern Washington University
Paulsen Building
Cheney, Washington 99004

Dental Hygiene Program
Pierce College
9401 Farwest Drive, S.W.
Tacoma, Washington 98498

Dental Hygiene Program
Shoreline Community College
16101 Greenwood Avenue
North Seattle, Washington 98133

Dental Hygiene Program
Yakima Valley Community College
16th Ave., South-Nob Hill Blvd.
Yakima, Washington 98907

WEST VIRGINIA

Dental Hygiene Program
West Liberty State College
West Liberty, West Virginia 26074

Dental Hygiene Program
West Virginia Institute of Technology
Montgomery, West Virginia 25136

Dental Hygiene Program
West Virginia University
School of Dentistry
Medical Center
Morgantown, West Virginia 26506

WISCONSIN

Dental Hygiene Program
Maidson Area Technical College
211 North Carroll Street
Madison, Wisconsin 53703

Dental Hygiene Program
Marquette University
School of Dentistry
604 North 16th Street
Milwaukee, Wisconsin 53233

Dental Hygiene Program
Milwaukee Area Technical College
1015 North Sixth Street
Milwaukee, Wisconsin 53203

Dental Hygiene Program
North Central Technical Institute
1000 Campus Drive
Wausau, Wisconsin 54401

Dental Hygiene Program
Northeast Wisconsin Tech. Institute
2740 W. Mason Street
P.O. Box 19042
Green Bay, Wisconsin 54307-9042

WYOMING

Dental Hygiene Program
Sheridan College
3059 Coffeen Avenue
Box 1500
Sheridan, Wyoming 82801

CANADA

Dental Hygiene Program
University of Alberta
Faculty of Dentistry
Edmonton, Alberta, Canada T6G 2N8

Dental Hygiene Program
University of Manitoba
780 Bannatyne Avenue
Winnipeg, Manitoba, Canada R3E 0W3

Dental Hygiene Program
Algonquin College-Applied Arts
1385 Woodroffe Avenue
Ottawa, Ontario, Canada K2G 1V8

Dental Hygiene Program
George Brown College-Applied Arts
P.O. Box 1015, Station B
Toronto, Ontario, Canada M5T 2T9

Dental Hygiene Program
Canadian Forces Dental School
Dental Therapist Level 6B
Camp Borden, Ontario, Canada

Dental Hygiene Program
Canadore College of AA&T
P.O. Box 5001
North Bay, Ontario, Canada P1B 8K9

Dental Hygiene Program
Seneca College
1255 Sheppard Avenue E.
Willowdale, Ontario, Canada M2K I2E

Dental Hygiene Program
College De Maisonneuve
3800 Est, Rue Sherbrooke
Montreal, Quebec, Canada H1X 2A2

Dental Hygiene Program
John Abbott College
P.O. Box 2000
Ste Anne De Bellevue, Quebec, Canada

Dental Hygiene Program
Cegep Francois Xavier Garneau
1660 Blvd. De L'Entente CP 63
Sillery, Quebec, Canada GLT 2S3

Dental Hygiene Program
College Regional Bourgchemin
3000 Rue Boulle, CP 9000
Ste Hyacinthe, Quebec, Canada J2S 7C7

Dental Hygiene Program
College Edouard Montpetit
945 - Chemin Chambly
Longeuil, Quebec, Canada J4H 3M6

Dental Hygiene Program
Dalhousie University
209 Forrest Building
Halifax, N.S., Canada B3H 3J5

Dental Hygiene Program
Wascana Institute of Applied Arts
4635 Wascana Parkway
Regina, Saskatchewan, Canada S4P 3A3

Dental Assistant

Under supervision the *dental assistant* assists the dentist with direct care of the dental patient. The responsibilities of the dental assistant vary widely depending upon the requirements of the dentist - employer and the extent of the dental assistant's education and experience. Duties of the dental assistant are governed by state law and may vary from state to state. The dental assistant can perform four types of functions: chairside assistance, clinical support, laboratory support duties, and office duties.

In chairside assistance the dental assistant, if qualified, can assist in all aspects of general dentistry and dental specialties. In clinical support the dental assistant may process X-rays and take and record dental and medical histories from patients. Laboratory support duties include pouring molds and making preliminary impressions for study casts. Finally the dental assistant can perform business office procedures such as maintaining an appointment schedule, acting as office receptionist, receiving payment from patients, and controlling office inventory. In a larger dental office a receptionist or office manager may take on these business office responsibilities allowing the dental assistant to perform dental work.

The dental assistant can be trained by a dentist - as many are - or complete a one-to-two-year postsecondary dental assisting program at a vocational-technical school or community college and receive a certificate, diploma, or associate degree. Those who have completed an accredited dental assisting program are eligible to take the certification examination by the Dental Assisting National Board. Certification is required in some states. For information on certification in dental assisting, contact the Dental Assisting National Board, Inc., 216 East Ontario Street, Chicago, Illinois 60611.

Application for a limited number of educational scholarships may be obtained from the American Dental Assistants Association at the address listed below.

According to a recent survey by the American Dental Assistants Association of the dental assistants who responded, 25% earned $10,000 and under a year; 30% earned $10,000 - $12,500, 35% earned $12,500 - $17,500 and the remainder earned $17,500 and over.

Below is a list of dental assisting programs accredited by the Commission on Dental Accreditation of the American Dental Association.

For more information on a career as a dental assistant, contact the American Dental Assistants Association, 666 North Lake Shore Drive, Suite 1130, Chicago, Illinois 60611.

SOURCES:

American Dental Assistants Association
Occupational Outlook Handbook

Dental Assistant Programs

ALABAMA

Dental Assisting Program
Bessemer State Technical College
P.O. Box 308
Bessemer, Alabama 35021

Dental Assisting Program
Council Trenholm State Tech. College
1225 Air Base Boulevard
Montgomery, Alabama 36108

Dental Assisting Program
James H. Faulkner State Jr. College
Hammond Circle
Bay Minnette, Alabama 36507

Dental Assisting Program
John C. Calhoun State Community College
P.O. Box 2216
Decatur, Alabama 35602

Dental Assisting Program
University of Alabama
School of Dentistry
1916 Ninth Avenue, South
Birmingham, Alabama 35294

Dental Assisting Program
Wallace State Community College
P.O. Box 250
Hanceville, Alabama 35077

ALASKA

Dental Assisting Program
Anchorage Community College
University of Alaska
2533 Providence Drive
Anchorage, Alaska 99408-4670

ARIZONA

Dental Assisting Program
Phoenix College
1202 West Thomas Road
Phoenix, Arizona 85013

Dental Assisting Program
Pima Community College
2202 West Anklam Road
Tucson, Arizona 85709

Dental Assisting Program
Cotton Boll Vocation Tech. School
Box 36
Burdette, Arizona 72321

Dental Assisting Program
Pulaski Vocational Tech. School
3000 West Scenic Road
North Little Rock, Arizona 72118-3399

CALIFORNIA

Dental Assisting Program
Abram Friedman Occupation Center
Paramedical Branch
3721 West Washington Blvd.
Los Angeles, California 90018

Dental Assisting Program
Andon College
1414 North Winchester Blvd.
San Jose, California 95128

Dental Assisting Program
Bakersfield College
1801 Panorama Drive
Bakersfield, California 93305

Dental Assisting Program
Cabrillo College
6500 Soquel Drive
Aptos, California 95003

Dental Assisting Program
Cerritos College
11110 East Alondra Boulevard
Norwalk, California 90650

Dental Assisting Program
Chabot College
25555 Hesperian Boulevard
Hayward, California 94545

Dental Assisting Program
Chaffey Community College
5885 Haven Avenue
Alta Loma, California 91701

Dental Assisting Program
Citrus College
18824 E. Foothill Blvd, P.O. RRR
Azusa, California 91702-1348

Dental Assisting Program
City College of San Francisco
50 Phelan Avenue
San Francisco, California 94112

Dental Assisting Program
College of Alameda
555 Atlantic Avenue
Alameda, California 94501

Dental Assisting Program
College of Marin
College Avenue
Kentfield, California 94904

Dental Assisting Program
College of the Redwoods
Tompkins Hill Road
Eureka, California 95501

Dental Assisting Program
College of San Mateo
1700 West Hillsdale Boulevard
San Mateo, California 94402

Dental Assisting Program
Contra Costa College
2600 Mission Bell Drive
San Pablo, California 94806

Dental Assisting Program
Cypress College
9200 Valley View Street
Cypress, California 90630

Dental Assisting Program
Diablo Valley College
321 Golf Club Road
Pleasant Hill, California 94523

Dental Assisting Program
East Los Angeles Occ Center
2100 Marengo Street
Los Angeles, California 90033

Dental Assisting Program
Foothill College
12345 El Monte Road
Los Altos Hills, California 94022

Dental Assisting Program
Kings River Community College
995 North Reed Avenue
Reedley, California 93654

Dental Assisting Program
La Puente Valley-Fairgrove
1110 Fickewirth Street
La Puente, California 91744

Dental Assisting Program
Loma Linda University
School of Dentistry
Prince Hall
Loma Linda, California 92350

Dental Assisting Program
Los Angeles City College
885 North Vermont Avenue
Los Angeles, California 90029

Dental Assisting Program
Merced College
3600 M Street
Merced, California 95340

Dental Assisting Program
Modesto Junior College
435 College Avenue
Modesto, California 95350

Dental Assisting Program
Monterey Peninsula College
98890 Fremont Avenue
Monterey, California 93940

Dental Assisting Program
North Valley Occ Center
11450 Sharp Avenue
Mission Hills, California 91345

Dental Assisting Program
Orange Coast College
2701 Fairview Road
Costa Mesa, California 92628-0120

Dental Assisting Program
Palomar Community College
1140 West Mission Road
San Marcos, California 92069

Dental Assisting Program
Pasadena City College
1570 East Colorado Boulevard
Pasadena, California 91106

Dental Assisting Program
Rio Hondo College
3600 Workman Mill Road
Whitter, California 90608

Dental Assisting Program
Sacramento City College
3835 Freeport Boulevard
Sacramento, California 95822

Dental Assisting Program
San Jose City College
2100 Moorpark Avenue
San Jose, California 95128

Dental Assisting Program
Santa Rosa Junior College
1501 Mendocino Avenue
Santa Rosa, California 95401

Dental Assisting Program
Simi Valley Adult School
3150 School Street
Simi Valley, California 93065

COLORADO

Dental Assisting Program
Emily Griffith Oppor. School
1250 Welton Street
Denver, Colorado 80204

Dental Assisting Program
Front Range Community College
3645 West 112th Avenue
Westminister, Colorado 80030

Dental Assisting Program
Larimer County Voc-Tech Center
4616 South Shields
Fort Collins, Colorado 80522

Dental Assisting Program
Mesa College
P.O. Box 2647
Grand Junction, Colorado 81501

Dental Assisting Program
Pikes Peak Community College
5765 South Academy Boulevard
Colorado Springs, Colorado 80906

Dental Assisting Program
T. H. Pickens Technical Center
Aurora Public School
500 Buckley Road
Aurora, Colorado 80011

CONNECTICUT

Dental Assisting Program
Albert I. Prince Voc-Tech School
500 Brookfield Street
Hartford, Connecticut 06106

Dental Assisting Program
Briarwood College
2279 Mount Vernon Road
Southington, Connecticut 06489

Dental Assisting Program
Eli Whitney Reg. Voc-Tech School
71 Jones Road
Hamden, Connecticut 06514

Dental Assisting Program
J.M. Wright Voc-Tech School
Box 1416
Stamford, Connecticut 06904

Dental Assisting Program
Tunxis Community College
Routes 6 & 177
Farmington, Connecticut 06032

Dental Assisting Program
Windham Reg. Voc-Tech School
210 Birch Street
Willimantic, Connecticut 06226

DELAWARE

Dental Assisting Program
Delaware Tech and Community College
333 Shipley Street
Wilmington, Delaware 19801

DISTRICT OF COLUMBIA

Dental Assisting Program
Margaret Murray Washington
Career Center
'O' Street, N.W.
Washington, DC 20001

FLORIDA

Dental Assisting Program
Brevard Community College
1519 Clear Lake Road
Cocoa, Florida 32922

Dental Assisting Program
Broward Community College
3501 Southwest Davie Road
Ft. Lauderdale, Florida 33314

Dental Assisting Program
Charlotte Voc-Tech Center
1468 Toledo Blade Blvd.
Port Charlotte, Florida 33952

Dental Assisting Program
Daytona Beach Community College
P.O. Box 1111-US92 Welch Blvd.
Daytona Beach, Florida 32019

Dental Assisting Program
Florida Junior College
4501 Capper Road
Jacksonville, Florida 32218

Dental Assisting Program
Gulf Coast Community College
5230 West Highway 98
Panama City, Florida 32401

Dental Assisting Program
Indian River Community College
3209 Virginia Avenue
Ft. Pierce, Florida 33450

Dental Assisting Program
Lindsey Hopkins Tech-Ed Center
750 N.W. 20th Street
Miami, Florida 33127

Dental Assisting Program
Manatee Area Voc-Tech Center
5603 34th St., West
Bradenton, Florida 33507

Dental Assisting Program
Orlando Vocational Technical Center
301 West Amelia Street
Orlando, Florida 32801

Dental Assisting Program
Palm Beach Junior College
4200 Congress Avenue
Lake Worth, Florida 33461

Dental Assisting Program
Pensacola Junior College
5555 W. Highway 98
Pensacola, Florida 32507

Dental Assisting Program
Robert Morgan Voc-Tech School
18180 S.W. 122 Avenue
Miami, Florida 33177

Dental Assisting Program
St. Petersburg Voc-Tech Institute
901 34th Street
St. Petersburg, Florida 33711

Dental Assisting Program
Santa Fe Community College
300 N.W. 83rd Street
Gainesville, Florida 32602

Dental Assisting Program
Southern College
5600 Lake Underhill Road
Orlando, Florida 32807

GEORGIA

Dental Assisting Program
Albany Area Voc-Tech School
1021 Lowe Road
Albany, Georgia 31708

Dental Assisting Program
Atlanta Area Technical School
1560 Stewart Avenue, SW
Atlanta, Georgia 30310

Dental Assisting Program
Augusta Area Voc-Tech School
Medical College of Georgia
1399 Walton Way
Augusta, Georgia 30901

Dental Assisting Program
Gwinnett Area Technical School
1250 Atkinson Road
P.O. Box 1505
Lawrenceville, Georgia 30246

Dental Assisting Program
Lanier Area Voc-Tech School
P.O. Box 58
Mundys Mill Road
Oakwood, Georgia 30566

Dental Assisting Program
Savannah Voc-Tech School
5717 White Bluff Road
Savannah, Georgia 31499

HAWAII

Dental Assisting Program
Kapiolani Community College
4303 Diamond Head Road
Honolulu, Hawaii 96816

IDAHO

Dental Assisting Program
Boise State University
1910 University Drive
Boise, Idaho 83725

Dental Assisting Program
Eastern Idaho Voc-Tech School
2299 East 17th Street
Idaho Falls, Idaho 83401

ILLINOIS

Dental Assisting Program
Black Hawk College
6600 34th Avenue
Moline, Illinois 61265

Dental Assisting Program
College of Lake County
19351 West Washington Blvd.
Grayslake, Illinois 60030

Dental Assisting Program
Elgin Community College
1700 Spartan Drive
Elgin, Illinois 60120

Dental Assisting Program
Illinois Central College
District 514
East Peoria, Illinois 61635

Dental Assisting Program
Illinois Valley Community College
Route One
Oglesby, Illinois 61348

Dental Assisting Program
John A. Logan College
Rural Route 2
Carterville, Illinois 62918

Dental Assisting Program
Kaskaskia Community College
Shattuc Road
Centralia, Illinois 62801

Dental Assisting Program
Lake Land College
South Route 45
Mattoon, Illinois 61938

Dental Assisting Program
Lewis and Clark Cmty. College
5800 Godfrey Road
Godfrey, Illinois 62035

Dental Assisting Program
Lincoln Land Community College
Shepard Road
Springfield, Illinois 62707

Dental Assisting Program
Loop College
City College System
64 East Lake Street
Chicago, Illinois 60601

Dental Assisting Program
Morton College
3801 South Central Avenue
Cicero, Illinois 60650

Dental Assisting Program
Olney Central College
305 North West Street
Olney, Illinois 62450

Dental Assisting Program
Parkland College
2400 West Bradley
Champaign, Illinois 61820

Dental Assisting Program
Prairie State College
202 South Halsted
Chicago Heights, Illinois 60411

Dental Assisting Program
Robert Morris College
College Avenue
Carthage, Illinois 62321

Dental Assisting Program
Rock Valley College
3301 North Mulford Road
Rockford, Illinois 61101

Dental Assisting Program
Triton College
2000 Fifth Avenue
River Grove, Illinois 60171

INDIANA

Dental Assisting Program
Indiana Univ.-Purdue Univ.
School of Dentistry
1121 West Michigan Street
Indianapolis, Indiana 46202

Dental Assisting Program
Indiana University Northwest
3223 Broadway
Gary, Indiana 46408

Dental Assisting Program
Indiana Univ.-Purdue Univ. at Fort Wayne
2101 Coliseum Boulevard
Fort Wayne, Indiana 46805

Dental Assistingt Program
Indiana University at South Bend
1700 Mishawaka Ave.-Box 7111
South Bend, Indiana 46634

Dental Assisting Program
Indiana Voc-Tech College
3208 Ross Rd.-Box 6299
Lafayette, Indiana 47905

Dental Assisting Program
Professional Careers Institute
2611 Waterfront Pkwy.-East Dr.
Indianapolis, Indiana 46224

Dental Assisting Program
University of Southern Indiana at Evansville
8600 University Boulevard
Evansville, Indiana 47712

IOWA

Dental Assisting Program
Des Moines Area Community College
2006 Ankeny Boulevard
Ankeny, Iowa 50021

Dental Assisting Program
Hawkeye Inst. of Technology
2800 Falls Avenue
Waterloo, Iowa 50701

Dental Assisting Program
Iowa Central Community College
300 Avenue 'M'
Fort Dodge, Iowa 50501

Dental Assisting Program
Iowa Western Community College
2700 College Road-Box 4C
Council Bluffs, Iowa 51502

Dental Assisting Program
Kirkwood Community College
Resident Program
6301 Kirkwood Blvd. SW-Box 2068
Cedar Rapids, Iowa 52406

Dental Assisting Program
Kirkwood Community College
Off-Campus Program
6301 Kirkwood Blvd. SW-Box 2068
Cedar Rapids, Iowa 52406

Dental Assisting Program
Marshalltown Community College
3700 South Center Street
Marshalltown, Iowa 50158

Dental Assisting Program
Northeast Iowa Tech Institute
Rural Route 1
Peosta, Iowa 52001

Dental Assisting Program
Western Iowa Tech Community College
4647 Stone Avenue
Sioux City, Iowa 51104

KANSAS

Dental Assisting Program
Flint Hills Area Voc-Tech
3301 West 18th Street
Emporia, Kansas 66801

Dental Assisting Program
Wichita Area Voc-Tech School
324 North Emporia
Wichita, Kansas 67202

KENTUCKY

Dental Assisting Program
Bowling Green State Voc-Tech
1845 Loop Drive
Bowling Green, Kentucky 42101-1059

Dental Assisting Program
Central Kentucky State
Voc-Tech School
104 Vo-Tech Road
Lexington, Kentucky 40511

Dental Assisting Program
Jefferson State Voc-Tech School
800 West Chestnut Street
Louisville, Kentucky 40203

Dental Assisting Program
Louisville College-Health Careers
1512 Crums Lane
Louisville, Kentucky 40216

Dental Assisting Program
Northern Kentucky Health Center
790 Thomas More Parkway
Edgewood, Kentucky 41017

Dental Assisting Program
Watterson College
4400 Breckenridge Lane
Louisville, Kentucky 40218

Dental Assisting Program
West Kentucky State Voc-Tech
Hwy 62 West, Blandville Rd.
Paducah, Kentucky 42001

MAINE

Dental Assisting Program
University of Maine-Orono
University College
Lincoln Hall
Bangor, Maine 04401

MARYLAND

Dental Assisting Program
Allegany Community College
Willow Brook Road
Cumberland, Maryland 21502

Dental Assisting Program
Community College of Baltimore
2901 Liberty Heights Avenue
Baltimore, Maryland 21215

Dental Assisting Program
Essex Community College
7201 Rossville Boulevard
Baltimore, Maryland 21237

Dental Assisting Program
Frederick Community College
7932 Opossumtown Pike
Frederick, Maryland 21701

Dental Assisting Program
Montgomery College
Takoma & Fenton Street
Takoma Park, Maryland 20012

MASSACHUSETTS

Dental Assisting Program
Boston University
School of Dentistry
100 East Newton Street
Boston, Massachusetts 02118

Dental Assisting Program
Cape Cod Community College
Route 132
West Barnstable, Massachusetts 02668

Dental Assisting Program
Charles H. McCann Tech School
Hodges Crossroad
North Adams, Massachusetts 01247

Dental Assisting Program
Diman Regional Technical Institute
Stonehaven Road
Fall River, Massachusetts 02723

Dental Assisting Program
Fanning School of Health Occupations
251 Belmont Street
Worcester, Massachusetts 01605

Dental Assisting Program
Massasoit Community College
One Massasoit Boulevard
Brockton, Massachusetts 02402

Dental Assisting Program
Middlesex Community College
Springs Road
Bedford, Massachusetts 01730

Dental Assisting Program
Mount Ida Junior College
777 Dedham Street
Newton Centre, Massachusetts 02159

Dental Assisting Program
Northeastern University
360 Huntington Avenue
Boston, Massachusetts 02115

Dental Assisting Program
Northern Essex Community College
100 Elliott Street
Haverhill, Massachusetts 01830

Dental Assisting Program
Southeastern Technical Institute
250 Foundry Street
South Easton, Massachusetts 02375

Dental Assisting Program
Springfield Tech. Community College
One Armory Square
Springfield, Massachusetts 01105

MICHIGAN

Dental Assisting Program
C.S. Mott Community College
1401 East Court Street
Flint, Michigan 48502

Dental Assisting Program
Delta College
University Center, Michigan 48710

Dental Assisting Program
Ferris State College
VFS Building 303
Big Rapids, Michigan 49307

Dental Assisting Program
Grand Rapids Junior College
143 Bostwick Avenue, N.E.
Grand Rapids, Michigan 49502

Dental Assisting Program
Lake Michigan College
2755 East Napier
Benton Harbor, Michigan 49022

Dental Assisting Program
Lansing Community College
419 N. Capital Ave.-Box 40010
Lansing, Michigan 48901-7211

Dental Assisting Program
Macomb Community College
44575 Garfield Road
Mount Clemens, Michigan 48044

Dental Assisting Program
Northwestern Michigan College
1701 East Front Street
Traverse City, Michigan 49684

Dental Assisting Program
Oakland Community College
7350 Cooley Lake Road
Union Lake, Michigan 48085

Dental Assisting Program
Washtenaw Community College
4800 East Huron River Drive
Ann Arbor, Michigan 48106

Dental Assisting Program
Wayne County Community College
Greenfield Center
8551 Grenfield
Detroit, Michigan 48228

MINNESOTA

Dental Assisting Program
Bemidiji Area Voc-Tech Institute
Roosevelt Road & Grant Avenue
Bemidiji, Minnesota 56601

Dental Assisting Program
Brainerd Area Voc-Tech Institute
300 Quince
Brainerd, Minnesota 58401

Dental Assisting Program
Hennepin Technical Centers
9000 77th Avenue North
Brooklyn Park, Minnesota 55455

Dental Assisting Program
Hibbing Area Voc-Tech Institute
2900 East Beltline
Hibbing, Minnesota 55746

Dental Assisting Program
Lakeland Medical-Dental Academy
1402 West Lake Street
Minneapolis, Minnesota 55408

Dental Assisting Program
Mankato Area Voc-Tech School
1920 Lee Boulevard
P.O. Box 1920
North Mankato, Minnesota 56001

Dental Assisting Program
Medical Institute of Minnesota
2309 Nicollet Avenue
Minneapolis, Minnesota 55404

Dental Assisting Program
Minneapolis Technical Institute
1415 Hennepin Ave. S.
Minneapolis, Minnesota 55404

Dental Assisting Program
Minnesota Institute
Medical & Dental Careers
2915 Wayzata Boulevard
Minneapolis, Minnesota 55405

Dental Assisting Program
Moorehead Area Voc-Tech Institute
1900 28th Avenue South
Moorehead, Minnesota 56560

Dental Assisting Program
916 Area Voc-Tech Institute
3300 Century Avenue North
White Bear Lake, Minnesota 55110

Dental Assisting Program
Normandale Community College
9700 France Avenue South
Bloomington, Minnesota 55431

Dental Assisting Program
Rochester Area Voc-Tech Institute
1926 Second Street, Southeast
Rochester, Minnesota 55904

Dental Assisting Program
SouthwesternVoc-Tech Institute
Canby Campus
1011 First Avenue West
Canby, Minnesota 56220

Dental Assisting Program
St. Cloud Area Voc-Tech Institute
1540 Northway Drive
St. Cloud, Minnesota 56301

MISSISSIPPI

Dental Assisting Program
Hinds Junior College District
3925 Sunset Drive
Jackson, Mississippi 39213

MISSOURI

Dental Assisting Program
East Central College
P.O. Box 529
Hwy 50 & Prairie Dell
Union, Missouri 63084

Dental Assisting Program
Graff Area Voc-Tech Center
815 North Sherman
Springfield, Missouri 63640

Dental Assisting Program
Mineral Area College
Flat River, Missouri 63640

Dental Assisting Program
Nichols Career Center
609 Union Street
Jefferson City, Missouri 65101

Dental Assisting Program
Penn Valley Community College
3201 Southwest Trafficway
Kansas City, Missouri 64111

Dental Assisting Program
Rolla Area Voc-Tech School
1304 East Tenth Street
Rolla, Missouri 65401

Dental Assisting Program
St. Louis Community College-Forest Park
5600 Oakland Avenue
St. Louis, Missouri 63110

Dental Assisting Program
St. Louis Community College-Meramec
11333 Big Bend Boulevard
Kirkwood, Missouri 63122

Dental Assisting Program
Three Rivers Community College
Three Rivers Boulevard
Poplar Bluff, Missouri 63901

MONTANA

Dental Assisting Program
Great Falls Voc-Tech Center
2100 16th Avenue South
Great Falls, Montana 59405

NEBRASKA

Dental Assisting Program
Central Technical Community College
Box 1024
Hastings, Nebraska 68901

Dental Assisting Program
Metropolitan Tech Community College
2909 Gomez Avenue
Omaha, Nebraska 68107

Dental Assisting Program
Mid-Plains Community College
Route 4, Box 1
North Platte, Nebraska 69101

Dental Assisting Program
Omaha College of Health Careers
1052 Park Avenue
Omaha, Nebraska 68105

Dental Assisting Program
Southeast Community College
Health Occupations Division
8800 'O' Street
Lincoln, Nebraska 68520

NEVADA

Dental Assisting Program
Truckee Meadows Community College
7000 Dandini Boulevard
Reno, Nevada 89512

NEW HAMPSHIRE

Dental Assisting Program
New Hampshire Tech Institute
Fan Road
Concord, New Hampshire 03301

NEW JERSEY

Dental Assisting Program
Berdan Institute
265 Route 46 West
Totowa, New Jersey 07512

Dental Assisting Program
Camden County College
Little Gloucester Road
Blackwood, New Jersey 08012

Dental Assisting Program
Camden County Voc-Tech School
P.O. Box 566
Cross Keys Road
Sicklerville, New Jersey 08081

Dental Assisting Program
County College of Morris
Center Grove Road & Route 10
Randolph, New Jersey 07801

Dental Assisting Program
Mercer County Community College
1200 Old Trenton Road
Trenton, New Jersey 08690

Dental Assisting Program
Union County College
1033 Springfield Avenue
Cranford, New Jersey 07016

Dental Assisting Program
Univ. of Medical & Dental of New Jersey
School of Health Professions
100 Bergen Street
Newark, New Jersey 07103

NEW MEXICO

Dental Assisting Program
Luna Voc-Tech Institute
P.O. Drawer K
Las Vegas, New Mexico 87701

Dental Assisting Program
University of New Mexico
Building B-2
Albuquerque, New Mexico 87131

NEW YORK

Dental Assisting Program
Dutchess Community College
Pendell Road
Poughkeepsie, New York 12601

Dental Assisting Program
Hudson Valley Community College
80 Vanderburgh Avenue
Troy, New York 12180

Dental Assisting Program
New York Univ. Dental Center
421 First Avenue
New York, New York 10010

Dental Assisting Program
Niagara County Community College
3111 Saunders Settlement Rd.
Sanborn, New York 14132

Dental Assisting Program
Rockland Community College
Office of Health Programs
145 College Road CS 57
Suffern, New York 10901

Dental Assisting Program
SUNY at Buffalo
Educ. Opportunity Center
485 Washington Street
Buffalo, New York 14203

Dental Assisting Program
Suffolk County Community College
Riverhead Bldg.
533 College Road
Selden, New York 11784

NORTH CAROLINA

Dental Assisting Program
Asheville-Buncombe Tech College
340 Victoria Road
Asheville, North Carolina 28801

Dental Assisting Program
Central Piedmont Community College
P.O. Box 35009
Charlotte, North Carolina 28235

Dental Assisting Program
Coastal Carolina Community College
444 Western Boulevard
Jacksonville, North Carolina 28540

Dental Assisting Program
Fayetteville Technical Institute
2201 Hull Road
P.O. Box 35236
Fayetteville, North Carolina 23328

Dental Assisting Program
Guilford Technical Community College
P.O. Box 309
Jamestown, North Carolina 27282

Dental Assisting Program
Rowan Technical College
I-85 Jake Alexander Blvd, Box 1595
Salisbury, North Carolina 28144

Dental Assisting Program
Technical College of Alamance
P.O. Box 623
Haw River, North Carolina 27258

Dental Assisting Program
University of North Carolina
School of Dentistry
Faculty Office Bld. 211H
Chapel Hill, North Carolina 27514

Dental Assisting Program
Wayne Community College
Caller Box 8002
Goldsboro, North Carolina 27530

Dental Assisting Program
Western Piedmont Community College
1001 Burkemont Avenue
Morganton, North Carolina 28655

NORTH DAKOTA

Dental Assisting Program
North Dakota State
School of Science
Dept. of Dental Auxiliaries
Wahpeton, North Dakota 58075

OHIO

Dental Assisting Program
Cuyahoga Community College
700 Carnegie Avenue
Cleveland, Ohio 44115

Dental Assisting Program
Jefferson Technical College
4000 Sunset Boulevard
Steubenville, Ohio 43952

OKLAHOMA

Dental Assisting Program
Rose State College
6420 Southeast 15th Street
Midwest City, Oklahoma 73110

OREGON

Dental Assisting Program
Blue Mountain Community College
2411 Northwest Carden
Pendleton, Oregon 97801

Dental Assisting Program
Chemeketa Community College
4000 Lancaster Dr. Northeast
Salem, Oregon 97309

Dental Assisting Program
Lane Community College
4000 East 30th Avenue
Eugene, Oregon 97405

Dental Assisting Program
Linn-Benton Community College
6500 Southwest Pacific Blvd.
Albany, Oregon 97321

Dental Assisting Program
Portland Community College
12000 Southwest 49th Avenue
Portland, Oregon 97219

PENNSYLVANIA

Dental Assisting Program
Community College of Philadelphia
1600 Spring Garden Street
Philadelphia, Pennsylvania 19130

Dental Assisting Program
Cumberland-Perry Voc-Tech School
110 Old Willow Mill Road
Mechanicsburg, Pennsylvania 17055

Dental Assisting Program
Harcum Junior College
Montgomery Avenue
Bryn Mawr, Pennsylvania 19010

Dental Assisting Program
Lehigh County Community College
2370 Main Street
Schnecksville, Pennsylvania 18078

Dental Assisting Program
Luzerne County Community College
Prospect St. & Middle Road
Nanticoke, Pennsylvania 18634

Dental Assisting Program
Manor Junior College
Fox Chase Road
Jenkintown, Pennsylvania 19046-3399

Dental Assisting Program
McCarrie Schools of Health Science & Technology
132 North 12th Street
Philadelphia, Pennsylvania 19107

Dental Assisting Program
Median School of Allied Health Careers
121 Ninth Street
Pittsburgh, Pennsylvania 15222-3691

Dental Assisting Program
Murrell DobbinsVoc-Tech School
22nd Street & Lehigh Avenue
Philadelphia, Pennsylvania 19132

Dental Assisting Program
National School of Health Technology
1819 John F. Kennedy Blvd.
Philadelphia, Pennsylvania 19103

Dental Assisting Program
National School of Health Technology
Northeast Location
2137 Welsh Road
Philadelphia, Pennsylvania 19115

Dental Assisting Program
Northampton County Community College
3835 Green Pond Road
Bethlehem, Pennsylvania 18017

Dental Assisting Program
Philadelphia College of Osteopathic Medicine
4190 City Avenue
Philadelphia, Pennsylvania 19131

Dental Assisting Program
University of Pittsburgh
School of Dental Medicine
Terrace and Darragh Streets
Pittsburgh, Pennsylvania 15261

PUERTO RICO

Dental Assisting Program
University of Puerto Rico
Medical-Science Campus
GPO Box 5067
San Juan, Puerto Rico 00936

RHODE ISLAND

Dental Assisting Program
Community College of Rhode Island
Louisquisset Pike
Lincoln, Rhode Island 02865

SOUTH CAROLINA

Dental Assisting Program
Florence-Darlington Tech
P.O. Drawer 8000
Florence, South Carolina 29501

Dental Assisting Program
Greenville Technical College
P.O. Box 5616, Station B
Greenville, South Carolina 29606-5616

Dental Assisting Program
McDuffie Vocational School
1225 South McDuffie Street
Anderson, South Carolina 29621

Dental Assisting Program
Midlands Technical College
P.O. Box 2408
Columbia, South Carolina 29202

Dental Assisting Program
Spartanburg Technical College
Highway I-85
Spartanburg, South Carolina 29305

Dental Assisting Program
Trident Technical College
P.O. Box 10367
Charleston, South Carolina 29411

Dental Assisting Program
York Technical College
Highway 21 By-Pass
Rock Hill, South Carolina 29730

SOUTH DAKOTA

Dental Assisting Program
Lake Area Voc-Tech Institute
230 Eleventh Street, N.E.
Watertown, South Dakota 57201

TENNESSEE

Dental Assisting Program
Chattanooga State Tech Community College
Dept. - Dental Auxiliaries
4501 Amnicola Highway
Chattanooga, Tennessee 37406

Dental Assisting Program
East Tennessee State University
Paramedical Center
1000 West E. Street
Elizabethton, Tennessee 37643

Dental Assisting Program
Knoxville City Schools
1807 East Vine Avenue
Knoxville, Tennessee 37915

Dental Assisting Program
Memphis Area Voc-Tech School
620 Mosby Street
Memphis, Tennessee 38105

Dental Assisting Program
Volunteer State Community College
Nashville Pike
Gallatin, Tennessee 37066

TEXAS

Dental Assisting Program
Del Mar College
Baldwin and Ayers Streets
Corpus Christi, Texas 78404

Dental Assisting Program
El Centro College
Main and Lamar Streets
Dallas, Texas 75202

Dental Assisting Program
El Paso Community College
P.O. Box 20500
El Paso, Texas 79998

Dental Assisting Program
Grayson County College
6101 Grayson Drive
Denison, Texas 75020

Dental Assisting Program
Houston Community College
3100 Shenandoah
Houston, Texas 77021

Dental Assisting Program
North Harris County College
2700 W.W. Thorne Drive
Houston, Texas 77073

Dental Assisting Program
San Antonio College
1300 San Pedro Avenue
San Antonio, Texas 78284

Dental Assisting Program
School of Health Care Science
MSDD 114
Sheppard AFB, Texas 76311

Dental Assisting Program
Tarrant County Junior College
828 Harwood Road, N.E. Campus
Hurst, Texas 76053

Dental Assisting Program
Texas State Tech Institute
Building 39-20
Waco, Texas 76705

Dental Assisting Program
Univ. of Texas-Health Sciences
6516 John Freeman Ave., #20068
Houston, Texas 77025

Dental Assisting Program
Univ. of Texas-Health Sciences
7703 Floyd Curl Drive
San Antonio, Texas 78284

UTAH

Dental Assisting Program
Utah Technical College
Provo Program
1395 North 150 E., Box 1609
Provo, Utah 84601

Dental Assisting Program
Utah Tech College-Salt Lake
4600 South Redwood Road
Salt Lake City, Utah 84107

VERMONT

Dental Assisting Program
Champlain College
163 South Willard Street
Burlington, Vermont 05401

VIRGINIA

Dental Assisting Program
J. Sargeant Reynolds College
2108 East Grace Street
Box 12084
Richmond, Virginia 23241

Dental Assisting Program
Northern Virginia Community College
Health Tech Division
8333 Little River Turnpike
Annandale, Virginia 22003

Dental Assisting Program
Old Dominion University
Technology Building
46th Street and Hampton Blvd.
Norfolk, Virginia 23508-8512

Dental Assisting Program
Virginia Western Community College
3095 Colonial Avenue, S.W.
Roanoke, Virginia 24015

Dental Assisting Program
Wytheville Community College
1000 East Main Street
Wytheville, Virginia 24382

WASHINGTON

Dental Assisting Program
Bellingham Voc-Tech Institute
3028 Lindbergh Avenue
Bellingham, Washington 98225

Dental Assisting Program
Clover Park Voc-Tech Institute
4500 Steilacoom Blvd., S.W.
Tacoma, Washington 98498-4098

Dental Assisting Program
Edmonds Community College
20000 68th Avenue West
Lynwood, Washington 98036

Dental Assisting Program
Highline Community College
South 240th & Pacific Hwy.
Midway, Washington 98032

Dental Assisting Program
Kinman Business University
North 214 Wall Street
Spokane, Washington 99201

Dental Assisting Program
Lake Washington Voc-Tech Institute
11605 132nd Avenue, N.E.
Kirkland, Washington 98034

Dental Assisting Program
L.H. Bates Voc-Tech Institute
1101 S. Yakima Avenue
Tacoma, Washington 98405

Dental Assisting Program
South Puget Sound Community College
2011 Mottman Road Southwest
Olympia, Washington 98502

Dental Assisting Program
Spokane Community College
North 1810 Green St. MS 2090
Spokane, Washington 99207

WISCONSIN

Dental Assisting Program
Blackhawk Technical Institute
1149 4th Street
Beliot, Wisconsin 53511

Dental Assisting Program
Fox Valley Technical Institute
1825 Bluemound Drive
Appleton, Wisconsin 54913

Dental Assisting Program
Gateway Technical Institute
3520 30th Avenue
Kenosha, Wisconsin 53141

Dental Assisting Program
Lakeshore Technical Institute
1290 North Avenue
Cleveland, Wisconsin 53015

Dental Assisting Program
Madison Area Technical College
211 North Carroll St., #643
Madison, Wisconsin 53703

Dental Assisting Program
Milwaukee Area Technical College
1015 North Sixth Street
Milwaukee, Wisconsin 53203

Dental Assisting Program
Northeast Wisconsin Tech Institute
2740 W. Mason Street
P.O. Box 19042
Green Bay, Wisconsin 54307-9042

Dental Assisting Program
Western Wisconsin Tech Institute
Sixth and Vine Streets
La Crosse, Wisconsin 54601

WYOMING

Dental Assisting Program
Sheridan College
3059 Coffeen Avenue
Sheridan, Wyoming 82801

Dental Laboratory Technician

The *dental laboratory technician* works in the field of dental laboratory technology. The dental laboratory technician constructs or repairs artificial teeth, fixed bridges, removable partial dentures, crowns, inlays, and orthodontic appliances, according to dentists' prescriptions. Using precision instruments and specialized equipment, the dental laboratory technician works with a range of material including gold, silver, stainless steel, porcelain and plastics.

Most dental laboratory technicians work in commercial dental laboratories while the remainder are employed by private dental practices or by federal and state agencies. There are also career opportunities available in education, research, and sales. Some technicians own their own commercial dental laboratories while others may work after hours in home dental labs.

There are two ways of becoming a dental laboratory technician, and both require a high school diploma. The apprenticeship program involves on-the-job training in a commercial dental laboratory and usually lasts for three-to-four years, depending upon the trainee's ability and previous experience. The trainee receives a salary during this apprenticeship. The academic program involves completion of a two-year certificate or associate degree program in a community or junior college, vocational-technical school or trade school. The academic programs provide both classroom instruction and "hands on" practical experience.

The National Association of Dental Laboratories states that high school students interested in a career in dental laboratory technology would be more qualified for apprenticeship or admission into a dental laboratory technician program if they have taken courses in ceramics, sculpture, chemistry, physiology, blue print reading, plastics and metal working. Also, employers and school admission officers more readily accept trainees or students who have a high degree of manual dexterity and a good sense of color perception as well as an affinity for accurate and detailed work.

Financial aid to those who qualify is available for study at accredited dental laboratory technician schools by applying to the American Fund for Dental Health, 211 East Chicago Avenue, Chicago, Illinois 60611.

As an acknowledgement of qualification, certification by the National Board for Certification of the National Association of Dental Laboratories is becoming increasingly important. Certification may be applied for after completion of five years of aggregate training and work experience and involves taking a general exam on dental laboratory technology and also written and practical exams on one or more of five laboratory specialties.

Recent starting salaries for trainees working for the federal government averaged $13,000 and those with greater experience earned in the low 20's. Dental laboratory technicians who work in commercial labs may earn in the mid - to high teens. A manager, supervisor, or owner of a dental laboratory may earn considerably more.

For additional information on educational programs or requirements for certification, contact the National Association of Dental Laboratories, 3801 Mt. Vernon Avenue, Alexandria, Virginia 22305.

Below is a list of schools that offer programs in dental laboratory technology accredited by the Commission on Dental Accreditation in conjunction with the American Dental Association.

SOURCES:

American Dental Association
National Association of Dental Laboratories
Occupational Outlook Handbook

ALABAMA

Dental Laboratory Technology Program
University of Alabama, VA Hospital
700 South 19th Street
Birmingham, Alabama 35233

ARIZONA

Dental Laboratory Technology Program
Pima Community College
2202 West Anklam Road
Tucson, Arizona 85709

CALIFORNIA

Dental Laboratory Technology Program
City College of San Francisco
50 Phelan Avenue
San Francisco, California 94112

Dental Laboratory Technology Program
Cypress College
9200 Valley View
Cypress, California 90630

Dental Laboratory Technology Program
Diablo Valley College
321 Golf Club Road
Pleasant Hill, California 94523

Dental Laboratory Technology Program
Los Angeles City College
855 North Vermont Avenue
Los Angeles, California 90029

Dental Laboratory Technology Program
Merced College
3600 'M' Street
Merced, California 95340

Dental Laboratory Technology Program
Orange Coast College
2701 Fairview Road
Costa Mesa, California 92626

Dental Laboratory Technology Program
Pasadena City College
1570 East Colorado Blvd.
Pasadena, California 91101

FLORIDA

Dental Laboratory Technology Program
Indian River Community College
3209 Virginia Avenue
Fort Pierce, Florida 33450

Dental Laboratory Technology Program
Lindsey Hopkins Education Center
750 N.W. 20th Street
Miami, Florida 33127

Dental Laboratory Technology Program
Palm Beach Junior College
4200 Congress Avenue
Lake Worth, Florida 33460

Dental Laboratory Technology Program
Pensacola Junior College
1000 College Boulevard
Pensacola, Florida 32504

Dental Laboratory Technology Program
Southern College
5600 Lake Underhill Road
Orlando, Florida 32807

GEORGIA

Dental Laboratory Technology Program
Atlanta Area Technical School
1560 Stewart Avenue, S.W.
Atlanta, Georgia 30310

Dental Laboratory Technology Program
Atlanta College
Medical and Dental Careers
1240 W. Peachtree St., N.W.
Atlanta, Georgia 30309

Dental Laboratory Technology Program
Augusta Area Technical School
Medical College of Georgia
Augusta, Georgia 30902

Dental Laboratory Technology Program
Gwinnett Area Technical School
1250 Atkinson Rd., Box 1505
Lawrenceville, Georgia 30246

ILLINOIS

Dental Laboratory Technology Program
Lewis & Clark Community College
Godfrey Road
Godfrey, Illinois 62035

Dental Laboratory Technology Program
Southern Illinois University
Dental Technology Department
Carbondale, Illinois 62901

Dental Laboratory Technology Program
Triton College
2000 N. Fifth Avenue
River Grove, Illinois 60171

INDIANA

Dental Laboratory Technology Program
Indiana University
Purdue University
2101 Coliseum Boulevard
Fort Wayne, Indiana 46805

Dental Laboratory Technology Program
University of Southern Indiana
8600 University Boulevard
Evansville, Indiana 47712

IOWA

Dental Laboratory Technology Program
Kirkwood Community College
6301 Kirkwood Blvd., S.W.
Box 2068
Cedar Rapids, Iowa 52406

KENTUCKY

Dental Laboratory Technology Program
Lexington Community College
Oswald Building
Cooper Drive
Lexington, Kentucky 40506

Dental Laboratory Technology Program
Louisville College of Medical and Dental Careers
1512 Crums Lane
Louisville, Kentucky 40216

LOUISIANA

Dental Laboratory Technology Program
Louisiana State University
School of Dentistry
1100 Florida Avenue
New Orleans, Louisiana 70199

MARYLAND

Dental Laboratory Technology Program
Community College of Baltimore
2901 Liberty Heights Avenue
Baltimore, Maryland 21215

Dental Laboratory Technology Program
Montgomery College
Takoma Ave. & Fenton St.
Takoma Park, Maryland 20012

MAINE

Dental Laboratory Technology Program
Middlesex Community College
Springs Road
Bedford, Maine 01730

MICHIGAN

Dental Laboratory Technology Program
Ferris State College
Swan Room 203
Big Rapids, Michigan 49307

MINNESOTA

Dental Laboratory Technology Program
916 Area Voc-Tech Institute
3300 Century Avenue North
White Bear Lake, Minnesota 55110

Dental Laboratory Technology Program
Hennepin Technical Centers
9000 North 77th Avenue
Brooklyn Park, Minnesota 55455

MISSOURI

Dental Laboratory Technology Program
St. Louis Community College-Meramec
11333 Big Bend Boulevard
St. Louis, Missouri 63122

NEBRASKA

Dental Laboratory Technology Program
Central Technical Community College
P.O. Box 1024
Hastings, Nebraska 68901

NEW JERSEY

Dental Laboratory Technology Program
Union County College
1033 Springfield Avenue
Cranford, New Jersey 07016

NEW YORK

Dental Laboratory Technology Program
Dutchess Community College
Pendell Road
Poughkeepsie, New York 12601

Dental Laboratory Technology Program
Erie Community College-South Campus
4140 Southwestern Boulevard
Orchard Park, New York 14127

Dental Laboratory Technology Program
New York City Technical College
300 Jay Street
Brooklyn, New York 11201

NORTH CAROLINA

Dental Laboratory Technology Program
Durham Technical Institute
1637 Lawson Street
Durham, North Carolina 27703

OHIO

Dental Laboratory Technology Program
Columbus Technical Institute
550 East Spring Street, Box 1609
Columbus, Ohio 43215

Dental Laboratory Technology Program
Cuyahoga Community College
4250 Richmond Road
Warrensville Township, Ohio 44122

OKLAHOMA

Dental Laboratory Technology Program
Rose State College
6420 Southeast 15th Street
Midwest City, Oklahoma 73110

OREGON

Dental Laboratory Technology Program
Portland Community College
12000 S.W. 49th Avenue
Portland, Oregon 97219

PENNSYLVANIA

Dental Laboratory Technology Program
Edinboro University of Pennsylvania
Edinboro, Pennsylvania 16444

Dental Laboratory Technology Program
Mastbaum Area Voc-Tech School
Frankford Ave. & Clementine St.
Philadelphia, Pennsylvania 19134

SOUTH CAROLINA

Dental Laboratory Technology Program
Trident Technical College
7000 Rivers Avenue
North Charleston, South Carolina 29411

SOUTH DAKOTA

Dental Laboratory Technology Program
Lake Area Voc-Tech School
230 11th Street, N.E.
Watertown, South Dakota 57201

TENNESSEE

Dental Laboratory Technology Program
Chattanooga State Tech Community College
4501 Amnicola Highway
Chattanooga, Tennessee 37406

Dental Laboratory Technology Program
East Tennessee State University
Paramed Center
1000 West E Street
Elizabethton, Tennessee 37643

TEXAS

Dental Laboratory Technology Program
School of Health Care Sciences
MSDD 114
Sheppard AFB, Texas 76311

Dental Laboratory Technology Program
Texas State Technical Institute
James Connally Campus
Waco, Texas 76705

Dental Laboratory Technology Program
Univ. of Texas-Health Sciences
7703 Floyd Curl Drive
San Antonio, Texas 78284

Dental Laboratory Technology Program
U.S. Army Academy of Health Sciences
Ft. Sam Houston, Texas 78234

VIRGINIA

Dental Laboratory Technology Program
J. Sargeant Reynolds Community College
2108 E. Grace Street
Box C-32040
Richmond, Virginia 23261-2040

Dental Laboratory Technology Program
Northern Virginia Community College
8333 Little River Turnpike
Annandale, Virginia 22003

WASHINGTON

Dental Laboratory Technology Program
L.H. Bates Voc-Tech Institute
1101 S. Yakima Avenue
Tacoma, Washington 98405

Dental Laboratory Technology Program
Seattle Central Community College
1717 Broadway
Seattle, Washington 98122

WISCONSIN

Dental Laboratory Technology Program
Milwaukee Area Technical College
1015 North Sixth Street
Milwaukee, Wisconsin 53203

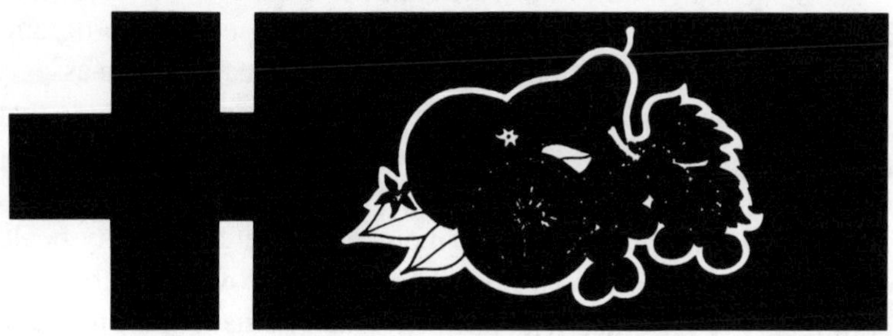

DIETETICS AND NUTRITIONAL CARE

Dietetics and nutritional care is the health profession concerned with human nutrition, that is, the study of the relationships between components of food and the body's needs. Quality nutritious food is essential in maintaining good health, in preventing or treating illness, and in aiding rehabilitation. Dietetics and nutritional care is one of the larger allied healthcare professions. It incorporates several career occupations including *dietitian, nutritionist, dietetic technician, dietetic manager, dietetic aide,* and *dietetic clerk.*

Dietitian

The *dietitian* is a food specialist responsible for nutritional care and food service. Generally speaking, the dietitian applies the principles of nutrition and management to the administration of institutional food service. He or she may also plan special diets for hospital patients and teach groups and individuals nutritional health, especially in food selection and eating habits. There are five specialized careers for dietitians: administrative, clinical, community work, education, and research.

The *administrative dietitian* supervises food service systems in large institutions by managing the large-scale planning, preparation and service of quality nutritious food. He or she establishes and maintains standards for food production, food service, sanitation, safety, and security and also budgets for and purchases food, equipment, and supplies. Large institutions where administrative dietitians are employed include hospitals; universities; schools; and government, commercial, and industrial establishments.

The *clinical dietitian,* who is also known as a *therapeutic dietitian,* assures that nutrition is incorporated as an integral part of a patient's recovery program from illness or injury. As a member of the hospital health team the clinical dietitian assesses the nutritional needs of patients, plans their diets, and provides dietary counseling to them and to their families so that special diets may be maintained after patients leave the hospital, clinic, or nursing home.

The *community dietitian* is the member of the community health team who plans and coordinates the nutritional component of improved health and preventive health in a community. Concerned with problems such as inadequate nutrients or overconsumption, the community dietitian assesses nutritional needs of the population-or portions of it, such as the elderly or adolescents- and then counsels individuals or families on nutrition, food selection, and economics in food purchasing. The community dietitian is usually employed by community or government agencies, such as day-care centers and public health facilities.

Working in a university, college, medical school, or vocational-technical institute, the *dietetic educator* plans and implements the educational curricula of dietetic students on the one hand and the teaching of nutrition to medical, dental, nursing, and other allied health students on the other.

The *research dietitian* conducts research for universities, medical centers, and food companies in nutrition, nutrition education, food management, food service, and also in the design of food processing equipment.

With experience a dietitian may also serve as a consultant on nutrition, nutritional care, or food service to hospitals, clinics, nursing homes, day care centers, restaurants, or food manufacturing companies.

The minimum education requirement for a dietitian is a bachelor's degree, preferably with a major in dietetics, nutrition, or institution or food systems management. These programs are primarily offered by departments of home economics or of nutritional sciences in colleges and universities. A graduate degree is usually required for teaching, research and public or community health nutrition.

Individuals who wish to take the national registration examination, administered by the American Dietetic Association must complete either (1) an approved six-to-twelve month clinical internship, or three years of approved experience after graduation from a bachelor's degree program, or (2) an approved coordinated undergraduate program which enables students to complete both their bachelor's degree program and clinical experience requirement in four years, or (3) an advanced degree program in nutrition or food service management plus six months of approved experience.

The credentials of Registered Dietitian (R.D.) are granted to individuals who complete the above prerequisites plus successfully pass the registration examination.

Recommended high school courses for students interested in dietetics are home economics, business administration, biology, health, mathematics, chemistry, English, and a second language.

Several scholarships are available from the American Dietetic Association for needy students enrolled in dietetic undergraduate and graduate programs, dietetic technician programs, and internships. For information on scholarships and financial aid, contact the American Dietetic Association, 216 West Jackson, Chicago, Illinois 60606. The American

Home Economic Foundation has fellowships available for dietitians at the graduate level who are also members of the Home Economic Foundation. Applications and membership information is available from the Foundation at 2010 Massachusetts Avenue, N.W., Washington, D.C. 20036-1028.

According to a national salary survey conducted by the University of Texas Medical Branch, entry level salaries of hospital dieticians average $20,900 annually. Salaries of experienced dietitians averaged $27,600 a year.

A list supplied by the American Dietetic Association contains over three hundred institutions throughout the United States that offer educational programs in dietetics. Most of these programs offered through departments of home economics or nutritional science offer the traditional bachelor's degree in dietetics; however, some of them which are listed below, also offer or only offer, the coordinated undergraduate program. Persons interested in attending a specific university or college should contact that school's registrar for complete information on its curriculum in dietetics.

To obtain a list of internships, or Plan IV and Plan V programs (programs approved by the American Dietetic Association which satisfy only the educational requirement for registration) can be obtained for a fee, by writing for the *Directory of Dietetic Programs*, The American Dietetic Association, 216 West Jackson, Chicago, Illinois 60606.

Further information on dietetic careers and registration requirements can also be obtained from the American Dietetic Association at the above listed address.

The following is a list of the coordinated undergraduate programs accredited by the American Dietetic Association.

SOURCES:

American Dietetic Association
American Home Economic Foundation
Occupational Outlook Handbook

Dietitian Programs

ALABAMA

Program in Dietetics
Auburn University
Dept. of Nutrition and Foods
School of Human Sciences
Auburn University, Alabama 36849

Program in Dietetics
The University of Alabama
Dept. of Food, Nutrition, and Institution Management
P.O. Box 1488
Tuscaloosa, Alabama 35487-1488

CALIFORNIA

Program in Dietetics
University of California, Berkeley
Dept. of Nutritional Sciences
119 Morgan Hall
Berkeley, California 94720

Program in Dietetics
Loma Linda University
School of Allied Health Professions
Dept. of Nutrition & Dietetics
Loma Linda, California 92350

Program in Dietetics
California State University, Los Angeles
5151 State University Drive
Los Angeles, California 90032

CONNECTICUT

Program in Dietetics
The University of Connecticut
358 Mansfield Road
Koons Hall, Box U-101
Storrs, Connecticut 06268

Program in Dietetics
Saint Joseph College
Dept. of Nutrition & Resource Management
1678 Asylum Avenue
W. Hartford, Connecticut 06117

DELAWARE

Program in Dietetics
University of Delaware
Dept. of Nutrition & Dietetics
244 Alison Hall
Newark, Delaware 19716

DISTRICT OF COLUMBIA

Program in Dietetics
Howard University
Dept. of Clinical Nutrition
6th & Bryant Sts. N.W., Annex 1
Washington, D.C. 20059

FLORIDA

Program in Dietetics
University of Florida
College of Health Related Professions
Box J-184 JHMHC
Gainesville, Florida 32610

Program in Dietetics
Florida International University
Dept. of Dietetics and Nutrition
Tamiami Campus, DM 212
Miami, Florida 33199

GEORGIA

Program in Dietetics
Georgia State University
Dept. of Nutrition and Dietetics
Box 873 University Plaza
Atlanta, Georgia 30303-3083

IDAHO

Program in Dietetics
University of Idaho-Eastern Washington
School of Home Economics
College of Agriculture
Moscow, Idaho 83843

ILLINOIS

Program in Dietetics
Chicago State University
College of Allied Health
95th St. and King Drive
Chicago, Illinois 60628

Program in Dietetics
University of Illinois at Chicago
Dept. of Nutrition & Medical Dietetics
808 S. Wood Street
Chicago, Illinois 60612

Program in Dietetics
Northern Illinois University
Dept. of Human & Family Resources
DeKalb, Illinois 60115

INDIANA

Program in Dietetics
Indiana State University
Home Economics Dept.
Terre Haute, Indiana 47809

Program in Dietetics
Purdue University
Dept. of Foods and Nutrition
Stone Hall
West Lafayette, Indiana 47907

IOWA

Program in Dietetics
Iowa State University
Dept. of Food & Nutrition
107 MacKay Hall
Ames, Iowa 50011

KANSAS

Program in Dietetics
Kansas State University
Manhattan, Kansas 66506

KENTUCKY

Program in Dietetics
University of Kentucky
Nutrition and Food Science
212 Funkhouser Building
Lexington, Kentucky 40506-0054

Program in Dietetics
Spalding University
851 S. Fourth Street
Louisville, Kentucky 40203

LOUISIANA

Program in Dietetics
Louisiana Tech University
College of Home Economics
Ruston, Louisiana 71272

MARYLAND

Program in Dietetics
Hood College
Home Economics Department
Rosemont Avenue
Frederick, Maryland 21701

MASSACHUSETTS

Program in Dietetics
Framingham State College
Dept. of Home Economics
Food & Nutrition, Box 2000
Framingham, Massachusetts 01701

MICHIGAN

Program in Dietetics
Andrews University
Dept. of Home Economics
Berrien Springs, Michigan 49104

Program in Dietetics
Mercy College of Detroit
8200 W. Outer Drive
Detroit, Michigan 48219

Program in Dietetics
Wayne State University
Dept. of Nutrition & Food Science
160 Old Main
Detroit, Michigan 48202

Program in Dietetics
Eastern Michigan University
Dept. of Human Environmental and Consumer Resources
Ypsilanti, Michigan 48197

MINNESOTA

Program in Dietetics
University of Minnesota
269 Food Science and Nutrition
1334 Eckles Avenue
St. Paul, Minnesota 55108

MISSISSIPPI

Program in Dietetics
University of Southern Mississippi
Dept. of Institutional Administration
Southern Station Box 100215
Hattiesburg, Mississippi 39406

MISSOURI

Program in Dietetics
University of Missouri-Columbia
Dietetic Education
318 Clark Hall
Columbia, Missouri 65211

NEW YORK

Program in Dietetics
State University College at Buffalo
Nutrition and Food Science Dept.
1300 Elmwood Avenue
Buffalo, New York 14222-1095

Program in Dietetics
Rochester Institute of Technology
One Lomb Memorial Drive
Rochester, New York 14623

Program in Dietetics
Syracuse University
Dept. of Human Nutrition
034 Slocum Hall
Syracuse, New York 13244-1250

NORTH CAROLINA

Program in Dietetics
The University of North Carolina
Department of Nutrition
315 Pittsboro Street, 325H
Chapel Hill, North Carolina 27514

Program in Dietetics
East Carolina University
School of Home Economics
Greenville, North Carolina 27858-4353

NORTH DAKOTA

Program in Dietetics
University of North Dakota
Dept. of Home Economics and Nutrition
Box 8273, University Station
Grand Fords, North Dakota 58202

OHIO

Program in Dietetics
The University of Akron
Dept. of Home Economics and Family Ecology
215 Schrank Hall South
Akron, Ohio 44325

Program in Dietetics
The Ohio State University
School of Allied Medical Professions
1583 Perry Street
Columbus, Ohio 43210

Program in Dietetics
Youngstown State University
410 Wick Avenue
Youngstown, Ohio 44555-0001

OKLAHOMA

Program in Dietetics
University of Oklahoma Health Sciences Center
Dept. of Clinical Dietetics
801 N.E. 13th St.
Oklahoma City, Oklahoma 73190

PENNSYLVANIA

Program in Dietetics
Edinboro University of Pennsylvania
Dept. of Biology and Health Services
Edinboro, Pennsylvania 16444

Program in Dietetics
Mercyhurst College
Dept. of Human Ecology
Glenwood Hills
Erie, Pennsylvania 16546

Program in Dietetics
Villa Maria College
Dept. of Science and Mathematics
2551 W. Lake Road
Erie, Pennsylvania 16505

Program in Dietetics
Immaculata College
Home Economics Dept.
Immaculata, Pennsylvania 19345

Program in Dietetics
Drexel University
Dept. of Nutrition and Food Sciences
32nd and Chestnut Sts.
Philadelphia, Pennsylvania 19104

Program in Dietetics
Marywood College
Dept. of Human Ecology
2300 Adams Avenue
Scranton, Pennsylvania 18509-1598

TEXAS

Program in Dietetics
The University of Texas at Austin
Dept. of Home Economics, GEA 115
Austin, Texas 78712

Program in Dietetics
University of Texas Health Science Center at
Dallas
Dept. of Clinical Nutrition
5323 Harry Hines Blvd.
Dallas, Texas 75235

Program in Dietetics
Pan American University
Dietetics Program NE 226
Edinburg, Texas 78539-2999

Program in Dietetics
Texas Christian University
Dept. of Nutrition & Dietetics
P.O. Box 32869
Fort Worth, Texas 76129

Program in Dietetics
University of Texas Health Science Center at Houston
John Freeman Bldg.
P.O. Box 20708
Houston, Texas 77225

UTAH

Program in Dietetics
Utah State University
Dept. of Nutrition and Food Sciences
Logan, Utah 84322-8700

Program in Dietetics
Brigham Young University
Food Science and Nutrition Dept.
2218 SFLC
Provo, Utah 84602

VIRGINIA

Program in Dietetics
Virginia Polytechnic Institute and State University
Dept. of Human Nutrition and Foods
Blacksburg, Virginia 24061

WASHINGTON

Program in Dietetics
Eastern Washington University-University of Idaho Consortium
Mail Stop 13
Cheney, Washington 99004

Program in Dietetics
Washington State University
401 White Hall
Pullman, Washington 99164-2032

WISCONSIN

Program in Dietetics
Viterbo College
815 S. 9th Street
LaCrosse, Wisconsin 54601-4797

Program in Dietetics
University of Wisconsin-Madison
Dept. of Nutritional Sciences
1415 Linden Drive
Madison, Wisconsin 53706

Program in Dietetics
Mount Mary College
Dept. of Dietetics
2900 N. Menomonee River Pkwy.
Milwaukee, Wisconsin 53222

Nutritionist

Although sometimes regarded as a general title for all food service science and nutrition occupations, including dietitians, home economists, and food technologists, the *nutritionist* is more specifically an educator of human nutrition. As a specialist, the nutritionist attempts to solve food problems, control disease, and maintain and promote health, all through education.

Although some may conduct research or teach nutrition to medical personnel while others act as consultants on health teams or in industry, most nutritionists work in the field of public health. Employed in government and voluntary health agencies, public health nutritionists are responsible for the nutritional aspects of community health care and preventive health services. They counsel and instruct the elderly, the poor, adolescents, and mothers with babies and young children, among other groups, on sound nutrition practices including special diets, meal planning and preparation, and food budgeting.

The nutritionist may also work for the media, conveying nutrition information on radio, television, or in newspapers. She or he may even help provide technical assistance in underdeveloped countries that are trying to improve their nutritional standards in food production.

Similar to a dietitian, the minimum educational requirement for nutritionists employed in healthcare facilities, business and industry is generally a bachelor's degree in dietetics, nutrition or institution or food systems management. A graduate degree is required for nutritionists employed in public or community health.

Consult the previous section on Dietitians for information on the similar wage scales, educational programs and opportunities for nutritionists.

SOURCES:

American Dietetic Association
Occupational Outlook Handbook

Dietetic Technician

The *dietetic technician* works on a healthcare team assisting the dietitian and specializing in either food service management or nutritional care services. In food service management the dietetic technician assists in the assessment, planning, implementation, and evaluation of food programs. In a large hospital he or she works under the supervision of an administrative dietitian. In a small hospital or extended care facility where he or she may be responsible for the daily food service operation, the dietetic technician is usually supervised by a consultant dietitian.

In nutritional services the dietetic technician works under the supervision of a clinical or community dietitian and provides nutrition education and care to individuals and groups in health and community facilities.

Training to become a dietetic technician involves completion of a two-year associate degree program offered by universities, colleges, community colleges and vocational-technical schools.

Dietetic technicians are employed in the same facilities that employ dietitians; such as hospitals, clinics, community or government agencies, day-care programs, and in school systems.

Registration as a Registered Dietetic Technician (D.T.R.) is available from the Commission on Dietetic Registration of the American Dietetic Association, to applicants who complete an approved dietetic technician program and successfully pass a credentialing examination.

Below is a list of education programs for dietetic technicians approved by the American Dietetic Association. Contact the American Dietetic Association, 216 West Jackson, Chicago, Illinois 60606, for registration and career information.

SOURCES:

American Dietetic Association
Occupational Outlook Handbook

Dietetic Technician Programs

ALABAMA

Dietetic Technician Program
University of Alabama at Birmingham
Webb Building
University Station
Birmingham, Alabama 35294

ARIZONA

Dietetic Technician Program
Central Arizona College
Woodruff at Overfield Road
Coolidge, Arizona 85228

CALIFORNIA

Dietetic Technician Program
Chaffey Community College
5885 Haven
Alta Loma, California 91701

Dietetic Technician Program
Orange Coast College
2701 Fairview Road
Costa Mesa, California 92628-0120

Dietetic Technician Program
Long Beach City College
Liberal Arts Campus
4901 E. Carson Street
Long Beach, California 90808

Dietetic Technician Program
Los Angeles City College
855 North Vermont Avenue
Los Angeles, California 90029

COLORADO

Dietetic Technician Program
Front Range Community College
3645 W. 112th Avenue
Westminster, Colorado 80030

CONNECTICUT

Dietetic Technician Program
South Central Community College
60 Sargent Drive
New Haven, Connecticut 06511

Dietetic Technician Program
Briarwood College
2279 Mount Vernon Road
Southington, Connecticut 06489

Dietetic Technician Program
University of New Haven
School of Hotel Restaurant and Tourism Administration
300 Orange Avenue
West Haven, Connecticut 06516

FLORIDA

Dietetic Technician Program
Broward Community College
3501 S.W. Davie Road
Fort Lauderdale, Florida 33314

Dietetic Technician Program
Florida Community College at Jacksonville-Kent Campus
3939 Roosevelt Boulevard
Jacksonville, Florida 32205

Dietetic Technician Program
Palm Beach Junior College
4200 Congress Avenue
Lake Worth, Florida 33461

Dietetic Technician Program
Miami-Dade Community College
Mitchell Wolfson-New World Ctr. Campus
300 N.E. 2nd Avenue
Miami, Florida 33132

Dietetic Technician Program
Orlando Vocational Technical Center
301 W. Amelia Avenue
Orlando, Florida 32801

Dietetic Technician Program
Pensacola Junior College
1000 College Boulevard
Pensacola, Florida 32504

ILLINOIS

Dietetic Technician Program
Malcolm X College
City Colleges of Chicago
1900 W. Van Buren
Chicago, Illinois 60612

Dietetic Technician Program
William Rainey Harper College
Algonquin and Roselle Roads
Palatine, Illinois 60067

INDIANA

Dietetic Technician Program
Marian College
3200 Cold Spring Road
Indianapolis, Indiana 46222

Dietetic Technician Program
Ball State University
Dept. of Home Economics
Muncie, Indiana 47306

KANSAS

Dietetic Technician Program
Butler County Community College and Wichita
Area Vocational-Tech School
Central Vocational Building
324 N. Emporia
Wichita, Kansas 67202

MAINE

Dietetic Technician Program
University of Maine at Farmington
Ricker Hall
Farmington, Maine 04938

Dietetic Technician Program
Southern Maine Vocational Technical Institute
Fort Road
South Portland, Maine 04106

MARYLAND

Dietetic Technician Program
Community College of Baltimore
Dept. of Health Technologies
2901 Liberty Heights Avenue
Baltimore, Maryland 21215

Dietetic Technician Program
Montgomery College
Department of Management
51 Mannakee Street
Rockville, Maryland 20850

MASSACHUSETTS

Dietetic Technician Program
Laboure College
2120 Dorchester Avenue
Boston, Massachusetts 02124-5698

Dietetic Technician Program
Holyoke Community College
303 Homestead Avenue
Holyoke, Massachusetts 01040

MICHIGAN

Dietetic Technician Program
Mercy College of Detroit
8200 W. Outer Drive
Detroit, Michigan 48219

Dietetic Technician Program
Wayne County Community College
801 W. Fort Street
Detroit, Michigan 48226

Dietetic Technician Program
Oakland Community College
27055 Orchard Lake Road
Farmington Hills, Michigan 48018

MINNESOTA

Dietetic Technician Program
Normandale Community College
9700 France Avenue, S.
Bloomington, Minnesota 55431

Dietetic Technician Program
University of Minnesota-Crookston
Div. of Hospitality and Home Economics
Crookston, Minnesota 56716

Dietetic Technician Program
Lakewood Community College-916
Northeast Metro Technical Institute
3401 Century Avenue, N.
White Bear Lake, Minnesota 55110

MISSOURI

Dietetic Technician Program
St. Louis Community College at Florissant Valley
3400 Pershall Road
St. Louis, Missouri 63135

NEBRASKA

Dietetic Technician Program
Central Community College
P.O. Box 1024
Hastings, Nebraska 68901-1024

Dietetic Technician Program
Southeast Community College
8800 "O" Street
Lincoln, Nebraska 68520

NEW JERSEY

Dietetic Technician Program
Camden County College
P.O. Box 200
Blackwood, New Jersey 08012

Dietetic Technician Program
Middlesex County College
155 Mill Road
P.O. Box 3050, CN-61
Edison, New Jersey 08818-3050

NEW YORK

Dietetic Technician Program
Erie Community College
North Campus
Main St. and Youngs Road
Buffalo, New York 14221

Dietetic Technician Program
State University of New York
Agriculture and Technical College
Cobleskill, New York 12043

Dietetic Technician Program
LaGuardia Community College
City University of New York
31-10 Thomson Avenue
Long Island City, New York 11101

Dietetic Technician Program
State University of New York
Agricultural and Technical College
Bailey Annex
Morrisville, New York 13408

Dietetic Technician Program
Dutchess Community College
Pendell Road
Poughkeepsie, New York 12601

Dietetic Technician Program
Suffolk County Community College
Eastern Campus
Speonk-Riverhead Road
Riverhead, New York 11901

Dietetic Technician Program
Rockland Community College
145 College Road
Suffern, New York 10901

Dietetic Technician Program
Westchester Community College
75 Grasslands Road
Valhalla, New York 10595

OHIO

Dietetic Technician Program
Cincinnati Technical College
Health Technologies Division
3520 Central Parkway
Cincinnati, Ohio 45223

Dietetic Technician Program
Cuyahoga Community College
2900 Community College Avenue
Cleveland, Ohio 44115

Dietetic Technician Program
Columbus State Community College
550 E. Spring Street
Columbus, Ohio 43215-9965

Dietetic Technician Program
Sinclair Community College
444 West Third Street
Dayton, Ohio 45402

Dietetic Technician Program
Kettering College of Medical Arts
3737 Southern Boulevard
Kettering, Ohio 45429

Dietetic Technician Program
Lima Technical College
4240 Campus Drive
Lima, Ohio 45804

Dietetic Technician Program
Hocking Technical College
Route 1
Nelsonville, Ohio 45764-9704

OREGON

Dietetic Technician Program
Portland Community College
12000 S.W. 49th
Portland, Oregon 97219

PENNSYLVANIA

Dietetic Technician Program
Luzerne County Community College
Prospect Street and Middle Rd.
Nanticoke, Pennsylvania 18634

Dietetic Technician Program
Bucks County Community College
Swamp Road
Newtown, Pennsylvania 18940

Dietetic Technician Program
Community College of Philadelphia
1700 Spring Garden Street
Philadelphia, Pennsylvania 19130

Dietetic Technician Program
Community College of Allegheny County
Allegheny Campus
808 Ridge Avenue
Pittsburgh, Pennsylvania 15212-6097

Dietetic Technician Program
The Pennsylvania State University
20 Human Development Bldg.
University Park, Pennsylvania 16802

TENNESSEE

Dietetic Technician Program
Shelby State Community College
P.O. Box 40568
Memphis, Tennessee 38174-0568

TEXAS

Dietetic Technician Program
El Paso Community College
P.O. Box 20500
El Paso, Texas 79998

Dietetic Technician Program
Tarrant County Junior College
5301 Campus Drive
Fort Worth, Texas 76119

Dietetic Technician Program
San Jacinto College Central
8060 Spencer Highway
Pasadena, Texas 77505

VIRGINIA

Dietetic Technician Program
Northern Virginia Community College
8333 Little River Turnpike
Annandale, Virginia 22003

Dietetic Technician Program
J. Sargeant Reynolds
Community College
P.O. Box C-32040
Richmond, Virginia 23261-2040

Dietetic Technician Program
Tidewater Community College
1700 College Crescent
Virginia Beach, Virginia 23456

WASHINGTON

Dietetic Technician Program
Shoreline Community College
16101 Greenwood Avenue, N.
Seattle, Washington 98133

WISCONSIN

Dietetic Technician Program
Madison Area Technical College
3550 Anderson Street
Madison, Wisconsin 53704

Dietetic Technician Program
Cardinal Stritch College
Dept. of Dietetics
6801 N. Yates Road
Milwaukee, Wisconsin 53217

Dietetic Technician Program
Milwaukee Area Technical College
1015 N. Sixth Street
Milwaukee, Wisconsin 53205

Dietary Manager

Also known as a *dietetic assistant* or *food service supervisor,* the *dietary manager* provides food service supervision and nutritional care under the direction of a dietitian or dietetic technician. She or he processes dietary orders by writing food menus following dietetic specifications, helps patients select menus, coordinates food service to patients, orders supplies, maintains sanitation, and supervises the work of food service employees.

Dietary managers work in hospitals and other healthcare facilities where food is served to patients.

Training to become a dietary manager requires high school graduation or the equivalent and completion of a one-year program offered at a community colleges, or vocational-technical school or on-the-job training in a hospital food service program. A certificate of completion is generally awarded to training program graduates.

Upon graduation from an approved program or approved full time food service management experience, the candidate is eligible to take the credentialing examination sponsored by the Dietary Managers Association, formerly the Hospital, Institution and Education Food Service Society, and if successfully passed use the letters C.D.M. (Certified Dietary Manager).

The following is a list of approved dietary manager training programs approved by the Dietary Managers Association. Several independent study courses are also included for individuals who are interested in continuing their education on-the-job.

For more information on certification or careers in dietary management, write to the Dietary Managers Association, 400 East 22nd Street, Lombard, Illinois 60148.

SOURCES:

Dietary Managers Association
Dictionary of Occupational Titles

Dietary Manager Programs

ALABAMA

Dietary Manager Program
Auburn University
Correspondence Course
Office of Continuing Ed., 100 Mell Hall
Auburn University, Alabama 36849

ALASKA

Dietary Manager Program
Anchorage Community College
2533 Providence Avenue
Anchorage, Alaska 99508

ARKANSAS

Dietary Manager Program
Black River Vocational Technical School
Highway 304 East
P.O. Box 468
Pocahontas, Arkansas 72455

CALIFORNIA

Dietary Manager Program
Bakersfield College
1801 Panorama Drive
Bakersfield, California 93305

Dietary Manager Program
Long Beach City College
Liberal Arts Campus
4901 East Carson Street
Long Beach, California 90808

Dietary Manager Program
Modesto Junior College
College Avenue
Modesto, California 93530

Dietary Manager Program
Merritt College
12500 Campus Drive
Oakland, California 94619

Dietary Manager Program
American River College
4700 College Oak Drive
Sacramento, California 95841

Dietary Manager Program
Santa Rosa Junior College
1501 Mendocino Avenue
Santa Rosa, California 95401

COLORADO

Dietary Manager Program
Front Range Community College
3645 W. 112th Avenue
Westminster, Colorado 80030

FLORIDA

Dietary Manager Program
Clearwater High School
Evening Adult Program
540 S. Hercules Avenue
Clearwater, Florida 33516

Dietary Manager Program
Atlantic Vocational Center
4700 Coconut Creek Parkway
Coconut Creek, Florida 33066

Dietary Manager Program
University of Florida
Correspondence Course
Box J-325
Gainesville, Florida 32601

Dietary Manager Program
Florida Junior College
Fred Kent Campus
Jacksonville, Florida 32205

Dietary Manager Program
Lindsey Hopkins Education Center
750 N.W. 20th Street
Miami, Florida 33127

Dietary Manager Program
Orlando Vocational Technical Center
301 W. Amelia
Orlando, Florida 32801

Dietary Manager Program
Gulf Coast Community College
5230 Highway 98
Panama City, Florida 32401

Dietary Manager Program
Pensacola Junior College
1000 College Boulevard
Pensacola, Florida 32504

Dietary Manager Program
North Technical Education Center
7071 Garden Road
Riviera Beach, Florida 33404

Dietary Manager Program
Sarasota County Vocational Center
4748 Beneva Road
Sarasota, Florida 33583

Dietary Manager Program
St. Petersburg Vocational-Technical Institute
901 34th Street South
St. Petersburg, Florida 33711

Dietary Manager Program
Lively Area Vocational-Technical Center
500 N. Appleyard Drive
Tallahassee, Florida 32304

Dietary Manager Program
Tampa Bay Vocational School
6410 Orient Road
Tampa, Florida 33610

HAWAII

Dietary Manager Program
University of Hawaii
Kapiolani Community College
620 Pensacola Street
Honolulu, Hawaii 96814

ILLINOIS

Dietary Manager Program
Chicago City-Wide College
30 East Lake Street
Chicago, Illinois 60601

Dietary Manager Program
Illinois Central College
East Peoria, Illinois 61635

Dietary Manager Program
John Wood Community College
150 S. 48th Street
Quincy, Illinois 62301

Dietary Manager Program
Rock Valley College
Health Care for Food Service Supervisors
3301 N. Mulford Road
Rockford, Illinois 61101

INDIANA

Dietary Manager Program
No. Lawrence Vocational Technical Center
P.O. Box 729
Bloomington, Indiana 47401

Dietary Manager Program
University of Southern Indiana
Dept. of Continuing Education
8600 University Boulevard
Evansville, Indiana 47712

Dietary Manager Program
Indiana Vocational Technical College
3800 North Anthony
Fort Wayne, Indiana 46805

Dietary Manager Program
J. Everett Light Career Center
1901 E. 86th Street
Indianapolis, Indiana 46240

Dietary Manager Program
Indiana Vocational Technical College at Lafayette
3208 Ross Road
P.O. Box 6299
Lafayette, Indiana 47903

Dietary Manager Program
Ball State University
PA 150, Dept. of Home Economics
2000 University
Muncie, Indiana 47306

Dietary Manager Program
Indiana Vocational Technical College at Richmond
2325 Chester Boulevard
Richmond, Indiana 47374

Dietary Manager Program
St. Mary of The Woods College
Science Hall
St. Mary of The Woods, Indiana 47876

Dietary Manager Program
Indiana Vocational Technical College-South Bend
1534 W. Sample Street
South Bend, Indiana 46619

Dietary Manager Program
Vincennes University
1002 N. 1st Street
Vincennes, Indiana 47591

Dietary Manager Program
Indiana Vocational Technical College-Warsaw
1534 W. Sample Street
South Bend, Indiana 46619

IOWA

Dietary Manager Program
Des Moines Area Community College
2006 S. Ankeny Boulevard
Ankeny, Iowa 50021

Dietary Manager Program
Eastern Iowa Community College District
Scott Community College
306 W. River Drive
Davenport, Iowa 52722

KANSAS

Dietary Manager Program
Southeast Kansas Area Vocational Technical School
6th and Roosevelt
Coffeyville, Kansas 67337

Dietetic Assistant Program
Barton County Community College
Great Bend, Kansas 67350

Dietary Manager Program
Washburn University
21st and Washburn
Topeka, Kansas 66621

Dietary Manager Program
Wichita Area Vocational Technical School
324 North Emporia
Wichita, Kansas 67202

KENTUCKY

Dietary Manager Program
University of Kentucky at Ashland
University of Kentucky C.E.D. Dept.
College of Allied Health
Lexington, Kentucky 40536

Dietary Manager Program
University of Kentucky at Covington
1913 Westminster Drive
Lexington, Kentucky 40504

Dietary Manager Program
University of Kentucky at Lexington
University of Kentucky C.E.D. Dept.
College of Allied Health
Lexington, Kentucky 40536

Dietary Manager Program
Spalding University
851 South Fourth Street
Louisville, Kentucky 40203

LOUISIANA

Dietary Manager Program
Alexandria Vocational Technical Institute
4311 South MacArthur Drive
Alexandria, Louisiana 71302

Dietary Manager Program
Jefferson Parish Vocational Technical
Food Service Training Program
5200 Blair Drive
Metairie, Louisiana 70001

MAINE

Dietary Manager Program
Southern Maine Vocational Technical Institute
Fort Road
South Portland, Maine 04106

MARYLAND

Dietary Manager Program
Community College of Baltimore
2901 Liberty Heights Avenue
Baltimore, Maryland 21215

Dietary Manager Program
Montgomery Community College
51 Mannakee Street
Rockville, Maryland 20850

MASSACHUSETTS

Dietary Manager Program
Bunker Hill Community College
Division of Continuing Education
New Rutherford Avenue
Charlestown, Massachusetts 02129

Dietary Manager Program
Berkshire Community College
West Street
Pittsfield, Massachusetts 01201

MICHIGAN

Dietary Manager Program
Wayne County Community College
8551 Greenfield Road
Detroit, Michigan 48228

Dietary Manager Program
Oakland Community College
27055 Orchard Lake Road
Farmington Hills, Michigan 48018

Dietary Manager Program
Lansing Community College
Health Careers Department
419 N. Capitol Avenue
Lansing, Michigan 48914

MINNESOTA

Dietary Manager Program
Alexandria Vocational Technical Institute
Food Service Supervisor Course
1601 Jefferson Street
Alexandria, Minnesota 56308

Dietary Manager Program
Granite Falls Area Vocational Technical Institute
Highway 23 West
Granite Falls, Minnesota 56241

Dietary Manager Program
Mankato Area Vocational Technical Institute
1920 Lee Boulevard
North Mankato, Minnesota 56001

Dietary Manager Program
St. Paul Vocational Technical Institute
235 Marshall Avenue
St. Paul, Minnesota 55102

MISSISSIPPI

Dietary Manager Program
Hinds Junior College
Jackson Branch
3925 Sunset Drive
Jackson, Mississippi 39204

MISSOURI

Dietary Manager Program
Columbia Public Schools
1104 Providence Road
Columbia, Missouri 65205-0874

Dietary Manager Program
Penn Valley Community College
Food Service Supervisor's Course
3201 S.W. Trafficway
Kansas City, Missouri 64111

Dietary Manager Program
St. Louis Community College at Florissant Valley
3400 Pershall Road
St. Louis, Missouri 63135

NEBRASKA

Dietary Manager Program
Central Technical Community College
P.O. Box 1024
Hastings, Nebraska 68901

Dietary Manager Program
Southeast Community College
Area Office
8800 O" Street"
Lincoln, Nebraska 68520

Dietary Manager Program
Mid-Plains Community College
Route 4, Box 1
I-80 and Highway 83
North Platte, Nebraska 69101

Dietary Manager Program
Metropolitan Technical Community College
2909 Gomez Avenue
Omaha, Nebraska 69107

NEW JERSEY

Dietary Manager Program
Bergen City Vocational Technical School
200 Hackensack Avenue
Hackensack, New Jersey 07601

Dietary Manager Program
Ocean City Vocational Technical
Adult Evening Program
Old Freehold & Bea Lea Roads
Toms River, New Jersey 07853

Dietary Manager Program
Passaic County Vocational School
45 Reinhardt Road
Wayne, New Jersey 07410

NEW YORK

Dietary Manager Program
Broome Community College
Office of Continuing Education
P.O. Box 1017, Upper Front St.
Binghamton, New York 13902

Dietary Manager Program
Erie Community College
Main & Youngs Road
Buffalo, New York 14221

Dietary Manager Program
Adelphi University
P.O. Box 516
Garden City, Long Island, New York 11530

Dietary Manager Program
La Guardia Community College
31-10 Thomson Avenue
Long Island City, New York 11101

Dietary Manager Program
New York University
Dept. of Home Economics & Nutrition
537 East Building
New York, New York 10003

Dietary Manager Program
Dutchess Community College
Pendell Road
Poughkeepsie, New York 12601

Dietary Manager Program
Westchester Community College
75 Grasslands Road
Valhalla, New York 10595

NORTH DAKOTA

Dietary Manager Program
University of North Dakota
Department of Correspondence Studies
Box 8277, University Station
Grand Forks, North Dakota 58202

OHIO

Dietary Manager Program
Cincinnati Technical College
3520 Central Parkway
Cincinnati, Ohio 45223

Dietary Manager Program
Columbus Technical Institute
Box 1609
550 E. Spring Street
Columbus, Ohio 43125

Dietary Manager Program
Sinclair Community College
444 W. Third Street
Dayton, Ohio 45402

Dietary Manager Program
Kent State University
Nixson Hall
Kent, Ohio 44242

Dietary Manager Program
Lima Technical College
4240 Campus Drive
Lima, Ohio 45804

Dietary Manager Program
Ohio State University
Dietetic Assistant Program
Lima Campus, 4240 Campus Drive
Lima, Ohio 45804

Dietary Manager Program
Hocking Technical College
Route 1
Nelsonville, Ohio 45764

Dietary Manager Program
North Central Technical College
2441 Kenwood Circle
P.O. Box 698
Mansfield, Ohio 44901

OKLAHOMA

Dietary Manager Program
Northeast Oklahoma Vocational Technical School
Drawer P
Afton, Oklahoma 74331

Dietary Manager Program
Kiamichi Area Vocational Technical School
P.O. Box 220
Atoka, Oklahoma 74525

Dietary Manager Program
Tulsa County Area Vocational Technical School
4600 South Olive
Broken Arrow, Oklahoma 74011-1706

Dietary Manager Program
Great Plains Area Vocational Technical School
4500 W. Lee Boulevard
Lawton, Oklahoma 73505

Dietary Manager Program
Moore-Norman Area Vocational Technical School
4701 N.W. 12th
Norman, Oklahoma 73069

Dietary Manager Program
Frances Tuttle Area Vocational Technical School
12777 N. Rockwell Avenue
Oklahoma City, Oklahoma 73142

Dietary Manager Program
Indian Meridian Area Vocational Technical School
1312 S. Sangre Road
Stillwater, Oklahoma 74074

Dietary Manager Program
High Plains Area Vocational Technical School
P.O. Box 5249
Woodward, Oklahoma 73803-5249

OREGON

Dietary Manager Program
Portland Community College
12000 S.W. 49th Avenue
Portland, Oregon 97219

PENNSYLVANIA

Dietary Manager Program
Harrisburg Area Community College
3300 Cameron Street
Harrisburg, Pennsylvania 17110

Dietary Manager Program
Immaculata College
Correspondence Course
Immaculata, Pennsylvania 19345

Dietary Manager Program
Luzerne County Community College
Prospect Street & Middle Road
Naticoke, Pennsylvania 18634

Dietary Manager Program
Bucks County Community College
Swamp Road
Newton, Pennsylvania 18940

Dietary Manager Program
Community College of Philadelphia
1700 Spring Garden Street
Philadelphia, Pennsylvania 19130

Dietary Manager Program
National School of Health Technology
801 Arch Street
Philadelphia, Pennsylvania 19103

Dietary Manager Program
Pennsylvania State University
Correspondence Course
College of Human Development
University Park, Pennsylvania 16802

RHODE ISLAND

Dietary Manager Program
University of Rhode Island
17 Woodward Hall
Kingston, Rhode Island 02881

SOUTH CAROLINA

Dietary Manager Program
Trident Technical College
Medical University of South Carolina
P.O. Box 10367
Charleston, South Carolina 29411

Dietary Manager Program
Florence-Darlington Technical College
P.O. Drawer F-8000
Florence, South Carolina 29501

Dietary Manager Program
Tri-County Technical College
P.O. Box 587
Pendleton, South Carolina 29670

Dietary Manager Program
Greenville Technical College
P.O. Box 5616
Greenville, South Carolina 29606-5616

SOUTH DAKOTA

Dietary Manager Program
South Dakota State University-Sioux Falls Site
SDSU, Box 2275A
Brookings, South Dakota 57007-0497

TEXAS

Dietary Manager Program
Austin Community College
P.O. Box 2285
Austin, Texas 78768

Dietary Manager Program
El Paso Community College
P.O. Box 20500
El Paso, Texas 79998

Dietary Manager Program
Tarrant County Junior College
5301 Campus Drive
Fort Worth, Texas 76119

Dietary Manager Program
North Harris County College
2700 W. Thorne Drive
Houston, Texas 77073

Dietary Manager Program
South Plains College
1302 Main
Lubbock, Texas 79405

Dietary Manager Program
San Jacinto College
8060 Spencer Highway
Pasadena, Texas 77505

Dietary Manager Program
Texarkana Community College
2500 N. Robison Road
Texarkana, Texas 75501

Dietary Manager Program
Texas State Technical Institute
Continuing Education Training Center
Building 44-10
Waco, Texas 76705

UTAH

Dietary Manager Program
Utah Technical College
1200 South 800 West
P.O. Box 1609
Orem, Utah 84603

Dietary Manager Program
Brigham Young University
401 12th Avenue
Salt Lake City, Utah 84103

VIRGINIA

Dietary Manager Program
North Virginia Community College
Annandale Campus
8333 Little River Turnpike
Annandale, Virginia 22003

Dietetic Assistant Program
J. Sargeant Reynolds Community College
P.O. Box 12084
Richmond, Virginia 23241

WASHINGTON

Dietary Manager Program
Bellingham Vocational Technical Institute
3028 Lindbergh Avenue
Bellingham, Washington 98225

Dietary Manager Program
Columbia Basin College
2600 N. 20th Avenue
Pasco, Washington 99301

Dietary Manager Program
Renton Vocational Technical Institute
3000 N.E. 4th Street
Renton, Washington 98055

Dietary Manager Program
Spokane Community College
N. 1810 Green Street
District 17
Spokane, Washington 99207

Dietary Manager Program
Clover Park Vocational Technical Institute
4500 Steliacoom Blvd., S.W.
Tacoma, Washington 98499

Dietary Manager Program
Yakima Valley College
P.O. Box 1647
16th and Nob Hill
Yakima, Washington 98802

WISCONSIN

Dietary Manager Program
Eau Claire Technical Institute
620 W. Clairemont Avenue
District 1, Vo-Tech. & Adult Education
Eau Clair, Wisconsin 54701

Dietary Manager Program
Moraine Park Technical Institute
235 N. National Avenue
Fond du Lac, Wisconsin 54935

Dietary Manager Program
Northeast Wisconsin Vocational
P.O. Box 19042
Green Bay, Wisconsin 54307-9042

Dietary Manager Program
Gateway Technical Institutes of Elkhorn, Kenosha, & Racine
3520 20th Avenue
Kenosha, Wisconsin 53140

Dietary Manager Program
Western Wisconsin Technical Institute
6th and Vine Streets
La Crosse, Wisconsin 54601

Dietary Manager Program
Milwaukee Area Technical College
1015 N. 6th Street
Milwaukee, Wisconsin 53203

Dietary Manager Program
Indianhead Technical Institute
1019 S. Knowles Avenue
New Richmond, Wisconsin 54017

Dietary Manager Program
Waukesha County Technical Institute
800 Main Street
Pewaukee, Wisconsin 52072

Dietetic Aide

The *dietetic aide* works in food service departments of hospitals or extended care facilities and assists in the preparation and serving of food to patients. High school graduation, or the equivalent, is the prerequisite for admittance into a three-month, on-the-job hospital training program. Those persons interested in becoming a dietetic aide should contact the Personnel Director or the Chief Dietitian of their local hospital.

SOURCE:

American Dietetic Association

Dietetic Clerk

Supervised by an administrative or a clinical dietitian, the *dietetic clerk* assists with the paperwork and inventory duties in the operation of the dietetic department. He or she examines diet orders, processes new diets, and informs kitchen personnel of food requirements. The clerk also keeps an inventory of food and equipment purchases and a record of costs and of total number of meals served. The dietetic clerk may also enter diet changes into patients' medical records.

Training to become a dietetic clerk requires high school graduation, or the equivalent, with recommended courses in bookkeeping and typing. One year of clerical experience or one year of business administration education is also required as a prerequisite for admittance into a one-month, on-the-job hospital training program.

For further information on career opportunities, salaries, and training, interested persons should contact the Personnel Director or the Chief Dietitian of their local hospital.

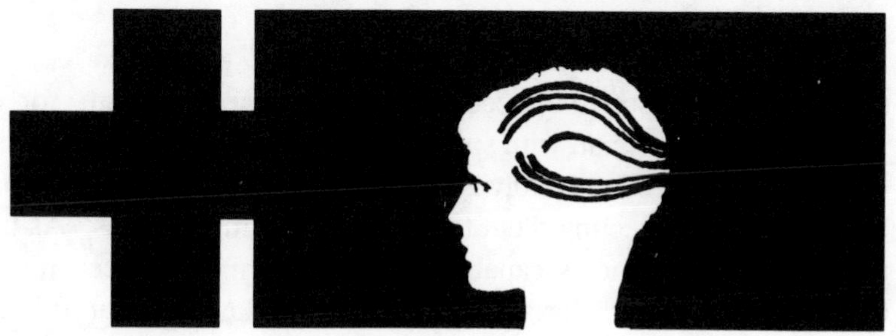

ELECTROENCEPHALOGRAPHIC TECHNOLOGY

Electroencephalographic (EEG) technology records and studies the electrical activity of the brain. As the brain controls breathing, heart rate, body temperature, and other essential bodily functions, it continually produces electrical impulses that can be amplified and measured by an EEG machine called the electroencephalograph. The written tracings of these electrical impulses are called electroencephalograms. By measuring impulse amplitude and frequency, EEG technology is used by neurologists and other physicians to diagnose brain diseases such as epilepsy, brain tumor, and stroke. It is also used to evaluate the effects of head trauma and infectious disease, as well as to indicate abnormal brain functions and pinpoint areas of the brain involved in disease processes.

EEG technology assists in determining the exact time that the body functions cease in a patient who is undergoing a vital organ transplantation. It is also used to diagnose any organic bases for serious adjustment problems or learning disabilities in children. Allied health personnel trained in EEG technology are referred to as EEG technologists or technicians. In some cases the terms EEG technologist and EEG technician refer to a similar skill level. In other cases, an EEG technologist refers to an individual with greater experience and possible supervisory responsibilities, while an EEG technician may denote an entry level position. The following chapter will refer to the *EEG technologist* position.

Electroencephalographic Technologist

Usually under the supervision of a department head or chief EEG technologist, the *EEG technologist* is responsible for the actual recording of a patient's EEG activity. With a thorough understanding of the EEG equipment and of common mental disorders, the EEG technologist selects the most appropriate combination of electrodes and instrument controls to produce the necessary electroencephalogram for interpretation by the neurologist (a physician with special training in the structure and diseases of the nervous system). The procedure involves placing small electrodes on the patient's scalp in standard locations and connecting them to the recording instruments. As the recording proceeds, the technologist, who is capable of distinguishing between normal brain activity and abnormal EEG characteristics, observes and keeps a careful record of the patient's behavior. The technologist must also be capable of handling basic medical emergencies in the laboratory; for example, he or she should be able to respond swiftly and wisely if a patient suffers an epileptic seizure.

Other duties of the EEG technologist may include taking medical histories, putting the patient at ease during the EEG recording, writing descriptive reports to accompany the EEG for use by the neurologist or other physicians, keeping accurate records, scheduling appointments, and ordering supplies.

Besides working in a hospital or clinic neurology department laboratory, EEG technologists may also work in neurologists' and neurosurgeons' offices, large medical centers, or health maintenance organizations, or with enough experience, they may conduct research or become members of a highly specialized neurosurgical team.

Advancement to administrative, supervisory, or training responsibilities in an EEG department may be available to EEG technologists with several years experience and a strong knowledge of the EEG technology field. Advanced on-the-job training may be available in larger facilities in other related neurological diagnostic techniques, including Evoked Potentials, ENG, EMG, and polysomnographic studies. Allied health personnel who perform numerous neurological diagnostic examinations are called *electroneurodiagnostic technologists*.

Training to become an EEG technologist involves the completion of a one-to-two year certificate or associate degree program offered by community and junior colleges, colleges and universities, vocational-technical institutes, or hospitals. Many EEG technologists learn their skill through on-the-job training in large hospitals and clinics.

After successful completion of an American Medical Association approved educational program, a required period of laboratory experience, and a comprehensive examination, an individual may apply for registration status. The title of Registered EEG Technologist (R.EEG.T.) is granted after meeting all requirements. Registration is also available to EEG technologists with on-the-job training, who have successfully completed the work experience requirement and successfully passed the registration examination.

Registration is not mandatory, but is advantageous for job placement, advancement, and higher salaries. For further information on registration requirements, write to the Psychological Corporation, American Board of Registration of Electroencephalographic Technologist's Exam, 555 Academic Street, San Antonio, Texas 78204.

Recommended high school courses for students interested in a career in EEG technology include health, biology, human anatomy, and mathematics.

According to a recent salary survey conducted by the University of Texas Medical Branch, starting salaries for electroencephalographic technologists ranged from $8,700 to $21,100, with average starting salaries equalling $15,000 annually. Experienced electroencephalographic technologists earned average salaries of $19,000 a year.

For more information on a career as an electroencephalographic technologist or for further information on other electroneurodiagnostic careers, contact the American Society of Electroneurodiagnostic Technologists (formerly the American Society of EEG Technologists) at Sixth at Quint, Carroll, Iowa 51401. For information about on-the-job training possibilities in EEG technology, students should contact the Personnel Director at large hospitals or clinics in their area. Below is a list of education programs in EEG technology, accredited by the Committee on Allied Health Education and Accreditation (CAHEA) of the American Medical Association.

SOURCES:

American Society of Electroneurodiagnostic Technologists
Occupation Outlook Handbook

EEG Technology Programs

ARIZONA

EEG Technology Program
Barrow Neurological Institute of St. Joseph's Hospital & Medical Center
P.O. Box 2071
Phoenix, Arizona 85001

CALIFORNIA

EEG Technology Program
Orange Coast College
2701 Fairview Road
Costa Mesa, California 92626-0120

FLORIDA

EEG Technology Program
Florida Neurological Institute, Inc.
5600 Spring Road
Jacksonville, Florida 32216

EEG Technology Program
V.A. Medical Center
S.W. Archer Road
Gainesville, Florida 32602

EEG Technology Program
Miami-Dade Community College
950 N.W. 20th Street
Miami, Florida 33127

EEG Technology Program
St. Joseph's Hospital
P.O. Box 4227
West Buffalo Avenue
Tampa, Florida 33677

ILLINOIS

EEG Technology Program
St. John's Hospital
800 East Carpenter Street
Springfield, Illinois 62769

IOWA

EEG Technology Program
Kirkwood Community College
6301 Kirkwood Boulevard, S.W.
P.O. Box 2068
Cedar Rapids, Iowa 52406

MASSACHUSETTS

EEG Technology Program
Children's Hospital Medical Center
300 Longwood Avenue
Boston, Massachusetts 02115

EEG Technology Program
Laboure College
2120 Dorchester Avenue
Boston Massachusetts 02124

MINNESOTA

EEG Technology Program
Annoka-Hennepin Vocational Technical Institute
1355 W. Main Street, Box 191
Annoka, Minnesota 55303

EEG Technology Program
Mayo Clinic Foundation
200 First Street, S.W.
Rochester, Minnesota 55905

NEW YORK

EEG Technology Program
Niagara County Community College
3111 Saunders Settlement Road
Sandborn, New York 14132

NORTH CAROLINA

EEG Technology Program
Duke University Medical Center
P.O. Box 3708
Durham, North Carolina 27710

PENNSYLVANIA

EEG Technology Program
Crozier-Chester Medical Center
15th Street & Upland Avenue
Chester, Pennsylvania 19013

EEG Technology Program
Philadelphia College of Osteopathic Medicine
4190 City Avenue
Philadelphia, Pennsylvania 19131

VIRGINIA

EEG Technology Program
Norfolk General Hospital
600 Gresham Avenue
Norfolk, Virginia 23507

WISCONSIN

EEG Technology Program
Western Wisconsin Technical Institute
Six and Vine Street
LaCrosse, Wisconsin 54601

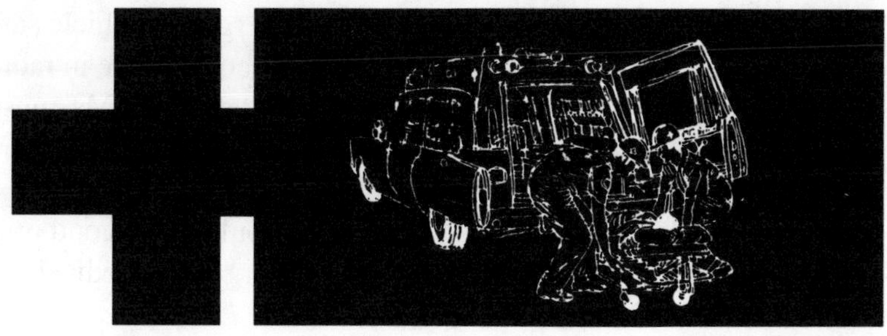

EMERGENCY MEDICAL SERVICES

When an accident or other medical emergency occurs, emergency medical services are employed to initially treat and transport the victims to the hospital. These services are regarded as an extension of a hospital's emergency department. A person employed in these services is known as an *emergency medical technician* (EMT). The career of dispatcher is summarized at the end of this chapter.

Emergency Medical Technician (EMT): EMT-Ambulance, EMT-Intermediate, EMT-Paramedic

Formerly referred to as ambulance attendants, *emergency medical technicians* are often the first qualified medical personnel to arrive at the scene of an emergency. Upon arrival they evaluate the nature and extent of the victims' illnesses or injuries and then administer specified diagnostic and emergency treatment procedures under standing orders or specific instructions of a physician. Emergency medical care may involve administering cardiac resuscitation, restoring breathing, controlling bleeding, treating for shock, immobilizing fractures, assisting in childbirth, or giving initial treatment to poison and burn victims. Using special equipment and techniques, EMT's may also have to extricate trapped victims.

The EMT is responsible for operating the emergency vehicle safely and efficiently and for maintaining continued medical care to the victims while in radio communication with the emergency departments en route to the hospital. The EMT must also transmit medical records and reports of each emergency to the hospital staff for their diagnostic purposes. The EMT must be alert and quick-thinking, especially in crucial situations. Finally, the EMT must maintain a clean, well-equipped ambulance in good operating condition.

There are three classifications of the emergency medical technician (EMT): the *EMT-Ambulance*, the *EMT-Intermediate* and the *EMT-Paramedic*.

The *EMT-Ambulance* is trained in basic life support and is certified to perform specific pre-hospital duties in emergency situations, including treating shock and poison victims, dressing and bandaging wounds, controlling bleeding, resuscitating heart attack victims, restoring breathing, maintaining a patient's airway, immobilizing fractures and providing obstetrical assistance.

The certified *EMT-Intermediate* provides the same care as the EMT-Ambulance, but because of additional training may also assess trauma patients, administer intravenous therapy, use antishock garments and airway maintenance equipment.

The certified *EMT-Paramedic* is the more highly trained technician who is qualified (subject to state law) to administer drugs, both orally and intravenously, and to operate more complicated equipment in an advanced life-support ambulance (intensive care vehicle), such as a defibrillator to shock a stopped heart into action. The EMT-Paramedic may also be required to assist in hospital emergency departments and intensive care units.

Training courses are available for all three levels of EMT. The basic national standard EMT-training course is a 100-plus hour program, offered throughout the country by police, fire and health departments, hospitals, colleges and universities. Applicants must be at least eighteen years of age, high school graduates or the equivalent, possess a valid driver's license, and be physically and emotionally capable to meet the rigors of the profession.

The training course for the EMT-Intermediate includes the same basic training course as the EMT-Ambulance but includes some of the EMT-Paramedic courses which cover patient assessment and use of the Esophageal Obturator Airway, intravenous fluids and antishock garments.

Training courses for the EMT-Paramedic include 600 to 1,000 hours of intensive classroom and clinical training. Some EMT-Paramedic programs are accredited by the American Medical Association's Committee on Allied Health Education and Accreditation.

Graduates of approved EMT-training programs, with the required amount of work experience, are qualified to take the written and practical certification examinations sponsored by the National Registry of Emergency Medical Technicians. All states have some form of certification requirement. Recertification is required every two-to-three years and refresher training in the latest techniques and equipment is available. Certification information can be obtained from the National Registry of Emergency Medical Technicians, P.O. Box 29233, Columbus, Ohio 43229.

A large percentage of basic EMT's (EMT-Ambulance) are non-paid volunteers for rescue squads that work closely with fire departments. Volunteer EMT's must still become certified and successfully complete the basic training course. Employed EMT's work for police and fire departments, private ambulance companies and hospital-based ambulance teams.

Overall average annual salaries were $18,710 for the EMT-Ambulance, $19,840 for the EMT-Intermediate and $24,100 for the EMT-Paramedic, according to a 1987 salary survey compiled by the *Journal of Emergency Medical Services.*

Students interested in a career in emergency medical services may find it helpful to talk with faculty at area EMT training sites or to arrange for an appointment at a local fire/rescue station for an observational meeting.

Hospitals; community colleges; and fire, health, and police departments throughout each state offer training programs. For further information on the location of these programs contact the State Emergency Medical Services Office listed at the end of this chapter.

For more information on a career as an emergency medical technician, write to the National Association of Emergency Medical Technicians, 9140 Ward Parkway, Kansas City, Missouri 64114.

SOURCES:

National Association of Emergency Medical Technicians
National Registry of Emergency Medical Technicians
Occupational Outlook Handbook

Dispatcher

Although not directly involved with emergency patients, the *dispatcher* provides a channel for communication among all aspects of emergency medical services. He or she receives calls for emergency medical help, dispatches the appropriate medical resources, and then acts as the communication link between the medical facility and the ambulance team. Besides working in emergency medical services, the dispatcher may also handle communication for public safety agencies such as police and fire departments. Training is generally provided on-the-job. Interested persons should contact their municipal fire-rescue departments or State Emergency Medical Services Office for more information on requirements and job opportunities.

SOURCE:

Occupational Outlook Handbook

State Emergency Medical Services Offices

ALABAMA

Emergency Medical Services Director
Department of Public Health
644 State Office Building
Montgomery, Alabama 36130

ALASKA

Emergency Medical Services Director
Emergency Medical Services Section
Division of Public Health
Pouch H-06C
Juneau, Alaska 99811

ARIZONA

Emergency Medical Services Director
Dept. of Health Services
701 E. Jefferson, 4th Floor
Phoenix, Arizona 85034

ARKANSAS

Emergency Medical Services Director
Arkansas Department of Health
Office of Emergency Medical Services
4815 West Markham Street
Little Rock, Arkansas 72205-3867

CALIFORNIA

Emergency Medical Services Director
Emergency Medical Services Authority
1030 15th Street, Suite 302
Sacramento, California 95814

COLORADO

Emergency Medical Services Director
Colorado Dept. of Health
Emergency Medical Services
4210 East 11th Avenue
Denver, Colorado 80220

CONNECTICUT

Emergency Medical Services Director
Dept. of Health Services
150 Washington Street
Hartford, Connecticut 06106

DELAWARE

Emergency Medical Services Director
EMS, Robbins Building
820 Silver Lake Blvd.
Dover, Delaware 19901

DISTRICT OF COLUMBIA

Emergency Medical Services Director
Office of Emergency Medical Services
1875 Connecticut Ave., N.W.
Washington, DC 20009

FLORIDA

Emergency Medical Services Director
Dept. of Health & Rehabilitative Services
1317 Winewood Boulevard
Room 267, Bldg. 6
Tallahassee, Florida 32301

GEORGIA

Emergency Medical Services Director
Emergency Health Unit
State Dept. of Human Resources
878 Peachtree St., N.E.
Atlanta, Georgia 30309

GUAM

Emergency Medical Services Director
Dept. of Health & Social Services
P.O. Box 2816
Agara, Guam 96912

HAWAII

Emergency Medical Services Director
Emergency Medical Services
State Dept. of Health
3627 Kilavea Avenue
Honolulu, Hawaii 96816

IDAHO

Emergency Medical Services Director
Emergency Medical Services Bureau
Dept. of Health and Welfare
450 West State Street
Boise, Idaho 83720

ILLINOIS

Emergency Medical Services Director
State Dept. of Public Health
Div. of EMS and Health Services
535 West Jefferson Street
Springfield, Illinois 62761

INDIANA

Emergency Medical Services Director
Emergency Medical Services Commission
State Office Bldg., Room 315
100 North Senate Avenue
Indianapolis, Indiana 46204

IOWA

Emergency Medical Services Director
Emergency Medical Services
State Dept. of Health
Lucas State Office Bldg.
Des Moines, Iowa 50319

KANSAS

Emergency Medical Services Director
Bureau of EMS
111 West 6th Street
Topeka, Kansas 66603

KENTUCKY

Emergency Medical Services Director
Dept. for Health Services
275 East Main Street
Frankfort, Kentucky 40601

LOUISIANA

Emergency Medical Services Director
Bureau of Emergency Medical Services
Department of Health & Human Resources
4550 North Blvd., 2nd Floor
Baton Rouge, Louisiana 70809

MAINE

Emergency Medical Services Director
Emergency Medical Services, Bureau of Health
295 Water Street
Augusta, Maine 04330

MARYLAND

Emergency Medical Services Director
Dept. of Health
31 South Greene St.
Baltimore, Maryland 21201

MASSACHUSETTS

Emergency Medical Services Director
Office of Emergency Medical Services
80 Boylston St., Suite 1040
Boston, Massachusetts 02116

MICHIGAN

Emergency Medical Services Director
Div. of Emergency Medical Services
Department of Public Health
P.O. Box 30035
Lansing, Michigan 48909

MINNESOTA

Emergency Medical Services Director
Emergency Medical Services Training
Minnesota Dept. of Health
717 Delaware St., S.E.
Minneapolis, Minnesota 55440

MISSISSIPPI

Emergency Medical Services Director
Emergency Medical Services
State Board of Health
P.O. Box 1700
Jackson, Mississippi 39215

MISSOURI

Emergency Medical Services Director
Bureau of Emergency Medical Services
Missouri Division of Health
P.O. Box 570
Jefferson City, Missouri 65102

MONTANA

Emergency Medical Services Director
Emergency Medical Services Bureau
Dept. of Health & Environmental Sciences
Cogswell Building
Helena, Montana 59620

NEBRASKA

Emergency Medical Services Director
Emergency Medical Services Division
State Department of Health
301 Centennial Mall, S. Box 95007
Lincoln, Nebraska 68509

NEVADA

Emergency Medical Services Director
State Department of Health
505 East King St.
Capital Complex
Carson City, Nevada 89710

NEW HAMPSHIRE

Emergency Medical Services Director
Division of Public Health Services
Health & Welfare Bldg.
Hazen Drive
Concord, New Hampshire 03301

NEW JERSEY

Emergency Medical Services Director
EMS, State Dept. of Health
CN 364
Trenton, New Jersey 08625

NEW MEXICO

Emergency Medical Services Director
Health Services Division
Emergency Medical Services
1100 St. Francis Drive
Sante Fe, New Mexico 87501

NEW YORK

Emergency Medical Services Director
Bureau of Emergency Health Services
State Department of Health
Tower Bldg. 7th Floor
Albany, New York 12237

NORTH CAROLINA

Emergency Medical Services Director
Office of Emergency Medical Services
701 Barbour Drive
Raleigh, North Carolina 27603

NORTH DAKOTA

Emergency Medical Services Director
Div. of Emergency Health Services
Department of Health
State Capitol Bldg.
Bismarck, North Dakota 58505

OHIO

Emergency Medical Services Director
Ohio EMS Agency
65 South Front St., Room 918
Columbus, Ohio 43215

OKLAHOMA

Emergency Medical Services Director
Oklahoma Department of Health
1000 N.E. 10th Street
Box 53551
Oklahoma City, Oklahoma 73152

OREGON

Emergency Medical Services Director
Emergency Medical Services
State Dept. of Human Resources
P.O. Box 231
Portland, Oregon 97207

PENNSYLVANIA

Emergency Medical Services Director
Div. of Emergency Health Services
Pennsylvania Dept. of Health
1033 Health & Welfare Bldg. Box 90
Harrisburg, Pennsylvania 17120

PUERTO RICO

Emergency Medical Services Director
Emergency Health Services
Department of Health
Ponce de Leon Avenue
San Juan, Puerto Rico 00908

RHODE ISLAND

Emergency Medical Services Director
Emergency Medical Services Division
State Department of Health
75 Davis Street, Room 301
Providence, Rhode Island 02908

SOUTH CAROLINA

Emergency Medical Services Director
Dept. of Health & Environ. Control
Div. of Emergency Medical Services
2600 Bull Street
Columbia, South Carolina 29201

SOUTH DAKOTA

Emergency Medical Services Director
Emergency Medical Services
State Dept. of Health
523 E. Capitol
Pierre, South Dakota 57501

TENNESSEE

Emergency Medical Services Director
State Department of Health & Environment
Division of EMS
287 Plus Park Blvd.
Nashville, Tennessee 37219-5407

TEXAS

Emergency Medical Services Director
Bureau of Emergency Medical Management
Division of EMS
1100 West 49th Street
Austin, Texas 78756

UTAH

Emergency Medical Services Director
Utah Department of Health
Emergency Medical Services
P.O. Box 16660
Salt Lake City, Utah 84116-0660

VERMONT

Emergency Medical Services Director
State Dept. of Health
60 Main St., Box 70
Burlington, Vermont 05402

VIRGIN ISLANDS

Emergency Medical Services Director
Department of Health
Government of Virgin Islands of the U.S.
P.O. Box 7304
St. Thomas, Virgin Islands 00801

VIRGINIA

Emergency Medical Services Director
Division of Emergency Medical Services
Department of Health
1001 James Madison Bldg.
Richmond, Virginia 23219

WASHINGTON

Emergency Medical Services Director
Emergency Medical Services
Dept. of Social & Health Services, ET-34
Olympia, Washington 98504

WEST VIRGINIA

Emergency Medical Services Director
Office of Emergency Medical Services
1800 Washington St., East
Building 3, Room 426
Charleston, West Virginia 25305

WISCONSIN

Emergency Medical Services Director
Emergency Medical Services Training
Division of Health
P.O. Box 309
Madison, Wisconsin 53701

WYOMING

Emergency Medical Services Director
Emergency Medical Services Program
Dept. of Health & Social Services
Hathaway Bldg.. Room 524
Cheyenne, Wyoming 82002

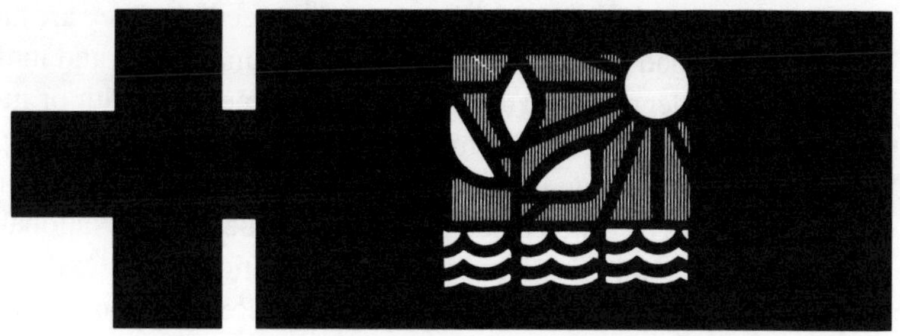

ENVIRONMENTAL HEALTH

As one of the many specialized professions in the field of public health, environmental health is concerned with the protection, maintenance, and improvement of the human environment. Environmental health occupations discussed below are those of the *sanitarian,* the *environmental health technician,* and the *executive housekeeper.*

Sanitarian

Also referred to as an *environmentalist* or *environmental specialist,* the sanitarian applies the principles of the physical, biological, and social sciences to a broad range of environmental management functions. The sanitarian plans, develops, directs, interprets, controls, and enforces comprehensive environmental health standards and programs in the following areas: air, water, land, and noise pollution; solid and hazardous waste management; food supply sanitation; consumer protection; epidemiology, and community sanitation. Other areas of concern to the sanitarian are occupational safety and health, health education, and radiologic health. Careers in these allied fields are discussed elsewhere in this handbook in their respective sections.

A sanitarian's specific duties might include the health inspection of food supplies; the sanitary inspection of restaurants, food processing plants, hospitals, nursing homes, recreation areas, and housing projects; the supervision of collection, treatment, and disposal of community wastes; or the monitoring of toxicant levels in public water supplies. Each location and process that the sanitarian inspects must comply with local, state, and federal public health regulations.

The range of job locations and types of employers for the sanitarian is almost as varied as the job responsibilities themselves. Sanitarians work for local, state and federal departments of health and of environmental protection. They are also employed in health-care facilities, food processing plants, chemical industries, and in the military.

A bachelor's degree, with a major in environmental health or in a related biological or physical science, is the minimum educational requirement for the professional sanitarian. Supervisory, research, and teaching positions require graduate degrees.

Credentials as a Registered Sanitarian are awarded by the National Environmental Health Association to applicants who meet all educational and experience requirements and satisfactorily pass the registration examination. Registration information is available from the National Environmental Health Association, 720 South Colorado Blvd., Suite 970, South Tower, Denver, Colorado 80222.

Below is a list provided by the National Environmental Health Association of bachelor degree programs specifically in environmental health. Programs marked with an asterisk (*) are accredited by the National Accreditation Council for Environmental Health. A list of schools that offer degrees in related science fields can be obtained from the National Environmental Health Association, as well as a list of schools of public health offering graduate degrees.

The National Environmental Health Association offers a scholarship award to needy students enrolled in these environmental health programs. For application information, write to them at the above listed address.

SOURCES:

National Environmental Health Association
Occupational Outlook Handbook

Sanitarian Programs

CALIFORNIA

Environmental Health Program
California State University at San Bernardino
5500 University Parkway
San Bernardino, California 92407

Environmental Health Program(*)
California State University at Northridge
Department of Health Science
18111 Nordhoff
Northridge, California 91330

Environmental Health Program(*)
California State University at Fresno
Department of Health Science
Fresno, California 93740-0001

Environmental Health Program
San Diego State University
Biology Department
San Diego, California 92182

Environmental Health Program
San Jose State University
Department of Biological Sciences
1 Washington Square
San Jose, California 95192-0100

COLORADO

Environmental Health Program(*)
Colorado State University
Dept. of Microbiology and Environmental Health
120 Microbiology Building
Fort Collins, Colorado 80521

GEORGIA

Environmental Health Science Program(*)
University of Georgia
Dairy Science Building.
Athens, Georgia 30602

IOWA

Environmental Health Program(*)
Boise State University
School of Health Science
1910 University Drive
Boise, Iowa 83725

ILLINOIS

Environmental Health Program(*)
Illinois State University
Moulton Hall
Normal, Illinois 61761

Community Health Program
Northern Illinois University
School of Allied Health Professions
DeKalb, Illinois 60115

Environmental Health Program
Western Illinois University
Department of Health Sciences
Macomb, Illinois 61455

INDIANA

Environmental Health Program(*)
Indiana State University
Environmental Health and Safety
Terre Haute, Indiana 47809

KENTUCKY

Environmental Health Program(*)
Eastern Kentucky University
Environmental Health Science Dept.
College of Allied Health
Richmond, Kentucky 40475

Environmental Health Program
University of Kentucky
Department of Community Health
UKMC, Annex 2
Lexington, Kentucky 40536-0080

LOUISIANA

Environmental Health Program
McNeese State University
Department of Biology and Environmental Science
P.O. Box 923
Lake Charles, Louisiana 70609

Environmental Health Program
Louisiana State University
Environmental Health Curricula
Department of Dairy Science
Baton Rouge, Louisiana 70803

MASSACHUSETTS

Environmental Health Program(*)
University of Massachusetts
Amherst, Massachusetts 01003

MICHIGAN

Environmental Health Program(*)
Ferris State College
Industrial and Environmental Health Management
School of Allied Health
Big Rapids, Michigan 49307

MISSISSIPPI

Environmental Health Program(*)
Mississippi Valley State University
Itta Bena, Mississippi 38941

MONTANA

Environmental Health Program(*)
Montana State University
Department of Microbiology
Bozeman, Montana 59717

NEW JERSEY

Environmental Health Program
Rutgers University
Department of Environmental Sciences
P.O. Box 231
New Brunswick, New Jersey 08903

NEW YORK

Environmental Studies Program
Alfred University
Alfred, New York 14802

Environmental Health Program
City University of New York
York College
Jamaica, New York 11433-1126

NORTH CAROLINA

Environmental Health Program(*)
East Carolina University
Department of Environmental Health
Greenville, North Carolina 27834

Environmental Health Program(*)
Western Carolina University
Cullowhee, North Carolina 28723

OHIO

Environmental Health Program(*)
Bowling Green State University
102 Health Center
Bowling Green, Ohio 43403

Environmental Health Program(*)
Wright State University
Biology Department
Dayton, Ohio 45431

OKLAHOMA

Environmental Health Program(*)
East Central State University
School of Environmental Science
Ada, Oklahoma 73019

OREGON

Environmental Health Program(*)
Oregon State University
Department of Health
311 Waldo Hall
Corvallis, Oregon 97331

TENNESSEE

Environmental Health Program(*)
East Tennessee State University
Department of Environmental Health
Johnson City, Tennessee 37604

TEXAS

Environmental Health Program
Lamar University
Environmental Science
P.O. Box 10022
Beaumont, Texas 77710

Environmental Science Program
Sam Houston State University
Huntsville, Texas 77341

UTAH

Environmental Health Program(*)
Brigham Young University
229 K-Richards Building
Provo, Utah 84601

Undergraduate Public Health Program
Utah State University
Department of Biology
Logan, Utah 84322-5305

VIRGINIA

Environmental Health Program(*)
Old Dominion University
College of Health Sciences
Norfolk, Virginia 23508

WASHINGTON

Environmental Health Program
Central Washington University
Department of Biological Science
Ellensburg, Washington 98926

Environmental Health Program(*)
University of Washington
Department of Environmental Health SC-34
Seattle, Washington 98195

WISCONSIN

Environmental Health Program(*)
University of Wisconsin-Eau Claire
Division of Allied Health, L2044
Eau Claire, Wisconsin 53701

Environmental Health Technician

The *environmental health technician* is a para-professional who assists and is supervised by a registered sanitarian or other environmental professional. Employed primarily in community sanitation, in such locations as solid waste collection and disposal facilities or water purification and waste water treatment plants, the environmental health technician obtains samples of air and water and tests their quality in relation to health standards. The technician also assists the sanitarian in the inspection and evaluation of procedures involved with most other public health programs.

Formal training programs for the environmental health technician are generally two year associate degree programs in either environmental health, environmental science, or a related field. These programs are usually entitled environmental health technology or sanitation technology and are offered by community colleges, universities, and vocational-technical schools. Students interested in such programs should contact postsecondary institutions in their area.

The National Environmental Health Association offers certification for the environmental health technician. Qualified applicants should have graduated from a recognized two-year college program in an environmental health field, or from a military technical school offering environmental health, preventive or veterinary medicine; or graduate with a high school diploma or equivalent plus a minimum of two years experience in an environmental health field.

For further information on the certification of environmental health technicians, interested persons should contact the National Environmental Health Association at 720 South Colorado Boulevard, Suite 970, South Tower, Denver, Colorado 80222.

SOURCE:

National Environmental Health Association

Executive Housekeeper

In hospitals and many other healthcare facilities the *executive housekeeper* is responsible for all environmental services, including cleaning, bacteriologic testing, and interior decorating. In some facilities the executive housekeeper is also responsible for the operation of the laundry and for security. His or her primary function is to maintain clean, antiseptic conditions in all the areas of the health facility that require a high degree of sanitation and sterilization especially patient wards, operating rooms, treatment rooms, and intensive care units.

Familiar with labor relations and safety/health regulations, the executive housekeeper also manages the housekeeping staff. He or she establishes work schedules and supervises the activities of the housekeeping department, so that its staff does not impede or interfere with the administration of healthcare by physicians, nurses, and other medical personnel. The housekeeper purchases cleaning supplies and equipment, forecasts future needs for the department, and prepares departmental budgets. He or she conducts continual research into new housekeeping products and into new healthcare facilities that will require housekeeping services.

In interior decorating the executive housekeeper selects furnishings, carpets, and wall coverings that provide pleasant yet utilitarian surroundings. If the housekeeping department supervises the facility's laundry, it is the executive housekeeper who maintains established sanitary standards and supervises the selection, laundering, and distribution of linens.

With experience, executive housekeepers move into positions as directors or assistant directors of housekeeping departments in healthcare facilities. They are employed by hotels, colleges and universities and private industry. In hospital situations executive housekeepers may advance to positions of administrative assistants or associate administrators.

On-the-job training is provided for the lower level jobs in hospital housekeeping. However, for those individuals interested in management positions there are certificate, associate and bachelor degree programs available in institutional housekeeping management. A degree in environmental science is also acceptable to many employers.

The credential of Certified Executive Housekeeper (C.E.H.) is awarded to those members of the National Executive Housekeepers Association who have successfully completed an approved educational program and have completed one year of management level experience in institutional housekeeping. The Registered Executive Housekeeper (R.E.H.) title is the highest level recognition awarded to certified members who meet more stringent requirements.

Recommended high school courses for students interested in a career in housekeeping include general science, biology, textiles, and business.

According to a survey published by *Executive Housekeeping Today,* most executive housekeepers responding earned salaries between $18,000 and $31,000 a year, while those who were highly qualified, trained and experienced earned over $32,000 a year. Nearly 80% of respondents worked in healthcare settings, such as hospitals and nursing homes.

Following is a list, supplied by the National Executive Housekeepers Association, Inc., of approved educational programs in institutional housekeeping management. Graduates must complete 330 subject hours, of which 270 are in required subjects such as housekeeping techniques, communications, environmental controls, management, behavioral sciences and business administration. Many of these programs offer financial aid to qualified students. Contact the school directly for financial aid application information, entrance requirements and type and length of program.

For additional information on a career as an executive housekeeper, write to the National Executive Housekeepers Association, 1001 Eastwind Drive, Suite 301, Westerville, Ohio 43081.

SOURCES:

National Executive Housekeeping Association, Inc.
Executive Housekeeping Today

Executive Housekeeper Programs

ARIZONA

Executive Housekeeper Program
Pima County Community College
P.O. Box 5027
Tucson, Arizona 85703

Executive Housekeeper Program
Rio Salado Community College
135 N. 2nd Avenue
Phoenix, Arizona 85003

ARKANSAS

Executive Housekeeper Program
Crowley's Ridge Vo-Tech School
P.O. Box 925
Forrest City, Arkansas 72335

CALIFORNIA

Executive Housekeeper Program
Fresno City College
1101 N. University Ave.
Fresno, California 93741

Executive Housekeeper Program
Palomar College
San Marcos, California 92069

Executive Housekeeper Program
Rancho Santiago Community College District
Continuing Education Division
541 N. Lemon Street
Orange, California 92667

Executive Housekeeper Program
Rio Salado Community College
St. Francis Medical Center
3630 E. Imperial Hwy.
Lynwood, California 90262

Executive Housekeeper Program
San Diego Community College District
3375 Camino del Rio South
San Diego, California 92108

Executive Housekeeper Program
Skyline College
3300 College Drive
San Bruno, California 94066

Executive Housekeeper Program
University of California Extension
Carriage House
Santa Cruz, California 95064

CANADA

Executive Housekeeper Program
Alberta Vocational Centre
10215 108th Street
Edmonton, Alberta, Canada T5J 1L6

FLORIDA

Executive Housekeeper Program
Collier County Vocational Technical Center
3702 Estey Avenue
Naples, Florida 33942

Executive Housekeeper Program
Daytona Beach Community College
P.O. Box 1111
Daytona Beach, Florida 32015-1111

Executive Housekeeper Program
Indian River Community College
3209 Virginia Avenue
Fort Pierce, Florida 33454-9003

Executive Housekeeper Program
Lee Vo-Tech
3800 Michigan Avenue
Ft. Myers, Florida 33901

Executive Housekeeper Program
Mid-Florida Technical Institute
2900 West Oak Ridge Road
Orlando, Florida 32809

Executive Housekeeper Program
Palm Beach Junior College
4200 Congress Avenue
Lake Worth, Florida 33461

Executive Housekeeper Program
Ridge Vocational Technical Center
7700 State Road 544 North
Winter Haven, Florida 33881

Executive Housekeeper Program
St. Petersburg Vocational Technical Institute
901 34th Street South
St. Petersburg, Florida 33711

Executive Housekeeper Program
Sarasota County Vocational Center
4748 Beneva Road
Sarasota, Florida 33583

Executive Housekeeper Program
Tampa Bay Evening Vocational School
6410 Orient Road
Tampa, Florida 33610

Executive Housekeeper Program
University of Florida
Division of Housing
S.W. 13th and Museum Road
Gainesville, Florida 32611

GEORGIA

Executive Housekeeper Program
Augusta Tech
3116 Deans Bridge Road
Augusta, Georgia 30906

Executive Housekeeper Program
Brunswick Junior College
Altama at Fourth Street
Brunswick, Georgia 31523

Executive Housekeeper Program
Savannah Area Vocational Technical School
107 Gignilliat Street
Savannah, Georgia 31408

HAWAII

Executive Housekeeper Program
Kapiolani Community College
4303 Diamond Head Road
Honolulu, Hawaii 96816

ILLINOIS

Executive Housekeeper Program
Black Hawk College
6600 34th Avenue
Moline, Illinois 61265

Executive Housekeeper Program
College of Lake County
19351 W. Washington St.
Grayslake, Illinois 60030

Executive Housekeeper Program
Lincoln Land Community College
Shepherd Road
Springfield, Illinois 62708

Executive Housekeeper Program
McHenry County College
Route 14 at Lucas Road
Crystal Lake, Illinois 60014

Executive Housekeeper Program
Parkland College
2400 W. Bradley Avenue
Champaign, Illinois 61821

Executive Housekeeper Program
William Rainey Harper College
Algonquin & Roselle Road
Palatine, Illinois 60067

INDIANA

Executive Housekeeper Program
Indiana Vocational Technical College
P.O. Box 1763
Indianapolis, Indiana 46206

Executive Housekeeper Program
University of Evansville
1800 Lincoln Avenue
Evansville, Indiana 47714

IOWA

Executive Housekeeper Program
Des Moines Area Community College
2006 South Ankeny Boulevard
Ankeny, Iowa 50021

Executive Housekeeper Program
Eastern Iowa Community College
2804 Eastern Avenue
Davenport, Iowa 52803

Executive Housekeeper Program
Hawkeye Institute of Technology
Box 8015
Waterloo, Iowa 51704

KENTUCKY

Executive Housekeeper Program
Hopkinsville Community College
P.O. Box 2100
Hopkinsville, Kentucky 42240

Executive Housekeeper Program
Jefferson Community College
109 East Broadway
Louisville, Kentucky 40204

Executive Housekeeper Program
Somerset Community College
808 Monticello Road
Somerset, Kentucky 42501

LOUISIANA

Executive Housekeeper Program
Georgia Military College
P.O. Drawer N
Barksdale AFB, Louisiana 71110

Executive Housekeeper Program
Jefferson Parish Vo-Tech School
5200 Blair Drive
Metairie, Louisiana 70001

Executive Housekeeper Program
Louisiana State University at Eunice
P.O. Box 1129
Eunice, Louisiana 70535

MAINE

Executive Housekeeper Program
University of Southern Maine
96 Fulmouth Street
Portland, Maine 04103

MARYLAND

Executive Housekeeper Program
Catonsville Community College
880 S. Rolling Road
Baltimore, Maryland 21228

Executive Housekeeper Program
Wor-Wic Tech Community College
Berlin-Ocean City Instructional Institute
Route 3, Box 79
Berlin, Maryland 21811

MICHIGAN

Executive Housekeeper Program
Henry Ford Community College
Dearborn Heights Center
22586 Ann Arbor Trail
Dearborn Heights, Michigan 48127

Executive Housekeeper Program
Lansing Community College
Dept. of Health Careers
P.O. Box 40010
Lansing, Michigan 48901

MINNESOTA

Executive Housekeeper Program
Normandale Community College
9700 France Avenue South
Bloomington, Minnesota 55431

Executive Housekeeper Program
Rochester Area Vo-Tech Institute
1926 Second Street, S.E.
Rochester, Minnesota 55904

MISSISSIPPI

Executive Housekeeper Program
Meridian Junior College
5500 Highway 19 North
Meridian, Mississippi 39305

Executive Housekeeper Program
Hinds Junior College
Jackson Campus
3925 Sunset Drive
Jackson, Mississippi 39213

MISSOURI

Executive Housekeeper Program
Maple Woods Community College
2601 N.E. Barry Road
Kansas City, Missouri 64156

Executive Housekeeper Program
University of Missouri - St. Louis
8001 Natural Bridge Road
St. Louis, Missouri 63121

NEBRASKA

Executive Housekeeper Program
Metro Tech Community College
P.O. Box 3777
Omaha, Nebraska 68103

NEVADA

Executive Housekeeper Program
Clark County Community College
3200 E. Cheyenne Avenue
N. Las Vegas, Nevada 89030

NEW JERSEY

Executive Housekeeper Program
Burlington County College
Pemberton-Browns Mill Road
Pemberton, New Jersey 08068

Executive Housekeeper Program
Center for Continuing Education
Montclair State College
Upper Montclair, New Jersey 07043

NEW MEXICO

Executive Housekeeper Program
National College
Albuquerque Branch
525 San Pedro, N.E.
Albuquerque, New Mexico 87108

NEW YORK

Executive Housekeeper Program
New York City Technical College
300 Jay Street
Brooklyn, New York 11201

Executive Housekeeper Program
Orange County Community College
115 South Street
Middletown, New York 10940

Executive Housekeeper Program
SUNY Agricultural & Technical College
Cobleskill, New York 12043

NORTH CAROLINA

Executive Housekeeper Program
Fayetteville Technical Institute
Horace Sisk Building
Fayetteville, North Carolina 28303

Executive Housekeeper Program
Forsyth Technical College
2100 Silas Creek Parkway
Winston-Salem, North Carolina 27103

Executive Housekeeper Program
Wake Technical College
9101 Fayetteville Road
Raleigh, North Carolina 27603

NORTH DAKOTA

Institutional Environmental Services Program
College of Home Economics
North Dakota State University
Fargo, North Dakota 58105

OHIO

Executive Housekeeper Program
Bowling Green State University
300 McFall Center
Bowling Green, Ohio 43403

Executive Housekeeper Program
Clark Technical College
P.O. Box 570
Springfield, Ohio 45501

Executive Housekeeper Program
Columbus Technical Institute
550 East Spring Street
Columbus, Ohio 43215

Executive Housekeeper Program
University of Akron
Continuing Education Department
Akron, Ohio 44325

OKLAHOMA

Executive Housekeeper Program
Oklahoma State University
Stillwater, Oklahoma 74078

OREGON

Executive Housekeeper Program
Lane Community College
1059 Willamette Street
Eugene, Oregon 97401

Executive Housekeeper Program
Portland Community College
12000 S.W. 49th Avenue
Portland, Oregon 97219

PENNSYLVANIA

Executive Housekeeper Program
Community College of Allegheny County
1130 Perry Highway
Pittsburgh, Pennsylvania 15237

Executive Housekeeper Program
Marywood College
2300 Adams Avenue
Scranton, Pennsylvania 18509

SOUTH CAROLINA

Executive Housekeeper Program
Horry Georgetown Technical College
Box 1966
Conway, South Carolina 29526

Executive Housekeeper Program
Spartanburg Technical College
Industry & Business Training
P.O. Drawer 4386
Spartanburg, South Carolina 29305

Executive Housekeeper Program
Trident Technical College
P.O. Box 10367
Charleston, South Carolina 29411

TENNESSEE

Executive Housekeeper Program
Nashville State Technical Institute
P.O. Box 90285
Nashville, Tennessee 37209

Executive Housekeeper Program
Shelby State Community College
P.O. Box 40568
Memphis, Tennessee 38174-0568

Executive Housekeeper Program
State Technical Institute at Memphis
5983 Macon Cove
Memphis, Tennesee 38134

Executive Housekeeper Program
Technical Education & Evening Trade School
Fulton High School
Knoxville, Tennessee 37917

Executive Housekeeper Program
Vanderbilt University
1161 21st Avenue South
AA-0210 MCN
Nashville, Tennessee 37232

TEXAS

Executive Housekeeper Program
Austin Community College
P.O. Box 2285
Austin, Texas 78767

Executive Housekeeper Program
Del Mar College
Baldwin & Ayers
Corpus Christi, Texas 78404

Executive Housekeeper Program
El Centro College
Main and Lamar Streets
Dallas, Texas 75202

Executive Housekeeper Program
El Paso Community College
9370 Gateway Blvd. North
El Paso, Texas 79924

Executive Housekeeper Program
Odessa College
201 West University
Odessa, Texas 79764

Executive Housekeeper Program
Houston Community College System
22 Waugh Drive
Houston, Texas 77270-7849

Executive Housekeeper Program
San Antonio College
1300 San Pedro
San Antonio, Texas 78284

Executive Housekeeper Program
Texas State Technical Institute - Harlingen
P.O. Box 2628
Harlingen, Texas 78551

UTAH

Executive Housekeeper Program
Utah Technical College
P.O. Box 1609
Provo, Utah 84603

Executive Housekeeper Program
Weber State College
Division of Continuing Education-3104
Ogden, Utah 84408

VERMONT

Executive Housekeeper Program
Norwich University
Vermont College Campus
Montpelier, Vermont 05602

VIRGINIA

Executive Housekeeper Program
Arlington Public Schools
2700 South Lang Street
Arlington, Virginia 22206

Executive Housekeeper Program
William Fleming High School
3649 Ferncliff Avenue
Roanoke, Virginia 24017

Executive Housekeeper Program
Thomas Nelson Community College
P.O. Box 9407
Hampton, Virginia 23670

Executive Housekeeper Program
Piedmont Virginia Community College
Route 6, Box 1-A
Charlottesville, Virginia 22901

WEST VIRGINIA

Executive Housekeeper Program
West Liberty State College
West Liberty, West Virginia 26074

WISCONSIN

Executive Housekeeper Program
District One Technical Institute
620 W. Clairemont Avenue
Eau Claire, Wisconsin 54701

Executive Housekeeper Program
Milwaukee Area Technical College
West Campus
1200 South 71st Street
West Allis, Wisconsin 53214

Executive Housekeeper Program
Northeast Wisconsin Technical Institute
2740 W. Mason Street
P.O. Box 19042
Green Bay, Wisconsin 54307

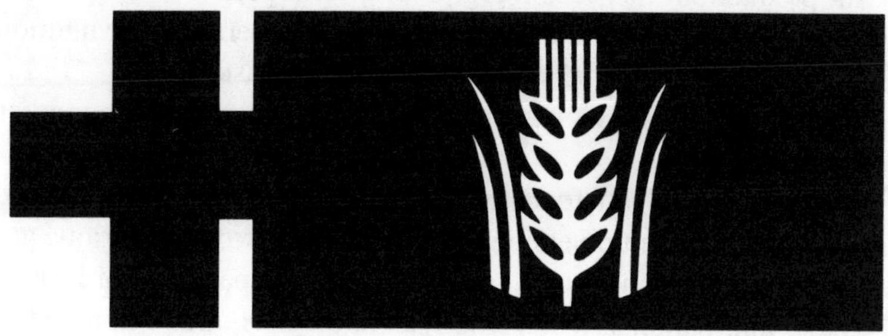

FOOD TECHNOLOGY

Food technology, also known as food science, is the application of chemistry, microbiology, and engineering to the production, processing, packaging, distribution, preparation, utilization and evaluation of foods. Food technology is of vital importance in less developed countries where it attempts to alleviate problems of malnutrition and lack of food. It is also of importance in developed countries where it, among other concerns, investigates food-processing methods and ingredients and attempts to provide greater varieties of nutritious foods that are easier to preserve and prepare. There are two career occupations in food technology: the *food technologist,* and the *food science technician.*

Food Technologist

Also known as a *food scientist,* the food technologist is a trained professional in the food industry who is concerned with the processing, preserving, sanitation, storage, and marketing of nutritious, wholesome, and economic foods. By researching the physical, chemical and biological nature of food, the technologist studies the changes that occur in the nutritional value and suitability of industrially prepared foods throughout their processing and storage.

In the research and development of new products, processes, and equipment, the food technologist may develop new foods or new factors that will improve the flavor, texture or appearance of existing foods.

In the assurance of quality control the technologist tests new ingredients for freshness and suitability for processing and tests finished products for purity and safety in storage. He or she checks for accurate package labeling.

In production the technologist prepares production specifications and schedules processing operations, maintains the proper temperature and humidity in storage areas, and supervises economic and sanitary disposal of wastes.

The food technologist may also teach or be involved with market research, advertising, or technical sales.

The majority of all food technologists are employed by private industry, while the remainder teach in universities and colleges or work in various government departments such as the Department of Agriculture or the Department of Health and Human Services. At the international level, food technologists are employed by the World Health Organization and the Food and Agriculture Organization of the United Nations.

The usual minimum educational requirement for employment as a food technologist is a bachelor's degree with a major in food science, chemistry or biology. An advanced degree is required for teaching and research positions.

Recommended high school courses for students preparing for a career in food science include biology, chemistry, mathematics and physics.

Current starting salaries for recent food technology graduates with some experience range from $20,000 to $27,000, while those employed by the federal government in entry level positions earn from $15,000 to $19,000 annually - those with several years experience may earn salaries in the mid-20's. Food technologists with graduate degrees earn considerably more.

Fellowships and scholarships for students entering universities in this field and students already enrolled in food science programs are administered by the Institute of Food Technologists. Information on the fellowship/scholarship program is available from the Institute of Food Technologists, 221 North La Salle Street, Chicago, Illinois 60601.

Below is a list of educational programs in food science and technology. As of September 1987, these programs are considered by the Institute of Food Technologists Education Committee to be teaching food science and technology in a manner that makes their students eligible for the IFT Undergraduate Scholarship Program. The Education Committee conducts continued surveillance of all programs, and changes are made annually. Graduate students applying for fellowships may attend any U.S. or Canadian school which conducts fundamental research in food science.

SOURCES:

Institute of Food Technologists
Occupational Outlook Handbook

Food Technologist Programs

ALABAMA

Food Technologist Program
Department of Nutrition and Foods
Auburn University
Auburn, Alabama 36830

Food Technologist Program
Department of Food Science and Technology
Alabama A&M University
Normal, Alabama 35762

ARKANSAS

Food Technologist Program
Department of Food Science
University of Arkansas
Route 11
Fayetteville, Arkansas 72701

CALIFORNIA

Food Technologist Program
Department of Food Science and Technology
University of California-Davis
Davis, California 95616

Food Technologist Program
Department of Food Science and Nutrition
Chapman College
333 North Glassell Street
Orange, California 92666

Food Technologist Program
Food Science and Nutrition Department
California Polytechnic State University
San Luis Obispo, California 93407

COLORADO

Food Technologist Program
Department of Food Science and Human Nutrition
Colorado State University
Fort Collins, Colorado 80523

DELAWARE

Food Technologist Program
Department of Food Science
University of Delaware
Newark, Delaware 19716

FLORIDA

Food Technologist Program
Food Science and Human Nutrition Department
University of Florida
Gainesville, Florida 32611

GEORGIA

Food Technologist Program
Food Science Division
University of Georgia
Athens, Georgia 30602

ILLINOIS

Food Technologist Program
Department of Food Science
University of Illinois
1304 Pennsylvania Avenue
Urbana, Illinois 61801

INDIANA

Food Technologist Program
Department of Food Science
Purdue University
West Lafayette, Indiana 47907

IOWA

Food Technologist Program
Department of Food Technology
Iowa State University
Ames, Iowa 50011

KANSAS

Food Technologist Program
Department of Food Science
Kansas State University
Manhattan, Kansas 66506

KENTUCKY

Food Technologist Program
Department of Animal Science
University of Kentucky
Lexington, Kentucky 40546

MARYLAND

Food Technologist Program
Department of Food Science
University of Maryland
College Park, Maryland 20742

MASSACHUSETTS

Food Technologist Program
Department of Food Science and Nutrition
University of Massachusetts
Amherst, Massachusetts 01003

MICHIGAN

Food Technologist Program
Department of Food Science and Human Nutrition
Michigan State University
East Lansing, Michigan 48824

MINNESOTA

Food Technologist Program
Department of Food Science and Nutrition
University of Minnesota
1334 Eckles Avenue
St. Paul, Minnesota 55108

MISSOURI

Food Technologist Program
Department of Food Science and Nutrition
University of Missouri
Columbia, Missouri 65211

NEBRASKA

Food Technologist Program
Department of Food Science and Technology
University of Nebraska
Lincoln, Nebraska 68583-0919

NEW JERSEY

Food Technologist Program
Department of Food Science Management
Rutgers-The State University
New Brunswick, New Jersey 08903

NEW YORK

Food Technologist Program
Department of Food Science
Cornell University
Ithaca, New York 14853

NORTH CAROLINA

Food Technologist Program
Department of Food Science
North Carolina State University
Box 7624
Raleigh, North Carolina 27695-7624

NORTH DAKOTA

Food Technologist Program
Cereal Science and Food Technology Department
North Dakota State University
P.O. Box 5728
Fargo, North Dakota 58105

OHIO

Food Technologist Program
Department of Food Science and Nutrition
Ohio State University
2121 Fyffe Road
Columbus, Ohio 43210

OREGON

Food Technologist Program
Department of Food Science and Technology
Oregon State University
Corvallis, Oregon 97331-6602

PENNSYLVANIA

Food Technologist Program
Department of Food Industry
Delaware Valley College
Doylestown, Pennsylvania 18901

Food Technologist Program
Department of Food Technology
Pennsylvania State University
University Park, Pennsylvania 16802

RHODE ISLAND

Food Technologist Program
Department of Food Science and Nutrition
University of Rhode Island
Kingston, Rhode Island 02881

SOUTH CAROLINA

Food Technologist Program
Department of Food Science
Clemson University
Clemson, South Carolina 29634-0371

TENNESSEE

Food Technologist Program
Department of Food Technology and Science
P.O. Box 1071
Knoxville, Tennessee 37901

TEXAS

Food Technologist Program
College of Agriculture
Texas A&M University
College State, Texas 77843

UTAH

Food Technologist Program
Department of Nutrition and Food Science
Utah State University
Logan, Utah 84322-8700

Food Technologist Program
Food Science and Nutrition Department
Brigham Young University
Provo, Utah 84622

VIRGINIA

Food Technologist Program
Department of Food Science and Technology
Virginia Polytechnic Institute and State University
Blacksburg, Virginia 24061

WASHINGTON

Food Technologist Program
Department of Food Science and Human Nutrition
Washington State University
Pullman, Washington 99164

Food Technologist Program
Division of Food Science and Technology
University of Washington
School of Fisheries
Seattle, Washington 98195

WISCONSIN

Food Technologist Program
Department of Food Science
University of Wisconsin
1605 Linden Drive
Madison, Wisconsin 53706

Food Technologist Program
Department of Animal and Food Science
University of Wisconsin-River Falls
River Falls, Wisconsin 54022

CANADA

Food Technologist Program
Department of Food Science
University of Alberta
Edmonton, Alberta, Canada T6G 2P5

Food Technologist Program
Department of Food Science
University of British Columbia
Vancouver, British Columbia, Canada V6T 2A2

Food Technologist Program
Department of Food Science
University of Guelph
Guelph, Ontario, Canada N1G 2W1

Food Technologist Program
Department of Food Science
University Laval
Quebec, P.Q., Canada G1K 7P4

Food Science Technician

Employed in the same locations as the food technologist, the food technician, who is also known as a *food processing technician,* assists the technologist in quality control and in laboratory research and development. The food science technician also assists in supervising the processing and packaging of foods and in the maintenance of sanitary conditions.

Community colleges, vocational technical schools, and technical divisions of universities offer curricula leading to an associate degree. Some programs offer concentrations in canning, dairy manufacturing and food quality control. One known school, the State University of New York-College of Agriculture and Technology at Morrisville offers hands-on experience at their on-campus pilot plant.

Salaries for food science technicians are lower than those for food technologists.

Below is a list of known educational programs in food technology for the food science and food processing technician. Other programs for the food science technician may exist throughout the country and it is recommended that interested students contact the educational institutions in their area for information.

SOURCES:

Institute of Food Technologists

Food Science Technician Programs

MASSACHUSETTS

Food Science Technician Program
Essex Agricultural and Technical Institute
Hawthorne, Massachusetts 01937

NEW YORK

Food Science Technician Program
Science Laboratory Technician Program
State University of New York
Canton, New York 13617
(concentration in milk and food quality control)

Food Science Technician Program
State University of New York
College of Agriculture and Technology at Morrisville
Morrisville, New York 13408

OREGON

Food Science Technician Program
Mount Hood Community College
26000 Southeast Stark Street
Gresham, Oregon 97030

WISCONSIN

Food Science Technician Program
Moraine Park Technical College
Fond du Lac Campus
235 North National Avenue
Fond du Lac, Wisconsin 54935

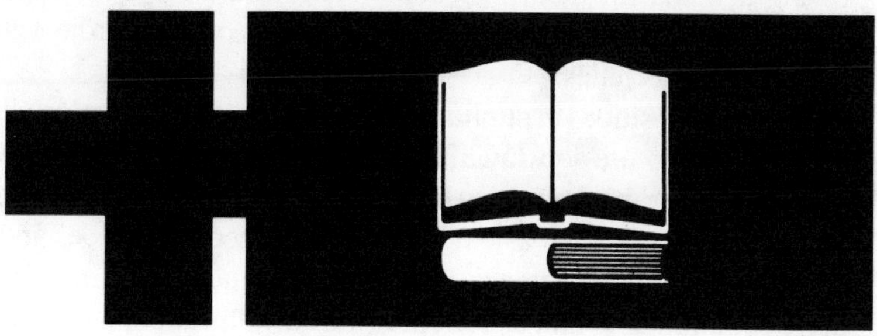

HEALTH EDUCATION

Health education teaches individuals and communities the methods of and the necessity for improving and maintaining optimum health practices. Health education is taught to the general public by *community health educators,* to students by *school health educators,* to the work force by *business* and *industry health educators* and to healthcare patients by *clinical health educators.* These four career classifications are listed below.

Community Health Educator

Also referred to as a *public health educator,* the *community health educator* works as a specialist on a community health team in the teaching and promoting of quality health. When people in a community, or the community as a whole, do not practice good health habits, the community health educator diagnoses why health information is lacking or why the information that is available is not utilized. She or he then implements appropriate educational programs that are designed to stimulate people to recognize and to rectify their own and the community's health inadequacies. Community health problems today include, among others, environmental pollution, drug and alcohol abuse, overpopulation, poor nutrition, and chronic disease.

The community health educator also acts as liaison between the community and professional health practitioners and their services, informing and advising the latter on how to plan and deliver healthcare in the most beneficial and useful ways. She or he also may consult on the development of training programs for community health workers, such as neighborhood health aides and citizen volunteers.

Job locations are varied for community health educators as there is a continual and growing demand for them in federal, state, and local health agencies; community and regional planning councils; healthcare facilities; poverty projects; teaching facilities; and in professional societies.

Professional positions in public or community health education usually require a master's degree, but there are jobs available in health agencies for those who have obtained a bachelor's degree in community health education. A bachelor's degree in health education with course emphasis in basic health sciences, social sciences and education is generally a prerequisite for application for admission to graduate school. Some graduate programs require community health experience prior to admission, while other schools incorporate such training into the curriculum.

Recommended high school courses for those students interested in a career as a community health educator include social sciences, biology, chemistry, communication and public speaking, and if possible, a second language.

Average annual salaries for public and community health educators vary because of education, work experience, type of employing agency or facility, individual job responsibility and geographic location. Earnings may start from the low-teens for bachelor degree graduates with minimal experience, to salaries reaching the mid-to-upper thirties for master degree graduates in professional positions.

For more information on a career as a community or public health educator contact the Society for Public Health Education, Inc., 2001 Addison Street, Suite 220, Berkeley, California 94704 or the Association for the Advancement of Health Education, 1900 Association Drive, Reston, Virginia 22091.

Below is a list of graduate degree programs in community health education provided by the Society for Public Health Education, Inc. and accredited by the Council on Education for Public Health.

A list of additional bachelor and master degree programs in community health education, supplied by the Association for the Advancement of Health Education, is included with those of school health educators listed at the end of this chapter.

SOURCES:

The Association for the Advancement of Health Education
Society for Public Health Education

Community Health Education Programs

CALIFORNIA

Community Health Education Program
School of Public Health
University of California at Berkeley
Berkeley, California 94720

Community Health Education Program
School of Public Health
Loma Linda University
Loma Linda, California 92350

Community Health Education Program
School of Public Health
University of California at Los Angeles
Los Angeles, California 90024

Community Health Education Program
Department of Health Sciences
California State University of Northridge
Northridge, California 91330

Community Health Education Program
Department of Health Sciences
San Jose State University
San Jose, California 95192

CONNECTICUT

Community Health Education Program
Department of Epidemiology and Public Health
Yale University
60 College Street
New Haven, Connecticut 06510

HAWAII

Community Health Education Program
School of Public Health
University of Hawaii
1960 East-West Road
Honolulu, Hawaii 96822

MARYLAND

Community Health Education Program
School of Hygiene and Public Health
Johns Hopkins University
615 North Wolfe Street
Baltimore, Maryland 21205

MASSACHUSETTS

Community Health Education Program
Department of Public Health
University of Massachusetts
Amherst, Massachusetts 01003

Community Health Education Program
School of Public Health
Harvard University
55 Shattuck Street
Boston, Massachusetts 02115

MICHIGAN

Community Health Education Program
School of Public Health
University of Michigan
Ann Arbor, Michigan 48104

MINNESOTA

Community Health Education Program
School of Public Health
University of Minnesota
1325 Mayo Memorial Building
Minneapolis, Minnesota 55455

MISSOURI

Community Health Education Program
Division of Community Health Education
University of Missouri
Columbia, Missouri 65211

NEW YORK

Community Health Education Program
School of Public Health
Columbia University
600 West 168th Street
New York, New York 10032

Community Health Education Program
Institute for Health Sciences
Hunter College
New York, New York 10021

Community Health Education Program
School of Education
New York University
Washington Square
New York, New York 10003

NORTH CAROLINA

Community Health Education Program
School of Public Health
University of North Carolina
Chapel Hill, North Carolina 27514

PUERTO RICO

Community Health Education Program
School of Public Health
University of Puerto Rico
General Post Office Box 5067
San Juan, Puerto Rico 00931

TENNESSEE

Community Health Education Program
College of Education
University of Tennessee
Knoxville, Tennessee 37996

School Health Educator

The *school health educator* teaches elementary, secondary, and college students the principles and methods of developing proper attitudes and skills toward the maintenance of optimal good health. In the classroom the school health educator teaches courses on family life, nutrition, safety education, first aid, personal hygiene, drug and alcohol abuse, mental health, human relations, disease prevention and control, community health, environmental pollution, and the use of health services and products. In addition to classroom instruction the school health educator actively cooperates with the rest of the school staff, including the school physician and nurse, other teachers, athletic coaches, and service personnel, in attempting to influence and instill the students with a sense of good healthcare judgment. They also represent the school in community health activities and use the latter's resources to supplement the school's health education program.

If not working in a single school the school health educator may act as the school health coordinator for a school district. As such, he or she coordinates the work and interests of community groups who are concerned with the health and health education of school children and assists in developing joint school and community health programs.

A four-year bachelor's degree in school health education with course emphasis in the biological, physical, behavioral, and social sciences, plus completion of the student teaching requirement is the minimum training criteria for the school health educator. The health educator must also meet the regular certification standards for teachers in the state in which he or she is seeking employment. Interested candidates should verify their own state's particular requirements. Graduate degrees in school health education are also available.

Starting salaries for school health educators are equal to those of other teachers with comparable training in the same school district.

For more information on a career as a school health educator contact the Association for the Advancement of Health Education, 1900 Association Drive, Reston, Virginia 22091.

A list, supplied by the Association for the Advancement of Health Education, of educational programs that offer bachelor's and master's degrees in school health education and public health education, follows this chapter.

SOURCE:

Association for the Advancement of Health Education

Health Educator In Business and Industry

The *health educator in business and industry* plans and conducts health maintenance programs for employees and executives in the work place. Utilizing numerous educational tools, including videotapes, slide presentations and informational brochures, the health educator directs workshops and group discussions on topics including nutrition, exercise, weight control, smoking cessation and stress management. The health education may also make recommendations to executives on health policies.

As a health promoter, the health educator is aware of the advantages to employees of beginning and maintaining healthy lifestyles: advantages such as improved appearance, emotional and physical well being and physiological improvements. The company benefits as well, through positive employee moral, improved absenteeism, and increased productivity.

Educational requirements for a career in Health Education in Business and Industry are either a bachelor's or master's degree in health education with course emphasis on business and industry programs. A list of schools in public, community and school health education follows this chapter.

SOURCES:

Association for the Advancement of Health Education

Clinical Health Educator

The *clinical health educator* develops and administers health maintenance and wellness programs in a healthcare setting. Clinical health educators mainly work in hospitals, but are also employed by clinics, health maintenance organizations, and with private physicians.

The clinical health educator can work one-on-one in a hospital setting, or may direct programs to groups of patients in an out-patient facility. On an individual basis, the clinical health educator deals with the patient, family and friends, and helps them better understand the patient's health condition. He or she explains the necessity of following the physicians's instructions and provides recommendations for avoiding recurrence of health problems in the future.

The clinical health educator also conducts educational programs on an out-patient basis for groups of patients with similar health conditions. Through the use of slide presentations, reading material and group discussions, the clinical health educator helps the patients develop ways to control their health situation.

The minimum educational requirement for a clinical health educator is a bachelor's degree in public or community health education plus a clinical internship. Graduate level degrees in health education are often required for professional level positions. Some clinical health educators have prior experience as registered nurses or related health professionals.

A list of schools in community or public health education is listed below.

For further information on a career as a clinical health educator write to the Association for the Advancement of Health Education, 1900 Association Drive, Reston, Virginia 22091.

KEY:

(1) Bachelor's degree in School Health Education

(2) Master's degree in School Health Education

(3) Bachelor's degree in Community Health Education

(4) Master's degree in Community Health Education

(5) Related program in school Health and/or Community Health Education

SOURCE:

Association for the Advancement of Health Education

Health Education Programs

ALABAMA

Health Education Program (1,2,3,4)
Auburn University
Auburn, Alabama 36830

Health Education Program (1)
Samford University
Birmingham, Alabama 35229

Health Education Program (1,2,3,4)
University of Alabama at Birmingham
Birmingham, Alabama 35294

Health Education Program (1)
Alabama A & M University
Huntsville, Alabama 35762

Health Education Program (1,2,3,4)
University of South Alabama
Mobile, Alabama 36688

Health Education Program (1,2,3,4)
University of Alabama
Tuscaloosa, Alabama 35486

ARIZONA

Health Education Program (1)
Northern Arizona University
Flagstaff, Arizona 86011

Health Education Program (1,2,3)
Arizona State University
Tempe, Arizona 85287

Health Education Program (1,2,3)
University of Arizona
Tuscon, Arizona 85719

ARKANSAS

Health Education Program (1,2,3)
University of Central Arkansas
Conway, Arkansas 72032

Health Education Program (1,2,3,4)
University of Arkansas
Fayetteville, Arkansas 72701

Health Education Program (1,3)
University of Arkansas at Little Rock
Little Rock, Arkansas 72204

CALIFORNIA

Health Education Program (4)
University of California
Berkeley, California 94720

Health Education Program (1,3)
California State University, Chico
Chico, California 95929

Health Education Program (1,2,3,4)
California State University, Fresno
Fresno, California 93740-0001

Health Education Program (3,4)
Loma Linda University
Loma Linda, California 92350

Health Education Program (1,2,3,4)
California State University, Long Beach
Long Beach, California 90840

Health Education Program (1,2,3,4)
California State University, Los Angeles
Los Angeles, California 90032

Health Education Program (1,2,4)
University of California
Los Angeles, California 90024

Health Education Program (1,2,3,4)
California State University, Northridge
Northridge, California 91330

Health Education Program (1,3)
California State University, Scaramento
Sacramento, California 95819

Health Education Program (3)
California State University, San Bernardino
San Bernardino, California 92407

Health Education Program (1,3)
San Diego State University
San Diego, California 92182

Health Education Program (1,2,3)
San Francisco State University
San Francisco, California 94132

Health Education Program (1,2,3,4)
San Jose State University
San Jose, California 95192

COLORADO

Health Education Program (3,4)
University of Northern Colorado
Greeley, Colorado 80639

CONNECTICUT

Health Education Program (1,3)
Western Connecticut State University
Danbury, Connecticut 06810

Health Education Program (1,2,3,4)
Southern Connecticut State University
New Haven, Connecticut 06515

DELAWARE

Health Education Program (1,3)
Delaware State College
Dover, Delaware 19901

DISTRICT OF COLUMBIA

Health Education Program (1,2)
American University
Washington, DC 20016

Health Education Program (1,2)
Howard University
Washington, DC 20059

Health Education Program (1,3)
University of the District of Columbia
Washington, DC 20008

FLORIDA

Health Education Program (1,2,3,4)
University of Florida
Gainesville, Florida 32611

Health Education Program (1,2,3,4)
University of North Florida
Jacksonville, Florida 32216

Health Education Program (1,2,3,4)
University of West Florida
Pensacola, Florida 32504

Health Education Program (1,2,3,4)
Florida State University
Tallahassee, Florida 32306

Health Education Program (1,3)
University of South Florida
Tampa, Florida 33620

GEORGIA

Health Education Program (1,2,3,4)
University of Georgia
Athens, Georgia 30602

Health Education Program (2,4)
Emory University School of Medicine
Atlanta, Georgia 30322

Health Education Program (1,2)
Georgia State University
Atlanta, Georgia 30303

Health Education Program (1,3)
Columbus College
Columbus, Georgia 31993

Health Education Program (1,3)
Georgia College
Milledgeville, Georgia 31061

IDAHO

Health Education Program (5)
University of Idaho
Moscow, Idaho 83843

Health Education Program (1,2)
Idaho State University
Pocatello, Idaho 83209

ILLINOIS

Health Education Program (1,2,3)
Southern Illinois University
Carbondale, Illinois 62901

Health Education Program (1,2,3,4)
University of Illinois
Champaign, Illinois 61820

Health Education Program (1,3)
Eastern Illinois University
Charleston, Illinois 61920

Health Education Program (1,3)
Chicago State University
Chicago, Illinois 60628

Health Education Program (2,3)
De Paul University
Chicago, Illinois 60614

Health Education Program (5)
University of Illinois at the Chicago Medical Center
Chicago, Illinois 60680

Health Education Program (1)
Northern Illinois University
DeKalb, Illinois 60115

Health Education Program (1)
Southern Illinois University
Edwardsville, Illinois 62026

Health Education Program (1,2,3,4)
Western Illinois University
Macomb, Illinois 61455

Health Education Program (1,2,3,4)
Illinois State University
Normal, Illinois 61761

INDIANA

Health Education Program (1,2,3,4)
Indiana University
Bloomington, Indiana 47405

Health Education Program (5)
St. Francis College
Ft. Wayne, Indiana 46808

Health Education Program (1,2)
Marian College
Indianapolis, Indiana 46222

Health Education Program (4)
Marion College
Marion, Indiana 46953

Health Education Program (1,2,3,4)
Ball State University
Muncie, Indiana 47306

Health Education Program (1)
Manchester College
North Manchester, Indiana 46962

Health Education Program (1,2,3)
Indiana State University
Terre Haute, Indiana 47809

Health Education Program (1,2,3,4)
Purdue University
West Lafayette, Indiana 47907

IOWA

Health Education Program (1,3)
Iowa State University
Ames, Iowa 50010

Health Education Program (1,2,3,4)
University of Northern Iowa
Cedar Falls, Iowa 50614

Health Education Program (1)
Luther College
Decorah, Iowa 52101

Health Education Program (1,2)
Drake University
Des Moines, Iowa 50311

Health Education Program (1)
Simpson College
Indianola, Iowa 50125

Health Education Program (1)
University of Iowa
Iowa City, Iowa 52242

Health Education Program (1)
Graceland College
Lamoni, Iowa 50140

KANSAS

Health Education Program (1)
Emporia State University
Emporia, Kansas 66801

Health Education Program (1,2,3)
University of Kansas
Lawrence, Kansas 66045

Health Education Program (1,3)
Kansas State University
Manhattan, Kansas 66506

KENTUCKY

Health Education Program (1,2)
Union College
Barbourville, Kentucky 40906

Health Education Program (1,2,3,4)
Western Kentucky University
Bowling Green, Kentucky 42101

Health Education Program (1,2,3)
University of Kentucky
Lexington, Kentucky 40506-0219

Health Education Program (1)
Morehead State University
Morehead, Kentucky 40351

Health Education Program (1)
Murray State University
Murray, Kentucky 42071

Health Education Program (1,2,3,4)
Eastern Kentucky University
Richmond, Kentucky 40475

Health Education Program (1,3)
Cumberland College
Williamsburg, Kentucky 40769

LOUISIANA

Health Education Program (1,2,3,4)
Louisiana State University
Baton Rouge, Louisiana 70803-7101

Health Education Program (1,2)
Southern University
Baton Rouge, Louisiana 70813

Health Education Program (1,2,3,4)
Southeastern Louisiana University
Hammond, Louisiana 70402

MAINE

Health Education Program (3)
University of Maine
Farmington, Maine 04938

Health Education Program (1,2)
University of Maine
Orono, Maine 04469

Health Education Program (1)
University of Maine
Presque Isle, Maine 04769

MARYLAND

Health Education Program (2,4)
Johns Hopkins University
Baltimore, Maryland 21205

Health Education Program (1,3)
Morgan State University
Baltimore, Maryland 21239

Health Education Program (1,2,3,4)
University of Maryland
College Park, Maryland 20742

Health Education Program (1,2,3,4)
Towson State University
Towson, Maryland 21204

MASSACHUSETTS

Health Education Program (1,2,3,4)
University of Massachusetts
Amherst, Massachusetts 01003

Health Education Program (1,2)
Boston University
Boston, Massachusetts 02215

Health Education Program (1,3)
Northeastern University
Boston, Massachusetts 02115

Health Education Program (2)
Bridgewater State College
Bridgewater, Massachusetts 02324

Health Education Program (1)
University of Lowell
Lowell, Massachusetts 01854

Health Education Program (1,3)
Springfield College
Springfield, Massachusetts 01109

Health Education Program (1,2)
Worcester State College
Worcester, Massachusetts 01602

MICHIGAN

Health Education Program (1,2)
Grand Valley State College
Allendale, Michigan 49401

Health Education Program (2,4)
University of Michigan
Ann Arbor, Michigan 48109-2029

Health Education Program (2,4)
Wayne State University
Detroit, Michigan 48202

Health Education Program (1,2)
Michigan State University
East Lansing, Michigan 48823

Health Education Program (1,3)
Western Michigan University
Kalamazoo, Michigan 49008

Health Education Program (1,2,3)
Northern Michigan University
Marquette, Michigan 49855

Health Education Program (1,2,3,4)
Central Michigan University
Mt. Pleasant, Michigan 48859

Health Education Program (1)
Eastern Michigan University
Ypsilanti, Michigan 48197

MINNESOTA

Health Education Program (1)
Bemidji State University
Bemidji, Minnesota 56601

Health Education Program (1,2,3,4)
University of Minnesota Duluth
Duluth, Minnesota 55812

Health Education Program (1,2,3,4)
Mankato State University
Mankato, Minnesota 56001

Health Education Program (1)
Southwest State University
Marshall, Minnesota 56258

Health Education Program (1)
Augsburg College
Minneapolis, Minnesota 55454

Health Education Program (4)
University of Minnesota
Minneapolis, Minnesota 55455

Health Education Program (1)
Concordia College
Moorhead, Minnesota 56560

Health Education Program (1,3)
Moorhead State University
Moorhead, Minnesota 56560

Health Education Program (1)
University of Minnesota, Morris
Morris, Minnesota 56267

Health Education Program (1)
St. Olaf College
Northfield, Minnesota 55057

Health Education Program (1,2,3)
St. Cloud State University
St. Cloud, Minnesota 56301

Health Education Program
Gustavus Adolphus College
St. Peter, Minnesota 56082

Health Education Program (1,2,3)
Winona State University
Winona, Minnesota 55987

MISSISSIPPI

Health Education Program (1,2,3,4)
University of Southern Mississippi
Hattiesburg, Mississippi 39406-5122

Health Education Program (1)
Jackson State College
Jackson, Mississippi 39217

MISSOURI

Health Education Program (1,2,3)
University of Missouri
Columbia, Missouri 65211

Health Education Program (1,3)
Northeast Missouri State University
Kirksville, Missouri 63501

Health Education Program (1,2)
Northeast Missouri State University
Maryville, Missouri 64468

Health Education Program (1)
Southwest Missouri State University
Springfield, Missouri 65802

Health Education Program (4)
St. Louis University Medical Center
St. Louis, Missouri 63104

Health Education Program (1)
Central Missouri State University
Warrensburg, Missouri 64093

MONTANA

Health Education Program (1)
Eastern Montana College
Billings, Montana 59101

Health Education Program (1,4)
University of Montana
Missoula, Montana 59801

NEBRASKA

Health Education Program (1)
Chadron State College
Chadron, Nebraska 69337

Health Education Program (1)
Kearney State College
Kearney, Nebraska 68849

Health Education Program (1,2,3,4)
University of Nebraska, Lincoln
Lincoln, Nebraska 68588

Health Education Program (1,3)
University of Nebraska, Omaha
Omaha, Nebraska 68182-0216

NEVADA

Health Education Program (1)
University of Nevada
Las Vegas, Nevada 89154

Health Education Program (1,2)
Plymouth State College
Plymouth, Nevada 03264

Health Education Program (1,3)
University of Nevada
Reno, Nevada 89557-0068

NEW HAMPSHIRE

Health Education Program (5)
Keene State College
Keene, New Hampshire 03431

Health Education Program (1,2)
Plymouth State College
Plymouth, New Hampshire 03264

NEW JERSEY

Health Education Program (1)
Glassboro State College
Glassboro, New Jersey 08028

Health Education Program (1,2,3,4)
Jersey City State College
Jersey City, New Jersey 07305

Health Education Program (1,3)
Rutgers, The State University of New Jersey
New Brunswick, New Jersey 08903

Health Education Program (1)
Seton Hall University
South Orange, New Jersey 07079

Health Education Program (1,2,3)
Trenton State College
Trenton, New Jersey 08625

Health Education Program (3)
Kean College of New Jersey
Union, New Jersey 07083

Health Education Program (1,2)
Montclair State College
Upper Montclair, New Jersey 07043

Health Education Program (1,3)
William Paterson College
Wayne, New Jersey 07470

NEW MEXICO

Health Education Program (1,2,3,4)
University of New Mexico
Albuquerque, New Mexico 87131

Health Education Program (1,2,3)
New Mexico State University
Las Cruces, New Mexico 88003

Health Education Program (5)
New Mexico Highlands University
Las Vegas, New Mexico 87701

NEW YORK

Health Education Program (1,2,3,4)
State University College
Brockport, New York 14420

Health Education Program (1,2)
Brooklyn College of City University of New York
Brooklyn, New York 11210

Health Education Program (3)
St. Francis College
Brooklyn, New York 11201

Health Education Program (2,4)
State University of New York at Buffalo
Buffalo, New York 14214

Health Education Program (1,2,3)
State University College
Cortland, New York 13045

Health Education Program (1,3)
Queens College of the City University of New York
Flushing, New York 11367

Health Education Program (2,4)
Adelphi University
Garden City, New York 11530

Health Education Program (1)
C.W. Post Center of Long Island University
Greenvale, New York 11548

Health Education Program (1,2,4)
Hofstra University
Hempstead, New York 11550

Health Education Program (1,3)
Ithaca College
Ithaca, New York 14850

Health Education Program (1,3)
York College of the City University of New York
Jamaica, New York 11451

Health Education Program (2)
City College of the City University of New York
New York, New York 10031

Health Education Program (4)
Columbia University School of Public Health
New York, New York 10032

Health Education Program (1,2,3,4)
Herbert H. Lehman College of City
University of New York
New York, New York 10468

Health Education Program (1,2)
Hunter College of City University of New York
New York, New York 10021

Health Education Program (1,2,4)
New York University
New York, New York 10003

Health Education Program (4)
Teachers College, Columbia University
New York, New York 10027

Health Education Program (1,3)
State University of New York at Old Westbury
Old Westbury, New York 11568

Health Education Program (1)
State University College
Plattsburgh, New York 12901

Health Education Program (1,3)
College of Mount Saint Vincent on Hudson
Riverdale, New York 10471

Health Education Program (1)
Manhattan College
Riverdale, New York 10471

Health Education Program (1,2,3,4)
Russell Sage College
Troy, New York 12180

Health Education Program (1,2)
Wagner College
Staten Island, New York 10301

Health Education Program (1,2)
Syracuse University
Syracuse, New York 13244

NORTH CAROLINA

Health Education Program (1,2)
Gardner-Webb College
Boiling Springs, North Carolina 28017

Health Education Program (1)
Appalachian State University
Boone, North Carolina 28608

Health Education Program (1,2,3,4)
University of North Carolina
Chapel Hill, North Carolina 27514

Health Education Program (2)
University of North Carolina
Charlotte, North Carolina 28223

Health Education Program (1,3)
Western Carolina University
Cullowhee, North Carolina 28723

Health Education Program (1,3)
North Carolina Central University
Durham, North Carolina 27707

Health Education Program (1,2,3,4)
University of North Carolina
Greensboro, North Carolina 27412

Health Education Program (1,2,3,4)
East Carolina University
Greenville, North Carolina 27834

Health Education Program (5)
University of North Carolina
Wilmington, North Carolina 28403

NORTH DAKOTA

Health Education Program (1)
Mayville State College
Mayville, North Dakota 58257

Health Education Program (1)
Minot State College
Minot, North Dakota 58701

Health Education Program (1)
Valley City State College
Valley City, North Dakota 58072

OHIO

Health Education Program (1)
Ohio Northern University
Ada, Ohio 45810

Health Education Program (1)
University of Akron
Akron, Ohio 44325

Health Education Program (1)
Mount Union College
Alliance, Ohio 44601

Health Education Program (1)
Ashland College
Ashland, Ohio 44805

Health Education Program (1,3)
Ohio University
Athens, Ohio 45701

Health Education Program (1,3)
Baldwin-Wallace College
Berea, Ohio 44017

Health Education Program (1)
Bluffton College
Bluffton, Ohio 45817

Health Education Program (1,2)
Bowling Green State University
Bowling Green, Ohio 43403

Health Education Program (1)
Malone College
Canton, Ohio 44709

Health Education Program (1)
College of Mt. St. Joseph
Cincinnati, Ohio 45051

Health Education Program (1,2,3,4)
University of Cincinnati
Cincinnati, Ohio 45221

Health Education Program (1)
Xavier University
Cincinnati, Ohio 45207

Health Education Program (1)
Notre Dame College
Cleveland, Ohio 44121

Health Education Program (1,3)
Capital University
Columbus, Ohio 43209

Health Education Program (1,2,3,4)
Ohio State University
Columbus, Ohio 43210

Health Education Program (1)
Defiance College
Defiance, Ohio 43512

Health Education Program (1,3)
University of Dayton
Dayton, Ohio 45469

Health Education Program (1,3)
Ohio Wesleyan University
Delaware, Ohio 43011

Health Education Program (1)
Findlay College
Findlay, Ohio 45840

Health Education Program (1)
Denison University
Granville, Ohio 43023

Health Education Program (1,2,3,4)
Kent State University
Kent, Ohio 44242

Health Education Program (1)
Marietta College
Marietta, Ohio 45750

Health Education Program (1)
Muskingham College
New Concord, Ohio 43762

Health Education Program (1,2)
Miami University
Oxford, Ohio 45056

Health Education Program (1)
Lake Erie College
Painesville, Ohio 44077

Health Education Program (1)
Rio Grande College
Rio Grande, Ohio 45674

Health Education Program (1)
Wittenberg University
Springfield, Ohio 45501

Health Education Program (1)
Heidelberg College
Tiffin, Ohio 44883

Health Education Program (1,2,3,4)
University of Toledo
Toledo, Ohio 43606

Health Education Program (1)
Urbana University
Urbana, Ohio 43078

Health Education Program (1)
Otterbein College
Westerville, Ohio 43081

Health Education Program (1)
Central State University
Wilberforce, Ohio 45384

Health Education Program (1)
Wilmington College
Wilmington, Ohio 45177

Health Education Program (1,3)
Youngstown State University
Youngstown, Ohio 44555

OKLAHOMA

Health Education Program (1,2,3)
Central State University
Edmond, Oklahoma 73034

Health Education Program (4)
University of Oklahoma
Oklahoma City, Oklahoma 73190

Health Education Program (1,2,3,4)
Oklahoma State University
Stillwater, Oklahoma 74078

OREGON

Health Education Program (1,2)
Southern Oregon State College
Ashland, Oregon 97520

Health Education Program (1,2,3,4)
Oregon State University
Corvallis, Oregon 97331

Health Education Program (1,2,3,4)
University of Oregon
Eugene, Oregon 97403-1273

Health Education Program (1)
Pacific University
Forest Grove, Oregon 97116

Health Education Program (1)
Eastern Oregon State College
LaGrande, Oregon 97850

Health Education Program (1)
Linfield College
McMinnville, Oregon 97128

Health Education Program (1,3)
Western Oregon State College
Monmounth, Oregon 97361

Health Education Program (1)
George Fox College
Newberg, Oregon 97132

Health Education Program (1,2)
Lewis and Clark College
Portland, Oregon 97219

Health Education Program (1,2,3)
Portland State University
Portland, Oregon 97207

Health Education Program (1)
Wagner Pacific College
Portland, Oregon 97215

PENNSYLVANIA

Health Education Program (1,2,3,4)
East Stroudsburg University
East Stroudsburg, Pennsylvania 18301

Health Education Program (5)
Gettysburg College
Gettysburg, Pennsylvania 17325

Health Education Program (1,2,3,4)
Temple University
Philadelphia, Pennsylvania 19122

Health Education Program (2)
University of Pittsburgh
Pittsburgh, Pennsylvania 15261

Health Education Program (1,2,3,4)
Slippery Rock University
Slippery Rock, Pennsylvania 16057

Health Education Program (1,2,3,4)
Pennsylvania State University
University Park, Pennsylvania 16802

Health Education Program (1,2,3,4)
West Chester University
West Chester, Pennsylvania 19383

RHODE ISLAND

Health Education Program (1,2)
Rhode Island College
Providence, Rhode Island 02908

SOUTH CAROLINA

Health Education Program (1)
Benedict College
Columbia, South Carolina 29204

Health Education Program (2,3,4)
University of South Carolina
Columbia, South Carolina 29208

SOUTH DAKOTA

Health Education Program (1,3)
South Dakota State University
Brookings, South Dakota 57007

Health Education Program (1)
University of South Dakota
Vermillion, South Dakota 57069

TENNESSEE

Health Education Program (2)
University of Tennessee at Chattanooga
Chattanooga, Tennessee 37402

Health Education Program (1,2,3,4)
Austin Peay State University
Clarksville, Tennessee 37040

Health Education Program (1,3)
Carson Newman College
Jefferson City, Tennessee 37760

Health Education Program (3,4)
East Tennessee State University
Johnson City, Tennessee 37601

Health Education Program (1,2,3,4)
University of Tennessee
Knoxville, Tennessee 37996-2700

Health Education Program (1,2,3,4)
Memphis State University
Memphis, Tennessee 38152

Health Education Program (1)
Middle Tennessee State University
Murfreesboro, Tennessee 37132

Health Education Program (1)
Tennessee State University
Nashville, Tennessee 37203

TEXAS

Health Education Program (1,3)
Abilene Christian University
Abilene, Texas 79699

Health Education Program (1)
University of Texas at Arlington
Arlington, Texas 76019

Health Education Program (1,2,3,4)
University of Texas at Austin
Austin, Texas 78712

Health Education Program (1)
Lamar University
Beaumont, Texas 77710

Health Education Program (1)
West Texas State University
Canyon, Texas 79016

Health Education Program (1,2,3,4)
Texas A & M University
College Station, Texas 77843

Health Education Program (1,2,3,4)
East Texas State University
Commerce, Texas 75428

Health Education Program (1,2,3,4)
North Texas State University
Denton, Texas 76203

Health Education Program (1,2,3,4)
Texas Woman's University
Denton, Texas 76204

Health Education Program (1)
Pan American University
Edinburg, Texas 78539

Health Education Program (1,2)
University of Texas at El Paso
El Paso, Texas 79968

Health Education Program (1)
Texas Christian University
Ft. Worth, Texas 76129

Health Education Program (2)
University of Texas Medical Branch at Galveston
Galveston, Texas 77550

Health Education Program (5)
Rice University
Houston, Texas 77251

Health Education Program (1,2)
Texas Southern University
Houston, Texas 77004

Health Education Program (1,2)
University of Houston at Clear Lake City
Houston, Texas 77058

Health Education Program (2,4)
University of Houston University Park
Houston, Texas 77004

Health Education Program (1,2,3,4)
Sam Houston State University
Huntsville, Texas 77341

Health Education Program (5)
Texas A & I University
Kingsville, Texas 78363

Health Education Program (1,2)
Texas Tech University
Lubbock, Texas 79409

Health Education Program (1,2,3)
Stephen F. Austin State University
Nacogdoches, Texas 75962

Health Education Program (1)
Prairie View A & M University
Prairie View, Texas 77446

Health Education Program (1)
University of Texas at San Antonio
San Antonio, Texas 78284

Health Education Program (1,2,3)
Southwest Texas State University
San Marcos, Texas 78666-4616

Health Education Program (1)
University of Texas at Tyler
Tyler, Texas 75701

Health Education Program (1,2)
Baylor University
Waco, Texas 76798

UTAH

Health Education Program (1,2)
Utah State University
Logan, Utah 84322

Health Education Program (1,2,3,4)
Brigham Young University
Provo, Utah 84602

Health Education Program (1,2,3,4)
University of Utah
Salt Lake City, Utah 84112

VERMONT

Health Education Program (1,3)
University of Vermont
Burlington, Vermont 05405

Health Education Program (1)
Norwich University
Northfield, Vermont 05663

VIRGINIA

Health Education Program (1,2,3,4)
Virginia Polytechnic Institute & State University
Blacksburg, Virginia 24061

Health Education Program (1)
Bridgewater College
Bridgewater, Virginia 22812

Health Education Program (5)
Averett College
Danville, Virginia 24541

Health Education Program (5)
Emory and Henry College
Emory, Virginia 24327

Health Education Program (1,2,3,4)
George Mason University
Fairfax, Virginia 22030

Health Education Program (5)
Longwood College
Farmville, Virginia 23901

Health Education Program (1,2)
Hampton Institute
Hampton, Virginia 23668

Health Education Program (1,2,3,4)
James Madison University
Harrisonburg, Virginia 22807

Health Education Program (1,3)
Liberty University
Lynchburg, Virginia 24506

Health Education Program (1,3)
Norfolk State University
Norfolk, Virginia 23504

Health Education Program (1,4)
Old Dominion University
Norfolk, Virginia 23508

Health Education Program (1)
Virginia State University
Petersburg, Virginia 23803

Health Education Program (1,3)
Radford University
Radford, Virginia 24142

Health Education Program (1,2)
University of Richmond
Richmond, Virginia 23173

Health Education Program (1)
Virginia Commonwealth University
Richmond, Virginia 23284

Health Education Program (5)
College of William and Mary
Williamsburg, Virginia 23185

WASHINGTON

Health Education Program (1,3)
Western Washington University
Bellingham, Washington 98225

Health Education Program (1,3)
Eastern Washington University
Cheney, Washington 99004

Health Education Program (1,3)
Walla Walla College
College Place, Washington 99324

Health Education Program (1,2,3)
Central Washington University
Ellensburg, Washington 98926

Health Education Program (1,2)
Whitworth College
Spokane, Washington 99251

WEST VIRGINIA

Health Education Program (1)
University of Charleston
Charleston, West Virginia 25304

Health Education Program (1)
Davis and Elkins College
Elkins, West Virginia 26241

Health Education Program (1,3)
Fairmont State College
Fairmont, West Virginia 27554

Health Education Program (1)
Marshall University
Huntington, West Virginia 25715

Health Education Program (1)
West Virginia State College
Institute, West Virginia 25112

Health Education Program (1)
West Virginia Institute of Technology
Montgomery, West Virginia 25136

Health Education Program (2,4)
West Virginia University
Morgantown, West Virginia 26505

Health Education Program (1)
Alderson Broaddus College
Philippi, West Virgina 26416

Health Education Program (1)
Shepherd College
Shepherdstown, West Virginia 25443

Health Education Program (1)
West Liberty State College
West Liberty, West Virginia 26074

WISCONSIN

Health Education Program (1,2)
University of Wisconsin
Eau Claire, Wisconsin 54701

Health Education Program (1,2,3,4)
University of Wisconsin
La Crosse, Wisconsin 54601

Health Education Program (1,2,3,4)
University of Wisconsin
Madison, Wisconsin 53706

WYOMING

Health Education Program (1)
University of Wyoming
Laramine, Wyoming 82071

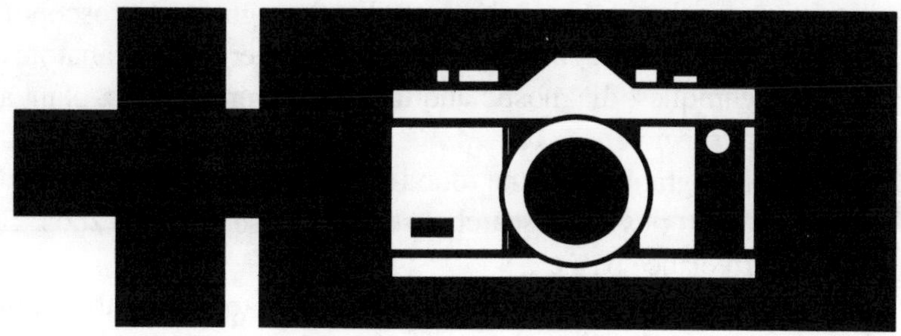

HEALTH SCIENCES COMMUNICATIONS

Healthcare professionals, students and the general public rely on accurate and up-to-date healthcare information in their jobs, education and everyday life. It is the field of *health sciences communications,* also referred to as *biocommunications,* that disseminates scientific, medical and healthcare information.

The *health sciences communicator* communicates healthcare data using a variety of educational media including photographs; medical books, texts and journals; information data bases; medical illustrations; films and television.

Seven major careers in health sciences communications are discussed in this chapter: the *biophotographer, medical writer/editor, health sciences librarian* and *health sciences library assistant, medical illustrator, medical television professional,* and the *biocommunications manager.*

Biophotographer

The biophotographer utilizes photography and other visual media, such as prints, transparencies and films, to aid in the biological and medical teaching and research of living and non-living things.

The *biophotographer,* also referred to as a *biomedical photographer,* is a trained specialist in optics, light theory, and the use of photosensitive materials and in the course of their work may utilize ultraviolet and infra-red light sources, high speed cinematography, X-ray photography, and slow motion/stop motion photography.

The biophotographer must possess a reasonable understanding of the subject matter being photographed. Techniques unique to the biophotography field include photomicrography (taking photographs through a microscope) and surgical motion pictures. Among other subjects, the photographer records anatomy, evidence of diseases, surgical techniques, diagnostic and therapeutic procedures, plant and animal tissues, and pathological specimens.

The biophotographer may be found working in hospitals; medical, veterinary and dental schools; laboratories and research institutes; museums; and zoos. Some biophotographers work on a freelance basis.

Two and four year degree programs in biophotography are offered at a limited number of universities and colleges and are listed below. Individual courses in biological and medical photography are offered at universities, colleges, community and junior colleges, and vocational-technical schools throughout the country. *A Survey, College Instruction in Photography,* a listing of such programs is available for a fee from the Eastman Kodak Company, Rochester, New York 14610. Through membership in the Biological Photographic Association, Inc., many professionals attend seminars and workshops to enhance their photographic skills.

Certification as a Registered Biological Photographer, (R.B.P.), is granted after successfully passing an intensive three-part examination sponsored by the Board of Registry of the Biological Photographic Association. For further information on certification or a career in biophotography, direct inquiries to the Biological Photographic Association, 115 Stoneridge Drive, Chapel Hill, North Carolina 27514.

Following is a list provided by the Health Sciences Communications Association of accredited institutions with programs in biophotography. Some programs in biophotography may require past experience or aptitude in science and/or in visual media. Prospective students may be asked to present a portfolio of photographs to show proficiency in photography. Contact the program directly for specific admission requirements, length of program, financial aid, and degree awarded.

SOURCES:

Biological Photographic Association, Inc.
Health Sciences Communication Association
Occupational Outlook Handbook

Biophotography Programs

INDIANA

Biophotography Program
Purdue University
Medical Illustration and Communications
School of Veterinary Medicine
West Lafayette, Indiana 47907

MICHIGAN

Biophotography Program
Grand Valley State College
School of Health Sciences
Allendale, Michigan 49401

WASHINGTON

Biophotography Program
Bellvue Community College
Office of Admission
3000 Landerholm Circle, S.E.
Bellvue, Washington 98007

In addition to these programs, the Biological Photographic Association also recommends the following programs which provide a background in biophotography:

CALIFORNIA

Biophotography Program
Brooks Institute of Photography
2190 Alston Road
Santa Barbara, California 93108

NEW YORK

Biophotography Program
Rochester Institute of Technology
One Lomb Memorial Drive
Rochester, New York 14623

Medical Writer And Editor

The medical writer or editor uses the written word to communicate scientific or technical information into language that is easily understood by the reader. The *medical writer* gathers information through research, interviewing, or personal experience. *Editors* usually rewrite or revise material, choose and arrange articles for publication, and supervise writers. Depending on the size of the publication, the writer may select his or her own topic.

Medical writers or editors are usually divided into two categories - those that provide health information to the public and those that make technical, medical, and scientific information available to healthcare professionals. Medical writers who provide information to the public on the latest, scientific developments are called *scientific writers,* and commonly work for newspapers, magazines, television, and radio stations. *Health information specialists* are employed by health organizations, such as the American Heart Association, to inform the public of their achievements and activities. Medical writers who provide technical information to healthcare professionals are called *technical writers,* and may be employed by pharmaceutical companies, research institutes, federal healthcare agencies, and universities. Medical writers or editors may also write for professional journals, newsletters, and health related books. Medical writers or editors may work on a freelance basis, or may be employed as part of an organization's writing staff.

Salaries for medical writers vary because of educational background, geographic location, and experience. Experienced medical writers could expect to earn $15,000 to $30,000 annually, although some may earn more. Salaries could be slightly higher for editors with supervisory experience. Freelance medical writers may hold other jobs, since income from freelancing is not guaranteed.

A bachelor's degree in journalism, reporting, writing, the biological sciences or physical sciences, with several years writing experience is the usual prerequisite to entry level positions in medical writing. Relatively few medical writers enter the occupation directly from college. Often many start as assistants, trainees, or come from medical, technical, or scientific backgrounds. Medical writers should have a solid background in the sciences and a working knowledge of medical and technical terminology. Continuing education programs in medical writing and editing are available through membership in the American Medical Writer's Association.

Employers of medical writers and editors usually request printed samples of an individual's writing that demonstrates the ability to communicate scientific and technical information. Interested students could gain writing experience by volunteering for high school and college newspapers or submitting articles to community or local newspapers. Recommended high school and college courses should include the physical and biological sciences, English composition, humanities, and computer science. It may also be helpful to learn to use basic office equipment, including typewriters, word processors, and computers.

For more information on a career as a medical writer or editor, contact the American Medical Writer's Association, 9650 Rockville Pike, Bethesda, Maryland 20814.

Below is a list provided by the Health Sciences Communications Association of accredited institutions offering programs in medical writing and editing. Degrees in the biological or physical sciences, writing, or journalism are available at numerous colleges and universities throughout the United States.

SOURCES:

American Medical Writer's Association
Health Sciences Communications Association
Occupational Outlook Handbook

Medical Writing and Editing Programs

MICHIGAN

Medical Writing and Editing Program
Grand Valley State College
School of Health Sciences
Allendale, Michigan 49401

OHIO

Medical Writing and Editing Program
Division of Biomedical Communications
School of Allied Medical Professions
Ohio State University
1583 Perry Street
Columbus, Ohio 43210

Health Sciences Librarian
Health Sciences Library Assistant

The *health sciences librarian,* also known as a *medical librarian,* is a highly trained specialist who manages the professional and technical services of a medical library. Healthcare facilities, departments of public health, medical schools, medical research institutions, and most pharmaceutical companies have libraries, and it is the responsibility of the health sciences librarian to assist physicians, researchers, and medical students to search for, and find, the information they require. Having a thorough knowledge of the kinds of medical books, journals, reports, films, microfiche, microfilm, computerized data-bases and other information resources that are available, the health sciences librarian selects publications to be purchased; classifies and catalogs new materials; issues materials to borrowers; prepares library material, such as bibliographies, abstracts, and reviews for teaching and research; teaches students and professionals how to use library resources; and manages the daily operations of the medical library.

In large institutions the duties of the health sciences librarian may be highly specialized, but in a small hospital library the health sciences librarian provides personalized services in all library functions.

The health sciences librarian must have a master's degree in library science from a program accredited by the American Library Association. A bachelor's degree with coursework in library science, the physical and life sciences, and management, is the usual prerequisite for admission to graduate level health sciences librarian programs. For specific graduate school prerequisites, contact the program director at the individual schools. Since many library functions are computerized, it is recommended that a student take courses in information and computer science.

The position of *health sciences library assistant,* on the other hand, is an entry-level position in the health sciences library that requires either on-the-job training or a bachelor's degree in the arts, sciences, or library sciences, depending upon the employer. Primarily responsible for carrying out routine library procedures under the supervision of a medical librarian, the assistant issues and receives books, compiles records, sorts and files publications and catalog cards, and provides non-technical assistance to library patrons.

Certification in health sciences librarianship is available through the Medical Library Association after graduating from an American Library Association accredited library science program, and successfully passing a competency examination.

According to recent salary data, beginning salaries for health sciences librarians ranged from $15,700 to $31,000, with average salaries equalling $22,000 annually. Experienced health sciences librarians earned average salaries in the high 20's. Salaries for health sciences library assistants are less than those of health sciences librarians.

For additional information on training and career opportunities in the health sciences library field, interested persons should contact the Medical Library Association, Inc., 6 North Michigan Avenue, Suite 300, Chicago, Illinois 60602, or the American Library Association, 50 East Huron Street, Chicago, Illinois 60611.

Below is a list of graduate library education programs accredited by the American Library Association. Those marked by an asterisk (*) indicate schools with courses in health sciences librarianship.

SOURCES:

Medical Library Association
Health Sciences Communications Association
Occupational Outlook Handbook

Graduate Library Education Programs

ALABAMA

Library Science Program*
University of Alabama
University, Alabama 35486

ARIZONA

Library Science Program
University of Arizona
Tucson, Arizona 85719

CALIFORNIA

Library Science Program*
University of California, Berkeley
Berkeley, California 94720

Library Science Program*
University of California, Los Angeles
Los Angeles, California 90024

Library Science Program
University of Southern California
Los Angeles, California 90089

Library Science Program
San Jose State University
San Jose, California 95192

CONNECTICUT

Library Science Program*
Southern Connecticut State University
New Haven, Connecticut 06515

DISTRICT OF COLUMBIA

Library Science Program*
Catholic University of America
Washington, D.C. 20064

FLORIDA

Library Science Program
Florida State University
Tallahassee, Florida 32306

Library Science Program*
University of South Florida
Tampa, Florida 33620

GEORGIA

Library Science Program
Atlanta University
Atlanta, Georgia 30314

Library Science Program*
Emory University
Atlanta, Georgia 30322

HAWAII

Library Science Program*
University of Hawaii
Honolulu, Hawaii 96822

ILLINOIS

Library Science Program
University of Chicago
Chicago, Illinois 60637

Library Science Program
Northern Illinois University
DeKalb, Illinois 60115

Library Science Program*
Rosary College
River Forest, Illinois 60305

Library Science Program*
University of Illinois
Urbana, Illinois 61801

INDIANA

Library Science Program*
Indiana University
Bloomington, Indiana 47405

IOWA

Library Science Program*
University of Iowa
Iowa City, Iowa 52242

KANSAS

Library Science Program
Emporia State University
Emporia, Kansas 66801

KENTUCKY

Library Science Program*
University of Kentucky
Lexington, Kentucky 40506

LOUISIANA

Library Science Program*
Louisiana State University
Baton Rouge, Louisiana 70803

MARYLAND

Library Science Program*
University of Maryland
College Park, Maryland 20742

MASSACHUSETTS

Library Science Program*
Simmons College
Boston, Massachusetts 02115

MICHIGAN

Library Science Program*
University of Michigan
Ann Arbor, Michigan 48109

MISSISSIPPI

Library Science Program*
University of Southern Mississippi
Hattiesburg, Mississippi 39406

MISSOURI

Library Science Program*
University of Missouri, Columbia
Columbia, Missouri 65211

NEW JERSEY

Library Science Program*
Rutgers University
New Brunswick, New Jersey 08903

NEW YORK

Library Science Program*
State University of New York, Albany
Albany, New York 12222

Library Science Program*
Pratt Institute
Brooklyn, New York 11205

Library Science Program*
State University of New York, Buffalo
Buffalo, New York 14260

Library Science Program*
Queens College, City University of New York
Flushing, New York 11367

Library Science Program*
Long Island University
Greenvale, New York 11548

Library Science Program*
St. John's University
Jamaica, New York 11439

Library Science Program*
Columbia University
New York, New York 10027

Library Science Program*
Syracuse University
Syracuse, New York 13244-2340

NORTH CAROLINA

Library Science Program*
University of North Carolina
Chapel Hill, North Carolina 27514

Library Science Program
North Carolina Central University
Durham, North Carolina 27707

Library Science Program
University of North Carolina at Greensboro
Greensboro, North Carolina 27412

OHIO

Library Science Program*
Kent State University
Kent, Ohio 44343

OKLAHOMA

Library Science Program*
University of Oklahoma
Norman, Oklahoma 73019

PENNSYLVANIA

Library Science Program
Clarion University
Clarion, Pennsylvania 16214

Library Science Program*
Drexel University
Philadelphia, Pennsylvania 19104

Library Science Program*
University of Pittsburgh
Pittsburgh, Pennsylvania 15260

SOUTH CAROLINA

Library Science Program*
University of South Carolina
Columbia, South Carolina 29208

TENNESSEE

Library Science Program
University of Tennessee, Knoxville
Knoxville, Tennessee 37996

Library Science Program*
Vanderbilt University
George Peabody College for Teachers
Nashville, Tennessee 37203

TEXAS

Library Science Program*
University of Texas at Austin
Austin, Texas 78712

Library Science Program*
North Texas State University
Denton, Texas 76203

Library Science Program*
Texas Women's University
Denton, Texas 76204

UTAH

Library Science Program
Brigham Young University
Provo, Utah 84602

WASHINGTON

Library Science Program*
University of Washington
Seattle, Washington 98195

WISCONSIN

Library Science Program*
University of Wisconsin, Madison
Madison, Wisconsin 53706

Library Science Program*
University of Wisconsin, Milwaukee
Milwaukee, Wisconsin 53201

Medical Illustrator

The *medical illustrator* produces a variety of artwork, including paintings, drawings, sketches and model designs, to visually communicate and teach complex medical and scientific data. Art mediums used by the medical illustrator may include watercolors, pen and ink, plaster, wax, plastics, airbrush and computer graphics. The medical illustrator has extensive training in both art and science. This knowledge is utilized through a variety of assignments such as painting or drawing the human anatomy for medical textbooks, sketching multi-dimensional models to illustrate a surgical procedure, sculpturing a three-dimensional model for medical students, or perhaps designing projects such as "moving" illustrations for television documentaries or films through the use of computer graphics.

The medical illustrator may be found working in a variety of settings, including hospitals; clinics; medical, dental and veterinary schools; large medical centers; as well as the private sector in medical publishing companies, advertising agencies, or in freelance work providing services to many facilities.

Degree programs in medical illustration are usually at the graduate level, with a bachelor's degree as a prerequisite.

Recommended course work at the bachelor's level should include the fine arts, pre-med biology, and the humanities. High school courses should also emphasize the arts and sciences. Graduate programs in medical illustration are usually two to three years in length. There are a limited number of programs in medical illustration, with limited enrollment in each. When applying to medical illustration schools, a prospective student may be asked to present a portfolio of art work and participate in a personal interview.

Salary information for medical illustrators will vary, based on quality of work, geographic location, type of employer and years of experience. Medical illustrators who freelance their work may not be guaranteed a steady income until they develop a reputation. They may hold other jobs to supplement their earnings.

In medical illustration, demonstrated ability and appropriate training are needed for success. Medical illustrators perform detail work and are relied upon to submit illustrations that are on time and precise. Medical illustrators may have to meet tight deadlines and sometimes work long or irregular hours.

Below is a list of graduate degree programs in medical illustration that are accredited by the Association of Medical Illustrators Accreditation Committee and Board of Governors. There are a limited number of scholarships available to students enrolled in accredited medical illustration programs. For more information on financial aid or a career as a medical illustrator, contact the Association of Medical Illustrators, 2692 Huguenot Springs Road, Midlothian, Virginia 23113.

SOURCES:

Health Sciences Communications Association
Association of Medical Illustrators

Medical Illustration Programs

CALIFORNIA

Medical Illustration Program
The University of California at San Francisco
1855 Folsom Street
San Francisco, California 94103

GEORGIA

Medical Illustration Program
Dept. of Medical Illustration
School of Graduate Studies
The Medical College of Georgia
Augusta, Georgia 30912

ILLINOIS

Medical Illustration Program
Dept. of Biocommunication Arts
University of Illinois at Chicago
1919 W. Taylor St.
Chicago, Illinois 60612

MARYLAND

Medical Illustration Program
Art as Applied to Medicine
The John Hopkins School of Medicine
Hampton House 546, 624 N. Broadway
Baltimore, Maryland 21205

MICHIGAN

Medical Illustration Program
The School of Medical & Biological Illustration
R4414, Kresge 1, Box 56
The University of Michigan Medical Center
Ann Arbor, Michigan 48109

TEXAS

Medical Illustration Program
Dept. of Biomedical Communications
The University of Texas Health Center at Dallas
5323 Harry Hines Boulevard
Dallas, Texas 75235

Medical Television Professional

A *medical television professional* uses visual "moving" media, such as film or video, to instruct. A large healthcare facility may employ a medical television team, including producers, directors, and camera personnel.

Most medical television producers receive their academic training in radio, television, broadcasting or educational media. For a list of schools offering programs in television and radio broadcasting, contact the Broadcast Education Association, 1771 "N" Street, N.W., Washington, D.C. 20036

Following the biocommunications manager chapter, is a list of programs accredited by the Health Sciences Communications Association, in medical television and instructional media.

Biocommunications Manager

The *biocommunications manager* supervises biocommunications professionals in a communications department, and coordinates their activities. Biocommunications managers assure that the department runs smoothly, and that high quality communications services are provided. They must be knowledgeable in a variety of biocommunications fields, including medical illustration, biophotography, medical writing and medical television/instructional media. Many managers start out in one of these biocommunications specialty areas.

Following is a list of programs accredited by the Health Sciences Communications Association, in medical television/instruction media and biocommunications management.

For more information on a career as a medical television/instructional media professional, or a biocommunications manager, contact the Health Sciences Communications Association, 6105 Lindell Boulevard, St. Louis, Missouri 63112.

SOURCES:

Health Sciences Communications Association,

Occupational Outlook Handbook

Medical Television/Instructional Media Programs

MICHIGAN

Medical Television/Instructional Media Program
Grand Valley State College
School of Health Sciences
Allendale, Michigan 49401

OHIO

Medical Television/Instructional Media Program
Division of Biomedical Communications
School of Allied Medical Professions
Ohio State University
1583 Perry Street
Columbus, Ohio 43210

TEXAS

Medical Television/Instructional Media Program
University of Texas Health Sciences Center at Dallas
5323 Harry Hines Blvd.
Dallas, Texas 75235

Biocommunications Management Programs

NEBRASKA

Biocommunications Management Program
University of Nebraska Medical Center
42nd and Dewey Avenue
Omaha, Nebraska 68105

NEW YORK

Biocommunications Management Program
Ithica College
Ithica, New York 14850

OHIO

Biocommunications Management Program
Division of Biomedical Communications
School of Allied Medical Professions
Ohio State University
1583 Perry Street
Columbus, Ohio 43210

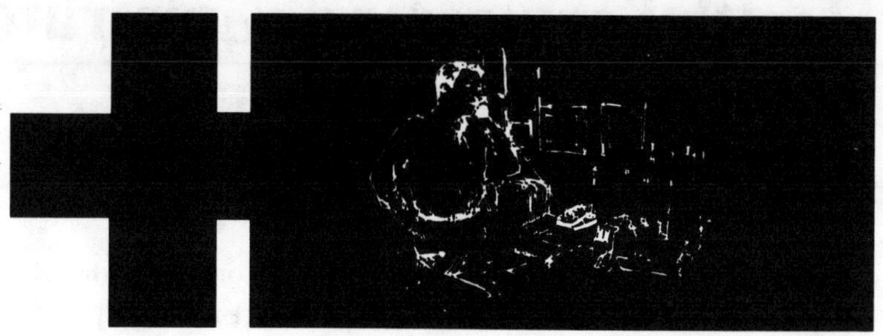

HEALTH SERVICES ADMINISTRATION

In general terms health services administration is that field responsible for the management of all aspects of healthcare including patient care, health education, and health research. Specifically, the planning, organization, and operation of all healthcare facilities, from large hospitals to small walk-in clinics, is the concern of each healthcare facility's office of administration. Administrators of health services work in every organization or institution that is connected to the health field, including general hospitals, extended care facilities, health maintenance organizations, nursing homes, psychiatric hospitals, rehabilitation institutes, group practice plans, outpatient clinics, private insurance programs, federal and state health departments, hospital associations, health education programs and research institutes. Approximately one-half of all health services administrators work in hospitals. Opportunities for upper level management and administrative positions in health services administration are most often granted to individuals with specialized graduate degrees in health services or hospital administration.

Below is general information on the careers involved with the overall administration of health services, including those of the *health services administrator,* the *associate administrator,* and the *administrative assistant*.

Health Services Administrator
Associate Administrator
Administrative Assistant

Under general supervision of a board of directors or similar governing body, the *health services administrator* occupies the senior-most executive position in the organization of the many complex components of a healthcare system. The primary responsibilities of the administrator lie in policy development, activity coordination, and procedural planning. Skilled in management decision making, the administrator decides on such matters as budget, personnel, equipment, and space allocations as well as taking an active role in labor relations and acting as a liaison between the governing bodies of the organization and its medical, health, and support staffs.

In a small health organization the administrator coordinates and administers all of its various functions and activities; while in a large organization or institution the administrator directs a staff of associate administrators in the operation of individual departments, which may number up to thirty in a large hospital. Besides overseeing the actual daily operation of the various departments the *associate administrator* (also referred to as an *assistant administrator*) acts as an advisor to the administrator interpreting hospital policies, assisting in budgeting and planning; resolving problems concerning staffing, equipment, and facilities; acting as a fund raiser and as a public relations officer; and finally recommending when and how changes in policy, physical plant, personnel, and equipment should be made.

The third administrative position, that of the *administrative assistant,* is considered an entry-level trainee position in health services administration. A hospital may employ several administrative assistants who work in specific projects that investigate, analyze and evaluate the various services and functions carried out within the hospital. Examples of these projects include the studying of the inter-relationships between specific hospital services; the recommending of alternatives for more efficient and less costly operating procedures; the comparing of cost structure of different institutions; and the determining of personnel work schedules, salaries and fringe benefits. All studies of these kinds are reported directly to the administrator.

Educational requirements for health services administrators vary according to the size of the health organization and the individual level of responsibility. Larger health institutions usually require their administrative personnel to have a higher degree of education than do smaller institutions. A graduate degree in health services administration is required for the senior-level positions of administrator, associate administrator, and department head while a bachelor's degree usually qualifies a candidate for the mid-level position of hospital administrative assistant, assistant department head, or unit manager or for the position of nursing home associate administrator.

Salaries in hospital administration vary considerably depending upon job responsibility, the size of the particular administration department, and the size and location of the health facility. Administrators of nursing homes usually earn less than those of hospitals with a comparable number of beds. Hospital chief administrators in 1987 averaged between $48,000 and $145,000 a year depending upon the size of the hospital, according to a survey conducted by *Modern Healthcare Magazine*. According to data from the *Occupational Outlook Handbook,* the associate administrator, who is directly under the chief administrator, may earn salaries in the mid-30's for small healthcare facilities to salaries in the high-60's for those employed in large facilities. Administrative assistants earned average annual starting salaries of $19,000, with experienced assistants earning average salaries of $27,000, according to a University of Texas Medical Branch survey.

Following is a list supplied by the Association of University Programs in Health Administration of schools that offer either bachelor's or master's degrees in health services administration. The association states that students can specialize in one of three areas including general administration; specialist training in a specific discipline such as financial management; or specialist training in a specific health setting such as a hospital, nursing home, or health planning department. Interested students should contact the schools of their choice for specific information on particular programs.

Sources for financial aid for students in health services administration may come from the university or college directly or students may inquire with the Association of University Programs in Health Administration/Citibank Student Loan Program about guaranteed student loans for eligible students in health services administration. Write to them for more information at AUPHA/Citibank Student Loan Program, 1911 North Fort Myer Drive, Suite 503, Arlington, Virginia 22209.

For further information on a career in health services administration, write to the American College of Hospital Administrators, 840 North Lake Shore Drive, Chicago, Illinois 60611 and the Association of University Programs in Health Administration, 1911 North Fort Myer Drive, Suite 503, Arlington, Virginia 22209. For individuals interested in a career in long-term care administration, write to the American College of Health Care Administrators, 325 South Patrick Street, Alexandria, Virginia 22314.

SOURCE:

American College of Hospital Administrators
American College of Health Care Administration
American Hospital Association
Association of University Programs in Health Administration
Modern Healthcare Magazine
Occupational Outlook Handbook

Health Services Administration Graduate Programs

ALABAMA

Health Services Administration
Graduate Program (*)
School of Community and Allied Health (SCAH)
University of Alabama-Birmingham
Susan Mott Webb Nutrition Sciences Building
Birmingham, Alabama 35294

ARIZONA

Health Services Administration
Graduate Program (*)
College of Business Administration
Arizona State University
Tempe, Arizona 85287

ARKANSAS

Health Services Administration
Graduate Program
University of Arkansas-Little Rock
33rd and University Avenue
Little Rock, Arkansas 72204

CALIFORNIA

Health Services Administration
Graduate Program (*)
School of Business Administration
University of California-Berkeley
Berkeley, California 94720

Health Services Administration
Graduate Program (*)
School of Public Health
University of California-Los Angeles
Los Angeles, California 90024

Health Services Administration
Graduate Program (*)
Graduate School of Public Health
San Diego State University
San Diego, California 92182

Health Services Administration
Graduate Program (*)
University of Southern California
663 West 34th Street
Bruce Hall
Los Angeles, California 90089-0662

CANADA

Health Services Administration
Graduate Program (*)
13-103 Clinical Sciences Building
University of Alberta
83rd Avenue and 112th Street
Edmonton, Alberta, Canada T6G 2G3

Health Services Administration
Graduate Program (*)
Department of Health Care and Epidemiology
University of British Columbia
5804 Fairview Crescent
Vancouver, British Columbia, Canada V6T 1W5

Health Services Administration
Graduate Program (*)
Département d'Administration de la Santé
University of Montreal
2375, Chemin de la Côte Ste-Catherine
Montreal, Quebec, Canada H3T 1A8

Health Services Administration
Graduate Program (*)
University of Ottawa
275 Nicholas Street
Faculty of Administration
Ottawa, Ontario, Canada K1N 9A9

Health Services Administration
Graduate Program (*)
University of Toronto
12 Queens Park Crescent West
McMurrich Building, 2nd Floor
Toronto, Ontario, Canada M5S 1A8

COLORADO

Health Services Administration
Graduate Program (*)
School of Business Administration
University of Colorado
1100 14th Street
Denver, Colorado 80202

CONNECTICUT

Health Services Administration
Graduate Program (*)
Department of Epidemiology and Public Health
Yale University
60 College Street, Box 3333 (LEPH)
New Haven, Connecticut 06510

DISTRICT OF COLUMBIA

Health Services Administration
Graduate Program (*)
Department of Health Services Administration
The George Washington University
600 21st Street, N.W.
Washington, DC 20052

Health Services Administration
Graduate Program (*)
School of Business and Public Administration
Howard University
2600 6th Street, N.W.
Washington, DC 20059

FLORIDA

Health Services Administration
Graduate Program (*)
Colleges of Business and Health Related Professions
University of Florida
Box J-195
Gainesville, Florida 32610

Health Services Administration
Graduate Program
Department of Health Services Administration
Florida International University-Bay Vista
North Miami, Florida 33181

GEORGIA

Health Services Administration
Graduate Program (*)
Institute of Health Administration
Georgia State University
1050 Lawyer's Title Building
Atlanta, Georgia 30303

ILLINOIS

Health Services Administration
Graduate Program (*)
Graduate School of Business
University of Chicago
1101 East 58th Street
Chicago, Illinois 60637

Health Services Administration
Graduate Program (*)
College of Health Professions
Governors State University
University Park, Illinois 60466

Health Services Administration
Graduate Program (*)
Northwestern University
2001 Sheridan Road
Nathaniel Levorone Hall
Evanston, Illinois 60201

Health Services Administration
Graduate Program (*)
Rush-Presbyterian-St. Luke's Medical Center
Rush University
600 South Paulina Street
Chicago, Illinois 60612

INDIANA

Health Services Administration
Graduate Program (*)
School of Public and Environmental Affairs
Indiana University
801 West Michigan Street
Indianapolis, Indiana 46223

IOWA

Health Services Administration
Graduate Program (*)
Center for Health Services Research
University of Iowa
2700 Steindler Building
Iowa City, Iowa 52242

KANSAS

Health Services Administration
Graduate Program
Department of Health Services Administration
University of Kansas-Lawrence
110 Watkins Home
Lawrence, Kansas 66045

KENTUCKY

Health Services Administration
Graduate Program
Program in Systems Science and Health Systems
Systems Science Institute
University of Louisville
Louisville, Kentucky 40292

LOUISIANA

Health Services Administration
Graduate Program (*)
Department of Health Systems Management
Tulane University
1430 Tulane Avenue
New Orleans, Louisiana 70112

MASSACHUSETTS

Health Services Administration
Graduate Program (*)
Division of Public Health
University of Massachusetts-Amherst
Arnold House
Amherst, Massachusetts 01003

Health Services Administration
Graduate Program (*)
School of Management
Boston University
704 Commonwealth Avenue
Boston, Massachusetts 02215

Health Services Administration
Graduate Program
Graduate School of Management
Clark University
University of Massachusetts Medical School
950 Main Street
Worcester, Massachusetts 01610

MICHIGAN

Health Services Administration
Graduate Program (*)
Department of Health Services Management
and Policy
University of Michigan
1420 Washington Heights
Ann Arbor, Michigan 48109

MINNESOTA

Health Services Administration
Graduate Program (*)
University of Minnesota
420 Delaware Street, S.E.
Box 97, Mayo Memorial Building
Minneapolis, Minnesota 55455

MISSOURI

Health Services Administration
Graduate Program (*)
School of Health Related Professions
University of Missouri-Columbia
324 Clarke Hall
Columbia, Missouri 65211

Health Services Administration
Graduate Program (*)
School of Medicine
Washington University
4547 Clayton Avenue
St. Louis, Missouri 63110

Health Services Administration
Graduate Program (*)
Department of Hospital and Health Care
Administration
Saint Louis University
3525 Caroline Street
St. Louis, Missouri 63104

NEW YORK

Health Services Administration
Graduate Program (*)
Baruch College
Mt. Sinai School of Medicine
City University of New York
17 Lexington Avenue
New York, New York 10010

Health Services Administration
Graduate Program
Division of Health Administration
Columbia University
600 West 168th Street, 6th Floor
New York, New York 10032

Health Services Administration
Graduate Program (*)
Sloan Program in Health Services Administration
Department of Human Services Studies
Cornell University
Ithaca, New York 14853

Health Services Administration
Graduate Program (*)
Health Studies Center
Union College
Union Avenue, Bailey Hall
Schenectady, New York 12308

Health Services Administration
Graduate Program (*)
Graduate School of Public Administration
New York University
Tisch Hall
New York, New York 10003

NORTH CAROLINA

Health Services Administration
Graduate Program
Department of Health Administration
Duke University
Box 3018
Durham, North Carolina 27710

Health Services Administration
Graduate Program (*)
Department of Health Policy and Administration
University of North Carolina-Chapel Hill
263 Rosenau Hall 201-H
Chapel Hill, North Carolina 27514

OHIO

Health Services Administration
Graduate Program (*)
Xavier University
2220 Victory Parkway
Becker House
Cincinnati, Ohio 45207

Health Services Administration
Graduate Program (*)
The Ohio State University
1583 Perry Street
Columbus, Ohio 43210

PENNSYLVANIA

Health Services Administration
Graduate Program (*)
Widener University
Chester, Pennsylvania 19013

Health Services Administration
Graduate Program (*)
Department of Health Administration
School of Business Administration
Temple University
Philadelphia, Pennsylvania 19122

Health Services Administration
Graduate Program (*)
University of Pennsylvania
3641 Locust Walk
Colonial Penn Center
Philadelphia, Pennsylvania 19104

Health Services Administration
Graduate Program (*)
College of Human Development
Pennsylvania State University
115 Human Development Building
University Park, Pennsylvania 16802

Health Services Administration
Graduate Program (*)
Department of Health Services Administration
University of Pittsburgh
130 DeSoto Street
Pittsburgh, Pennsylvania 15261

PUERTO RICO

Health Services Administration
Graduate Program (*)
University of Puerto Rico
G.P.O. Box 5067
Medical Sciences Campus Building
San Juan, Puerto Rico 00936

SOUTH CAROLINA

Health Services Adminstration
Graduate Program
College of Health Related Professions
Medical University of South Carolina
171 Ashley Avenue
Charleston, South Carolina 29425

TENNESSEE

Health Services Administration
Graduate Program
Division of Community Health Sciences
Meharry Medical College
1005 Todd Boulevard
Nashville, Tennessee 37208

Health Services Administration
Graduate Program
Department of Political Science
Memphis State University
Memphis, Tennessee 38152

TEXAS

Health Services Administration
Graduate Program (*)
University of Houston-Clear Lake
2700 Bay Area Boulevard
Bayou Building
Houston, Texas 77058

Health Services Administration
Graduate Program (*)
Academy of Health Sciences, USA
Health Care Administration Division
Army-Baylor University
Fort Sam Houston, Texas 78234-6100

Health Services Administration
Graduate Program
Departments of Allied Health Sciences and
Health Care Administration
Health Science Center
Southwest Texas State University
San Marcos, Texas 78666

Health Services Administration
Graduate Program (*)
Trinity University
715 Stadium Drive, TU Box 58
San Antonio, Texas 78284

UTAH

Health Services Administration
Graduate Program
Graduate School of Management
Brigham Young University
760 TNRB
Provo, Utah 84602

VIRGINIA

Health Services Administration
Graduate Program (*)
Medical College of Virginia
Virginia Commonwealth University
MCV Station, Box 203
Richmond, Virginia 23298

WASHINGTON

Health Services Administration
Graduate Program (*)
Department of Health Services SC 37
University of Washington-Seattle
Seattle, Washington 98195

WISCONSIN

Health Services Administration
Graduate Program (*)
University of Wisconsin-Madison
1300 University Avenue
Madison, Wisconsin 53706

Health Services Administration
Graduate Program
School of Business Administration
University of Wisconsin-Milwaukee
P.O. Box 742
Milwaukee, Wisconsin 53201

(*) Accredited by the Accrediting Commission on Education for Health Services Administration.

Health Services Administration Bachelor Degree Programs

CALIFORNIA

Health Services Administration Bachelor
Degree Program
Health Science Department, Eng. 220
California State University-Northridge
1811 Nordhoff Street
Northridge, California 91330

Health Services Administration Bachelor
Degree Program
The Consortium of the California State University
400 Golden Shore
Long Beach, California 90802-4275

Health Services Administration Bachelor
Degree Program
Saint Mary's College of California
P.O. Box 397
Moraga, California 94575

COLORADO

Health Services Administration Bachelor
Degree Program
Metropolitan State College
1006 11th Street
California Building
Denver, Colorado 80204

CONNECTICUT

Health Services Administration Bachelor Degree Program
Center for Health Systems Management
School of Business Administration, U-41
University of Connecticut
Storrs, Connecticut 06268

Health Services Administration Bachelor Degree Program
Department of Health Services Administration and Long-Term Care Administration
Quinnipiac College
Mount Carmel Avenue
Hamden, Connecticut 06518

FLORIDA

Health Services Administration Bachelor Degree Program
School of Allied Health Sciences
Florida A and M University
Ware-Rhaney Building
Tallahassee, Florida 32307

ILLINOIS

Health Services Administration Bachelor Degree Program
College of Health Sciences Professions
Governors State University
University Park, Illinois 60466

Health Services Administration Bachelor Degree Program
Health Science Professions Cluster
Sangamon State University
Shepherd Road, A-13
Springfield, Illinois 62708

KANSAS

Health Services Administration Bachelor Degree Program
College of Health Professions
Wichita State University
Health Sciences Building
Wichita, Kansas 67208

KENTUCKY

Health Services Administration Bachelor Degree Program
College of Allied Health Professions
University of Kentucky
103 Medical Center, Annex 2
Lexington, Kentucky 40536-0080

MAINE

Health Services Administration Bachelor Degree Program
External Degree Program
Saint Joseph's College
White's Bridge Road
North Windham, Maine 04062

MASSACHUSETTS

Health Services Administration Bachelor Degree Program
Duffy Academic Center
Stonehill College
Washington Street
North Easton, Massachusetts 02357

MICHIGAN

Health Services Administration Bachelor Degree Program
Eastern Michigan University
327 King Hall
Ypsilanti, Michigan 48197

MISSOURI

Health Services Administration Bachelor Degree Program
School of Health Related Professions
University of Missouri-Columbia
324 Clark Hall
Columbia, Missouri 65211

NEW HAMPSHIRE

Health Services Administration Bachelor Degree Program
School of Health Studies
University of New Hampshire
211 Hewitt Hall
Durham, New Hampshire 03824

NEW JERSEY

Health Services Administration Bachelor Degree Program
Urban Studies Department
Rutgers University
Lucy Stone Hall
New Brunswick, New Jersey 08903

NEW YORK

Health Services Administration Bachelor Degree Program
College of Business and Administration
Alfred University
Alfred, New York 14802

Health Services Administration Bachelor
Degree Program
School of Allied Health Professions
Ithaca College
New Academic Building
Ithaca, New York 14850

Health Services Administration Bachelor
Degree Program
Herbert H. Lehman College-City University
of New York
Bedford Park Boulevard West
Gillet Hall
Bronx, New York 10468

NORTH CAROLINA

Health Services Administration Bachelor
Degree Program
John A. Walker College of Business
Appalachian State University
221 John Walker Hall
Boone, North Carolina 28608

Health Services Administration Bachelor
Degree Program
University of North Carolina-Asheville
One University Heights
Owen Building
Asheville, North Carolina 28804-3299

Health Services Administration Bachelor
Degree Program
University of North Carolina-Chapel Hill
263 Rosenau Hall 201-H
Chapel Hill, North Carolina 27514

Health Services Administration Bachelor
Degree Program
School of Nursing and Health Sciences
Western Carolina University
141 Moore Hall
Cullowhee, North Carolina 28723

OHIO

Health Services Administration Bachelor
Degree Program
School of Planning, DAAP ML 16
College of Design, Architecture, Art and Planning
University of Cincinnati
Cincinnati, Ohio 45221

OREGON

Health Services Administration Bachelor
Degree Program
Oregon State University
Waldo Hall, 304
Corvallis, Oregon 97331

PENNSYLVANIA

Health Services Administration Bachelor
Degree Program
College of Human Development
Pennsylvania State University
Human Development Bldg.
University Park, Pennsylvania 16802

RHODE ISLAND

Health Services Administration Bachelor
Degree Program
Providence College
River Avenue and Eaton Street
Howley Hall
Providence, Rhode Island 02918

SOUTH DAKOTA

Health Services Administration Bachelor
Degree Program
School of Business
University of South Dakota
Patterson Hall
Vermillion, South Dakota 57069

TENNESSEE

Health Services Administration Bachelor
Degree Program
Meharry Medical College-Fisk and Tennessee
State Universities
T.B. Todd Boulevard
P.O. Box 63-A
Nashville, Tennessee 37208

TEXAS

Health Services Administration Bachelor
Degree Program
Departments of Allied Health Sciences and
Health Administration
Health Science Center
Southwest Texas State University
San Marcos, Texas 78666

VIRGINIA

Health Services Administration Bachelor
Degree Program
Medical College of Virginia
Virginia Commonwealth University
MCV Station, Box 203
Richmond, Virginia 23298

UTAH

Health Services Administration Bachelor
Degree Program
School of Allied Health Sciences
Weber State College
3750 Harrison Boulevard
Ogden, Utah 84408

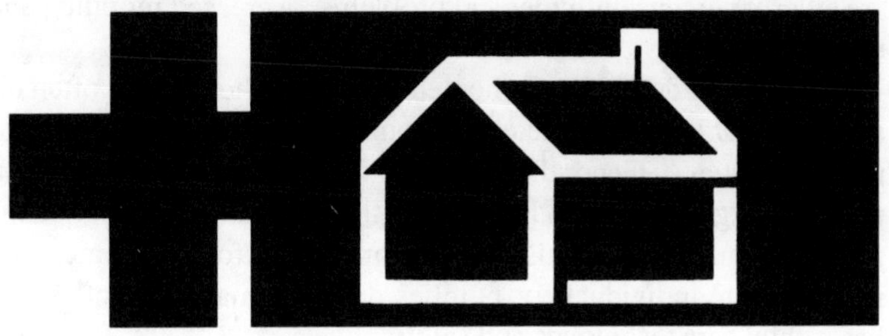

HOMEMAKER - HOME HEALTH AIDE SERVICES

Based on the principle that family solidarity is essential to family and community life, homemaker-home health aide services involve domestic and social services and healthcare. They are provided by public, private, and voluntary health or welfare agencies and offer a variety of "in-home" services for families or individuals who are experiencing disruptions in normal living habits because of illness, disability, or social disadvantage. The primary concern of homemaker-home health aide services is the maintenance and improvement of the health and well-being of those who must, or choose to, live at home instead of remaining in, or entering a hospital or institution. The advantage of these services is that they allow the ill or disabled individual to benefit from the familiar surroundings of home and community in relative independence. Examples of when these services are needed include situations when the mother of a family is ill or incapacitated, when discharged surgery patients are permitted to recuperate at home, or when handicapped or elderly persons require personal care and domestic assistance. The individual who performs these services in the home is the *homemaker-home health aide*.

Homemaker - Home Health Aide

As the recruited, trained and supervised staff member of a health or welfare agency, the *homemaker-home health aide* may provide homemaking and personal services, instructions, emotional support, and some minimal healthcare to clients in their own homes. Although also caring for children and the handicapped, most of the aide's clients are elderly persons with medical problems, decreased mobility, and/or little or no family to care for them.

Job titles and duties for the homemaker-home health aide often differ between agencies and states. Often, homemaker and home-health aide are separate positions with varied job responsibilities. Generally, the position of homemaker refers to an individual who performs light homemaking duties that include cleaning, laundering, planning and preparing nutritious meals, and shopping for food. Homemakers may also provide instruction to individuals or families on home management skills, including budgeting, basic child care techniques and safety.

A home-health aide often performs personal care duties such as bathing, feeding, and helping the client move about the home. With training and supervision from a registered nurse, the home-health aide performs basic nursing tasks which may include changing bandages, reminding clients to take medications, and assisting with prescribed exercises or with special therapies. The aide also offers instruction in how to adapt both physically and mentally to illness or disability, and how to cope with daily tasks that are difficult for the client to perform, such as caring for children or cooking meals. Finally, the aide provides emotional support and understanding when the client is depressed, frustrated, or lonely.

Homemaker-home health aide services may be used on an "as needed" basis or may be one part of a longer term home healthcare plan that may include a physician, nurse, social worker, therapist and dietician. If complex medical treatments are required, a client may employ a home healthcare nurse or visiting nurse service. Registered nurses (RN's) can provide hospital-type care in the comfort of home. Licensed practical nurses (LPN's) usually provide more routine treatment and care. For more details on a career as a registered nurse or licensed practical nurse, refer to the chapter in this book titled, "Nursing".

Although there are few restrictions on the age of homemaker-home health aides, most agencies prefer to employ mature women and men who have had some experience in homemaking.

Although high school graduation is not always required, courses in home economics are advisable for younger persons who wish to become aides and who have little to no experience in family living and meal planning. Some agencies do require that their aides have previous training and experience as nursing aides or orderlies. Aides should be above average in physical strength and be able to show compassion and responsibility.

The homemaker-home health aide is expected to be responsible, dependable and resourceful. The aide is generally supervised by a registered nurse, social worker or a professional with a four year degree in a related field, who visits the client's home on a regular basis. During these meetings with the supervisor, the homemaker-home health aide can report on the client's condition and make recommendations for a change in services.

Homemaker-home health aides should undergo a sixty-hour training program as recommended by the National Home Caring Council. Depending on state practices, training may be administered at the home healthcare agency or in the school system through secondary schools, vocational-technical institutes, or community colleges. This training should include basic home nursing, personal care, food and nutrition, safety, budgeting, child care and family relations, and is taught by registered nurses, licensed practical nurses and other healthcare professionals. In addition, on-the-job training is often provided by the home healthcare agency so that the aide will feel comfortable in a greater variety of situations.

One way to gain a better understanding of the home healthcare field is through volunteering. Some social service organizations provide supplementary home health services and need volunteers to provide companionship to homebound individuals, to deliver nutritious meals, and to assist with transportation. For more information on volunteering, contact The United Way, American Red Cross, or other social service organizations (generally listed under "Social Service Organizations", in the local telephone directory).

Salaries for homemaker-home health aides vary considerably depending upon the type and location of health or welfare agency. Benefits such as guaranteed hours, sick leave, health insurance, and pension plans also vary greatly between agencies. Persons interested in becoming aides should compare these factors in accepting various salaries.

The major benefit to this occupation is that most of the work is part-time and persons may use the job to supplement income from another job or from their Social Security.

Those interested in additional information on a career as a homemaker-home health aide should contact the secondary public schools, vocational-technical institutes, and community colleges in their area, or refer to telephone listings under "Home Health Aide Agencies", "Home Health Care", or "Social Service Organization". Potential employment opportunities may also be found in the classified advertising section of local newspapers under the heading "Medical" or "Domestic".

Additional reading material on homemaker-home health aide services can be obtained from the National Home Caring Council, A Division of the Foundation for Hospice and Home Care, 591 "C" Street, N.E., Stanton Park, Washington, D.C. 20002.

SOURCES:

Dictionary of Occupational Titles
Foundation for Hospice and Home Care
National Home Caring Council
Occupational Outlook Handbook

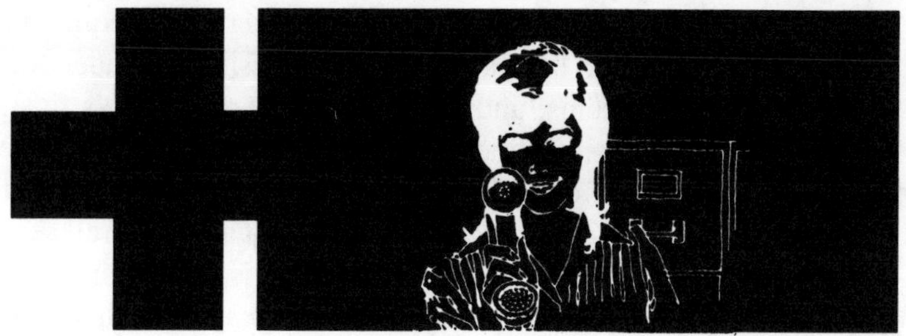

MEDICAL ASSISTING

Medical assisting is the allied health profession that provides administrative and clinical support for physicians in the efficient operation of their office practices as well as in hospitals, clinics and other healthcare facilities. In a small, one-employee office the *medical assistant* performs all the necessary supportive duties for the physician, but in a large office or medical practice these duties are differentiated among two or more medical assistants.

Medical assisting employs mostly women, although some positions are filled by men, and the career provides an excellent opportunity for mature persons to reenter the work force on either a full-or-part-time basis.

The various job functions of medical assisting are discussed under the heading of medical assistant. The occupations of medical assisting in dentistry, optometry, and ophthalmology are discussed in their respective chapters elsewhere in this handbook.

Medical Assistant

Most often employed in a physician's office the *medical assistant* serves as the direct link between the physician and his or her patients, professional associates, and suppliers of medical drugs and equipment. Nearly every practicing physician requires at least one medical assistant.

Depending on degree of training and working conditions the medical assistant may perform either administrative and/or clinical duties.

The responsibilities of a medical assistant who performs administrative duties include scheduling appointments; receiving patients; answering the telephone; operating office machinery; handling correspondence; taking medical dictation; transcribing shorthand;

typing medical reports; maintaining patients' files and medical records; receiving representatives of pharmaceutical companies and medical equipment suppliers; arranging hospital admissions and laboratory tests; processing the paperwork involved with health insurance data and claims; and finally handling the office's financial records including patients' fees. If responsibilities are limited to secretarial and receptionist functions, the medical assistant may often be referred to as a *medical secretary.* If the assistant is employed solely as an office receptionist and not as an overall secretary, a high degree of training and knowledge in medical terminology is not required.

In a small office, advancement opportunities may be limited, however, in a large office or clinic, medical assistants may be promoted to office manager after several years experience plus demonstrated leadership ability.

With sufficient formal or on-the-job training, however, the medical assistant can go beyond office management and perform clinical duties that include preparing patients for examination; taking blood pressures and temperatures; recording medical histories; performing diagnostic and routine laboratory procedures; and assisting the physician with examinations and treatment.

Training in medical assisting varies with specific job responsibilities. For medical secretaries, general secretarial programs of one-to-two years are offered by most community colleges and vocational-technical schools. More comprehensive training is available from formal medical assistant educational programs offered by community colleges, vocational-technical and specialized schools of medical assisting, which also include practical experience in physicians' offices or hospitals.

Certification as a Certified Medical Assistant (CMA) is available from the American Association of Medical Assistants for candidates who successfully complete the association's examination and satisfy the educational and/or experience requirements. Credentials are also granted by the American Medical Technologists for the Registered Medical Assistant (RMA) status. For information on certification or registration awards write to the American Association of Medical Assistants, 20 North Wacker Drive, Suite 1575, Chicago, Illinois 60606 or the American Medical Technologists, 710 Higgins Road, Park Ridge, Illinois 60068, respectively.

Recommended high school courses include typing, business, mathematics, secretarial skills, biology, chemistry, and psychology.

Financial aid is available upon application for needy high school graduates who are seriously interested in and have the aptitude for becoming a medical assistant. Interested students should contact the American Association of Medical Assistants' Endowment, 20 North Wacker Drive, Suite 1575, Chicago, Illinois 60606. The American Medical Technologists also offers undergraduate and graduate scholarship awards to its members.

Salaries for medical assistants are usually equal to those of other office personnel with comparable degrees of training. Average starting salaries for medical assistants equal $11,000 per year, although some medical assistants who become office managers can earn significantly more.

For more information on careers as a medical assistant contact the American Association of Medical Assistants, 20 North Wacker Drive, Suite 1575, Chicago, Illinois 60606, or the American Medical Technologists, 710 Higgins Road, Park Ridge, Illinois 60068.

Two agencies are recognized by the U.S. Department of Education to accredit medical assisting programs. They are the Committee on Allied Health Education and Accreditation (CAHEA) of the American Medical Association and the Accrediting Bureau of Health Education Schools (ABHES).

Below is the list of accredited programs in medical assisting. As they are either one-year certificate or diploma programs or two-year associate degree programs, with some schools offering both, interested persons should contact the schools directly for specific information on the type and length of their programs(s).

KEY:

(1) Accredited by the American Medical Association's Committee on Allied Health Education and Accreditation in collaboration with the American Association of Medical Assistants.

(2) Program or institution accredited by the Accrediting Bureau of Health Education Schools.

SOURCES:

American Association of Medical Assistants
Accrediting Bureau of Health Education Schools
American Association of Medical Assistants' Endowment
American Medical Technologists
Occupational Outlook Handbook

Medical Assistant Programs

ALABAMA

Medical Assistant Program (1)
University of Alabama at Birmingham
University Station
Birmingham, Alabama 35294

Medical Assistant Program (2)
Birmingham College of Allied Health
916 South 18th Street
Birmingham, Alabama 35205

Medical Assistant Program (2)
Capps College
2970 Cottage Hill Road
P.O. Box 6553
Mobile, Alabama 36606

ARIZONA

Medical Assistant Program (2)
Apollo College of Medical and Dental Careers
630 West Southern Avenue
Mesa, Arizona 85202

Medical Assistant Program (2)
Pima Medical Institute (Branch)
2815 South Alma School Rd., Suite 121
Mesa, Arizona 85202

Medical Assistant Program (2)
Apollo College of Medical and Dental Careers
8503 North 27th Avenue
Phoenix, Arizona 85021

Medical Assistant Program (2)
Arizona College of Medical-Dental Careers
4020 North 19th Avenue
Phoenix, Arizona 85015

Medical Assistant Program (1)
National Education Ctr.-Bryman Campus
9215 N. Black Canyon Hwy.
Phoenix, Arizona 85006

Medical Assistant Program (2)
Southwestern Medical Society Academy
2100 N. Central Avenue
Phoenix, Arizona 85001

Medical Assistant Program (2)
Arizona Academy of Medical and Dental Assistants
1020 Sandretto Drive, Suite A
Prescott, Arizona 86301

Medical Assistant Program (2)
Crestwood Career Academy
2103 E. Southern Avenue
Tempe, Arizona 85282

Medical Assistant Program (2)
Apollo College of Medical and Dental Careers
(Branch)
13 West Wetmore
Tucson, Arizona 85705

Medical Assistant Program (2)
3975 N. Tucson Blvd.
Tucson, Arizona 85716

Medical Assistant Program (2)
Pima Medical Institute
3350 East Grant Road
Tucson, Arizona 85716

ARKANSAS

Medical Assistant Program (1)
Capital City College
7723 Asher Avenue
Little Rock, Arkansas 72204

Medical Assistant Program (2)
Eastern College of Health Vocations
6423 Forbing Road
Little Rock, Arkansas 72209

Medical Assistant Program (1)
Arkansas Tech University
Russellville, Arkansas 72801

CALIFORNIA

Medical Assistant Program (1)
National Education Ctr.-Bryman College
1120 N. Brookhurst St.
Anaheim, California 92801

Medical Assistant Program (2)
Southern California College of Medical
& Dental Careers
1717 South Brookhurst Street
Anaheim, California 92804

Medical Assistant Program (2)
National Education Center
20835 Sherman Way
Canoga Park, California 91306

Medical Assistant Program (2)
Apollo College of Medical and Dental Careers
(Branch)
310 Third Avenue, Suite C22
Chula Vista, California 92010

Medical Assistant Program (1)
Orange Coast College
2701 Fairview Road
Costa Mesa, California 92628

Medical Assistant Program (1)
De Anza College
21250 Stevens Creek Blvd.
Cupertino, California 95014

Medical Assistant Program (2)
Southland Career Institute-South Campus
8022 East Florence Avenue
Downey, California 90241

Medical Assistant Program (1)
Ohione College
43600 Mission Bend, Box 3909
Fremont, California 94539

Medical Assistant Program (2)
Glendale College of Business and Paramedical
335 North Brand Boulevard
Glendale, California 91203

Medical Assistant Program (1)
Chabot College
25555 Hesperian Blvd.
Hayward, California 94545

Medical Assistant Program (2)
Southland Career Institute-Main Campus
846 South Union Avenue
Los Angeles, California 90017

Medical Assistant Program (2)
Technical Health Careers School, Inc.
1843 West Imperial Highway
Los Angeles, California 90047

Medical Assistant Program (2)
Webster Career College
222 South Hill Street, Suite 400
Los Angeles, California 90012

Medical Assistant Program (2)
California Institute
4365 Atlantic Avenue
Long Beach, California 90807

Medical Assistant Program (2)
California Paramedical and Technical College
3745 Long Beach Boulevard
Long Beach, California 90807

Medical Assistant Program (1)
National Education Ctr.-Bryman Campus
5350 Atlantic Avenue
Long Beach, California 90805

Medical Assistant Program (2)
Andon College at Modesto
1314 "H" Street
Modesto, California 95354

Medical Assistant Program (1)
Modesto Junior College
435 College Avenue
Modesto, California 95350

Medical Assistant Program (2)
Southland Career Institute-East Campus
512 West Beverly Blvd.
Montebello, California 90640

Medical Assistant Program (2)
Lawton School (Branch)
1330 Broadway, Suite 1200
Oakland, California 94612

Medical Assistant Program (2)
MTD Business College
2148 Broadway
Oakland, California 94612

Medical Assistant Program (1)
Pasadena City College
1570 E. Colorado Blvd.
Pasadena, California 91106

Medical Assistant Program (2)
North-West College of Medical and Dental Assistants
134 West Holt Avenue
Pomona, California 91768

Medical Assistant Program (2)
California Paramedical and Technical College
4550 LaSierra Avenue
Riverside, California 92505

Medical Assistant Program (1)
National Education Ctr.-Bryman Campus
3505 North Hart Avenue
Rosemead, California 91770

Medical Assistant Program (1)
Cosumnes River College
8401 Center Parkway
Sacramento, California 95823

Medical Assistant Program (1,2)
Western Career College
4000 El Camino Avenue
Sacramento, California 95821

Medical Assistant Program (1)
United Health Careers Institute
600 North Sierra Way
San Bernandino, California 92401

Medical Assistant Program (2)
Apollo College of Medical and Dental Careers (Branch)
1333 Camino Del Rio South, Suite 313
San Diego, California 92108

Medical Assistant Program (2)
Maric College of Medical Careers
7202 Princess View Drive
San Diego, California 92120

Medical Assistant Program (1)
San Diego Mesa College
7250 Mesa College Drive
San Diego, California 92111

Medical Assistant Program (2)
Bay City College of Dental-Medical Assistants
211 Sutter Street, 10th Floor
San Francisco, California 94108

Medical Assistant Program (1)
City College of San Francisco
50 Phelan Avenue
San Francisco, California 94112

Medical Assistant Program (1)
National Education Ctr.-Bryman Campus
731 Market Street
San Francisco, California 94103

Medical Assistant Program (1,2)
Clayton Career College
1414 N. Winchester Blvd.
San Jose, California 95128

Medical Assistant Program (2)
Lawton School
950 South Bascom, Suite 2011
San Jose, California 95128

Medical Assistant Program (1)
National Education Ctr.-Bryman Campus
2015 Naglee Avenue
San Jose, California 95128

Medical Assistant Program (2)
Western Career College (Branch)
170 Bay Fair Mall
San Leandro, California 94578

Medical Assistant Program (2)
Maric College of Medical Careers
1300 Rancheros Drive
San Marcos, California 92069

Medical Assistant Program (1)
West Valley Comm. College District
14000 Fruitvale Avenue
Saratoga, California 95070

Medical Assistant Program (1)
National Education Ctr.-Bryman Campus
4212 W. Artesia Blvd.
Torrance, California 90504

Medical Assistant Program (2)
Valley College of Medical & Dental Careers
6850 Van Nuys Blvd., Suite 210
Van Nuys, California 91405

Medical Assistant Program (2)
San Joaquin Valley College
8400 West Mineral King Avenue
Visalia, California 93291

Medical Assistant Program (2)
North-West College of Medical and Dental Assistants
2121 West Garvey Avenue
West Covina, California 91790

COLORADO

Medical Assistant Program (1)
T.H. Pickens Technical Center
500 Buckley Road
Aurora, Colorado 80011

Medical Assistant Program (1)
Boulder Valley Area Voc Tech Ctr.
805 Gillaspie Drive
Boulder, Colorado 80303

Medical Assistant Program (2)
PPI Health Careers School
820 Arcturus Drive
Colorado Springs, Colorado 80906

Medical Assistant Program (2)
Colorado College of Medical and Dental Careers
770 Grant Street
Denver, Colorado 80203

Medical Assistant Program (1)
Emily Griffith Opportunity School
1250 Welton Street
Denver, Colorado 80204

Medical Assistant Program (1)
Parks College, Inc.
7350 N. Broadway
Denver, Colorado 80221

CONNECTICUT

Medical Assistant Program (1)
Morse School of Business
275 Asylum Street
Hartford, Connecticut 06103

DELAWARE

Medical Assistant Program (2)
National Institute of Careers
301 B East Lea Blvd.
Wilmington, Delaware 19802

DISTRICT OF COLUMBIA

Medical Assistant Program (2)
Georgetown School of Science and Arts, Ltd.
2461 Wisconsin Avenue, N.W.
Washington, D.C. 20007

FLORIDA

Medical Assistant Program (1)
Broward Community College
3501 S.W. Davie Road
Fort Lauderdale, Florida 33301

Medical Assistant Program (2)
Florida College of Medical and Dental Careers
6250 North Andrews Avenue
Fort Lauderdale, Florida 33309

Medical Assistant Program (2)
Keiser College of Technology
1401 West Cypress Creek Road
Fort Lauderdale, Florida 33309

Medical Assistant Program (2)
Southern Technical Institute
2200 North-West 9th Avenue
Fort Lauderdale, Florida 33305

Medical Assistant Program (2)
National School of Technology, Inc. (Branch)
4355 West 16th Avenue
Hialeah, Florida 33012

Medical Assistant Program (2)
Vocational Institute
3810 West 12th Avenue, 2nd Floor
Hialeah, Florida 33012

Medical Assistant Program (2)
Medical Arts Training Center
1801 South State Road 7 (U.S. 441)
Hollywood, Florida 33023

Medical Assistant Program (2)
Florida College of Medical and Dental Careers
7960 Arlington Expressway
Jacksonville, Florida 32211

Medical Assistant Program (2)
American Medical Training Institute
10700 Caribbean Boulevard, Suite 301
Miami, Florida 33189

Medical Assistant Program (1)
Lindsey Hopkins Tech Education Center
750 N.W. 20th Street
Miami, Florida 33132

Medical Assistant Program (2)
Prospect Hall College
3218 South University Drive
Miramar, Florida 33025

Medical Assistant Program (2)
National School of Technology, Inc.
16150 N.E. 17th Avenue
North Miami Beach, Florida 33162

Medical Assistant Program (2)
Southern Technical Institute (Branch)
19928 North-West 2nd Avenue
North Miami, Florida 33169

Medical Assistant Program (1)
Sarasota County Voc Tech Center
4748 Beneva Road
Sarasota, Florida 33583

Medical Assistant Program (1)
St. Petersburg Voc Tech Institute
901 34th Street South
St. Petersburg, Florida 33711

Medical Assistant Program (2)
Charron-Williams College
Sunrise Executive Building
6289 W. Sunrise Blvd., Suite 265
Sunrise, Florida 33313

Medical Assistant Program (2)
Florida College of Medical and Dental Careers
2700 West Buffalo Avenue, Suite 100
Tampa, Florida 33607

Medical Assistant Program (2)
MBC Medical Education Center
8313 W. Hillsborough Avenue
Building 3, Suite 1
Tampa, Florida 33615

Medical Assistant Program (2)
United College
9203 North Florida Avenue
Tampa, Florida 33612

Medical Assistant Program (2)
Ross Technical Institute
1490 South Military Trail, Suite 11
West Palm Beach, Florida 33415

Medical Assistant Program (1)
Winter Park Adult Vocational Center
901 Webster Avenue
Winter Park, Florida 32789

GEORGIA

Medical Assistant Program (1)
Atlanta College of Med & Dental Careers
1240 W. Peacktree St., N.W.
Atlanta, Georgia 30309

Medical Assistant Program (2)
Georgia Medical Institute Education Preparation Center
42 Spring Street, Suite 295
Atlanta, Georgia 30303

Medical Assistant Program (1)
National Educational Center-Bryman Campus
1789 Peachtree Road
Atlanta, Georgia 30309

Medical Assistant Program (1)
Augusta Area Technical School
1399 Walton Way
Augusta, Georgia 30901

Medical Assistant Program (1)
Savannah Area Vocational Technical School
5717 White Bluff Road
Savannah, Georgia 31499

Medical Assistant Program (1)
South College
709 Mall Boulevard
Savannah, Georgia 31406

HAWAII

Medical Assistant Program (1)
Kapiolani Community College
4303 Diamond Head Road
Honolulu, Hawaii 96816

Medical Assistant Program (2)
Med-Assist School of Hawaii, Inc.
1164 Bishop Street, Suite 912
Honolulu, Hawaii 96813

IDAHO

Medical Assistant Program (2)
American Institute of Health Technology, Inc.
6600 Emerald Street
Boise, Idaho 83704

ILLINOIS

Medical Assistant Program (1)
Belleville Area College
2500 Carlyle Road
Belleville, Illinois 62221

Medical Assistant Program (1)
Robert Morris College
College Avenue
Carthage, Illinois 62321

Medical Assistant Program (2)
Apollo College of Medical and Dental Careers (Branch)
20 North Michigan Avenue
Chicago, Illinois 60602

Medical Assistant Program (2)
Illinois Medical Training Center
162 North State Street
Chicago, Illinois 60601

Medical Assistant Program (2)
Medical Careers Institute
116 S. Michigan Avenue, 2nd Floor
Chicago, Illinois 60603

Medical Assistant Program (2)
National Technical College
909 West Montrose Street
Chicago, Illinois 60613

Medical Assistant Program (1)
Midstate College
224 S.W. Jefferson Street
Peoria, Illinois 61602

Medical Assistant Program (2)
Gem City College
Seventh and State Streets
P.O. Box 179
Quincy, Illinois 62306

Medical Assistant Program (1)
William Rainey Harper College
Algonquin & Rosell Roads
Palatine, Illinois 60067

Medical Assistant Program (1)
Triton College
2000 Fifth Avenue
River Grove, Illinois 60171

INDIANA

Medical Assistant Program (1)
Indiana Voc Technical College SW
3501 First Avenue
Evansville, Indiana 47710

Medical Assistant Program (2)
Aristotle College of Medical & Dental Technology (Branch)
1000 North Madison Avenue
Greenwood, Indiana 46142

Medical Assistant Program (2)
Aristole College of Medical & Dental Technology (Branch)
5255 Hohman Avenue
Hammond, Indiana 46320

Medical Assistant Program (1)
Indiana Vo-Tech College
3800 N. Anthony Blvd.
Fort Wayne, Indiana 46805

Medical Assistant Program (1)
Indiana Voc Technical College NW Region
5727 Sohl Avenue
Hammond, Indiana 46420

Medical Assistant Program (2)
Aristotle College of Medical & Dental Technology
3833 North Meridian
Indianapolis, Indiana 46205

Medical Assistant Program (1)
Clark College
1840 N. Meridian Street
Indianapolis, Indiana 46202

Medical Assistant Program (1)
Indiana Vocational Technical College
1 West 26th Street, P.O. Box 1763
Indianapolis, Indiana 46202

Medical Assistant Program (1)
Professional Careers Institute
2611 Waterfront Pkwy East
Indianapolis, Indiana 46224

Medical Assistant Program (1)
Indiana Voc Tech College Kokomo
1815 E. Morgan Street
Kokomo, Indiana 46901

Medical Assistant Program (1)
Indiana Voc Tech College
3208 Ross Road
P.O. Box 6299
Lafayette, Indiana 47903

Medical Assistant Program (1)
Indiana Voc Tech College SE
Ivy Tech Drive
Madison, Indiana 47250

Medical Assistant Program (2)
Davenport College (Branch)
8200 Georgia Street
Merrillville, Indiana 46410

Medical Assistant Program (1)
Indiana Voc Tech College
4100 Cowan Road
Muncie, Indiana 47302

Medical Assistant Program (1)
Indiana Vocational Technical College
8204 Highway 311
Sellersburg, Indiana 47172

Medical Assistant Program (2)
Davenport College
6327 State Road 23
South Bend, Indiana 46635

Medical Assistant Program (1)
Indiana Voc Tech College N Ctrl
1534 W. Sample Street
South Bend, Indiana 46619

Medical Assistant Program (1)
Indiana Voc Technical College
7377 S. Dixie Bee Road
Terre Haute, Indiana 47802

IOWA

Medical Assistant Program (1)
Des Moines Area Community College
2006 Ankeny Boulevard
Ankeny, Iowa 50021

Medical Assistant Program (1)
Kirkwood Community College
6301 Kirkwood Blvd. S.W.
Cedar Rapids, Iowa 52406

Medical Assistant Program (1)
Iowa Western Community College
2700 College Rd., Box 4-C
Council Buffs, Iowa 51501

Medical Assistant Program (1)
Iowa Central Community College
330 Avenue M
Fort Dodge, Iowa 50501

Medical Assistant Program (1)
Marshalltown Community College
3700 S. Center Street
Marshalltown, Iowa 50158

Medical Assistant Program (1)
Southeastern Community College
Drawer F 1015 S. Gear Avenue
West Burlington, Iowa 52655

KANSAS

Medical Assistant Program (2)
American Business College
8800 Blue Ridge Boulevard
Kansas City, Kansas 64138

Medical Assistant Program (2)
Kansas City College of Medical and Dental Careers
6600 College Blvd., Suite 100
Overland Park, Kansas 66211

Medical Assistant Program (2)
Bryan Institute
1004 South Oliver
Wichita, Kansas 67218

Medical Assistant Program (2)
United Technical Institute
2015 South Meridian
Wichita, Kansas 67213

KENTUCKY

Medical Assistant Program (2)
Bowling Green Junior College of Business
1141 State Street
Bowling Green, Kentucky 42101

Medical Assistant Program (2)
Southwestern College of Business (Branch)
2929 South Dixie Highway
Crestview Hills, Kentucky 41017

Medical Assistant Program (1)
Fugazzi College
406 Lafayette Avenue
Lexington, Kentucky 40502

Medical Assistant Program (2)
Health Careers Institute
1202 South Third Street
Louisville, Kentucky 40203

Medical Assistant Program (2)
Louisville College
1512 Crums Lane
Louisville, Kentucky 40216

Medical Assistant Program (1)
Spencerian College
914 E. Broadway
Louisville, Kentucky 40204

Medical Assistant Program (1)
Watterson College
4400 Breckinridge Lane
Louisville, Kentucky 40218

Medical Assistant Program (1)
Eastern Kentucky University
Begley 419
Richmond, Kentucky 40475

LOUISIANA

Medical Assistant Program (2)
Eastern College of Health Vocations (Branch)
3540 I-10 Service Road, South
Metairie, Louisiana 70001

Medical Assistant Program (1)
Phillips College
1333 S. Clearview Pkwy.
New Orleans, Louisiana 70121

MAINE

Medical Assistant Program (1)
Beal College
629 Main Street
Bangor, Maine 04401

Medical Assistant Program (1)
Westbrook College
716 Stevens Avenue
Portland, Maine 04103

MARYLAND

Medical Assistant Program (1)
The Medix School
1406 Crain Hwy. South
Glen Burnie, Maryland 21061

Medical Assistant Program (1)
The Medix School
1306 Bellona Avenue
Lutherville, Maryland 21093

Medical Assistant Program (1)
The Medix School
8719 Colesville Road
Silver Springs, Maryland 20912

Medical Assistant Program (1)
Montgomery College
Takoma Ave. & Fenton St.
Takoma Park, Maryland 20912

Medical Assistant Program (2)
National Education Center
Temple School Campus
8635 Colesville Road
Silver Springs, Maryland 20910

MASSACHUSETTS

Medical Assistant Program (1)
Middlesex Community College
Springs Road
Bedford, Massachusetts 01730

Medical Assistant Program (2)
Bay State Junior College
Allied Health Studies
122 Commonwealth Avenue
Boston, Massachusetts 02115

Medical Assistant Program (1)
Fisher Junior College
118 Beacon Street
Boston, Massachusetts 02116

Medical Assistant Program (1)
Dean Junior College
99 Main Street
Franklin, Massachusetts 02038

Medical Assistant Program (1)
Bay Path Junior College
588 Longmeadow Street
Longmeadow, Massachusetts 01106

Medical Assistant Program (1)
Aquinas Junior College
303 Adams Street
Milton, Massachusetts 02186

Medical Assistant Program (1)
Lasell Junior College
1844 Commonwealth Avenue
Newton, Massachusetts 02166

Medical Assistant Program (1)
Mount Ida College
777 Dedham Street
Newton Centre, Massachusetts 02159

Medical Assistant Program (1)
Springfield Tech Community College
1 Amory Square
Springfield, Massachusetts 01105

Medical Assistant Program (1)
Becker Junior College
61 Sever Street
Worcester, Massachusetts 01609

MICHIGAN

Medical Assistant Program (1)
Henry Ford Community College
22586 Ann Arbor Trail
Dearborn, Michigan 48128

Medical Assistant Program (2)
Ross Medical Education Center (Branch)
14110 Telegraph Road
Detroit, Michigan 48239

Medical Assistant Program (2)
The Ross Medical Education Center
1553 Woodward, Suite 650
Detroit, Michigan 48226

Medical Assistant Program (2)
Ferndale Medical Careers, Inc.
22720 Woodward Avenue
Ferndale, Michigan 48220

Medical Assistant Program (1)
Baker College
1110 Eldon Baker Drive
Flint, Michigan 48507

Medical Assistant Program (2)
The Ross Medical Education Center
1012 Gilbert
Flint, Michigan 48532

Medical Assistant Program (1)
Davenport College
415 E. Fulton Street
Grand Rapids, Michigan 49503

Medical Assistant Program (2)
Grand Rapids Educational Center for Medical & Dental Assistants
Northbrook Park, Bldg. 2
2922 Fuller Avenue, N.E.
Grand Rapids, Michigan 49505

Medical Assistant Program (2)
Davenport College
4123 West Main Street
Kalamazoo, Michigan 49007

Medical Assistant Program (1)
Kalamazoo Valley Community College
6767 West "O" Avenue
Kalamazoo, Michigan 49009

Medical Assistant Program (2)
The Ross Medical Education Center
913 West Holmes, Suite 260
Lansing, Michigan 48910

Medical Assistant Program (1)
Macomb Community College
4475 Garfield Road
Mt. Clemens, Michigan 48044

Medical Assistant Program (1)
Muskegon Business College
141 Hartford
Muskegon, Michigan 48442

Medical Assistant Program (2)
Michigan Para-Professional Training Institute
21800 Greenfield Road
Oak Park, Michigan 48237

Medical Assistant Program (2)
The Ross Medical Education Center (Branch)
20820 Greenfield Road
Oak Park, Michigan 48237

Medical Assistant Program (2)
Michigan Para-Professional Training Institute
(Branch)
298114 Smith Road
Romulus, Michigan 48174

Medical Assistant Program (2)
Michigan Para-Professional Training Institute
(Branch)
18600 Florence Avenue, B-3
Roseville, Michigan 48066

Medical Assistant Program (2)
National Technical Institute
410 Cambridge
Royal Oak, Michigan 48067

Medical Assistant Program (2)
The Ross Medical Education Center
4054 Bay Road
Saginaw, Michigan 48603

Medical Assistant Program (1)
Carnegie Institute
550 Stephenson Hwy, 100
Troy, Michigan 48083

Medical Assistant Program (1)
Oakland Community College
7350 Cooley Lake Road
Union Lake, Michigan 48085

Medical Assistant Program (2)
The Ross Medical Education Center
26417 Hoover Road
Warren, Michigan 48089

Medical Assistant Program (1)
Cleary College
2170 Washtenaw Ave.
Ypsilanti, Michigan 48197

MINNESOTA

Medical Assistant Program (1)
Anoka Voc-Tech Institute
1355 W. Main St., Box 191
Anoka, Minnesota 55303

Medical Assistant Program (1)
Normandale Community College
9700 France Avenue S.
Bloomington, Minnesota 55431

Medical Assistant Program (1)
E. Grand Forks Area Voc Tech Inst.
Highway 220 North
East Grand Forks, Minnesota 56721

Medical Assistant Program (1)
Lakeland Medical Dental Academy
1402 W. Lake Street
Minneapolis, Minnesota 55408

Medical Assistant Program (1,2)
Medical Institute of Minnesota
2309 Nicollet Avenue
Minneapolis, Minnesota 55404

Medical Assistant Program (1)
Rochester Community College
East Highway 14
Rochester, Minnesota 55904

Medical Assistant Program (1)
Northeast Metro Tech. Inst.
3300 Century Avenue N.
White Bear Lake, Minnesota 55110

Medical Assistant Program (1)
Willmar Area Voc Tech Institute
P.O. Box 1097
Willmar, Minnesota 56201

MISSISSIPPI

Medical Assistant Program (1)
N.E. Mississippi Junior College
Cunningham Boulevard
Booneville, Mississippi 38829

MISSOURI

Medical Assistant Program (2)
Eastern Jackson County College of Allied Health
808 South 15th Street
Blue Springs, Missouri 64015

Medical Assistant Program (2)
Bryan Institute
12184 Natural Bridge Road
Bridgeton, Missouri 63044

Medical Assistant Program (2)
Kansas City College of Medical & Dental Careers
Penn Park Medical Center
2928 Main Street
Kansas City, Missouri 64108

Medical Assistant Program (2)
Midwest Institute for Medical Assistants
112 West Jefferson, Suite 120
Kirkwood, Missouri 63122

Medical Assistant Program (1)
Rutledge Junior College
625 Benton, POB 3275
Springfield, Missouri 65806

Medical Assistant Program (2)
Al-Med Academy
10963 St. Charles Rock Road
St. Louis, Missouri 63074

Medical Assistant Program (2)
Missouri School for Doctors' Assistants, Inc.
10121 Manchester Road
Laboratory Sciences Building
St. Louis, Missouri 63122

Medical Assistant Program (2)
Medical Professions Institute
9100 Lackland Road
St. Louis, Missouri 63114

Medical Assistant Program (1)
St. Louis Comm. College at Forest Park
5600 Oakland Avenue
St. Louis, Missouri 63110

NEBRASKA

Medical Assistant Program (1)
Central Community College Hastings Campus
P.O. Box 1024
Hastings, Nebraska 68901

Medical Assistant Program (1)
Southeast Community College
8800 O" Street"
Lincoln, Nebraska 68520

Medical Assistant Program (1)
Omaha College of Health Careers
1052 Park Avenue
Omaha, Nebraska 68105

NEW HAMPSHIRE

Medical Assistant Program (1)
New Hampshire Voc Tech College
Hanover Street Extension
Claremont, New Hampshire 03743

NEW JERSEY

Medical Assistant Program (2)
Omega Institute
Cinnaminson Mall
Route 130 South
Cinnaminson, New Jersey 08077

Medical Assistant Program (2)
Lyons Institute
10 Commerce Place
Clark, New Jersey 07066

Medical Assistant Program (1)
Union County College
1033 Springfield Avenue
Cranford, New Jersey 07016

Medical Assistant Program (1)
National Education Ctr. Bryman Campus
Branco Estates Route 18
East Brunswick, New Jersey 08816

Medical Assistant Program (2)
Lyons Institute
320 Main Street
Hackensack, New Jersey 07601

Medical Assistant Program (1)
Hudson Community College
94 Audubon Avenue
Jersey City, New Jersey 07305

Medical Assistant Program (1)
Bergen County Community College
400 Paramus Road
Paramus, New Jersey 07652

Medical Assistant Program (1)
Camden City Voc Tech Schools
Cross Keys Rd., P.O. Box 566
Sicklerville, New Jersey 08081

NEW MEXICO

Medical Assistant Program (2)
Pima Medical Institute (Branch)
5509 Menaul Boulevard, N.E.
Albuquerque, New Mexico 87110

NEW YORK

Medical Assistant Program (2)
The Stratford School (Branch)
845 Central Avenue
Albany, New York 12206

Medical Assistant Program (1)
Broome Community College
P.O. Box 1017
Binghamton, New York 13902

Medical Assistant Program (1)
Byrant & Stratton Business Institute
P.O. Box 1299
Buffalo, New York 14240

Medical Assistant Program (1)
Erie Community College-North Campus
Main Street & Youngs Road
Buffalo, New York 14221

Medical Assistant Program (2)
American Career Schools, Inc.
1707-8 Veterans Highway
Central Islip, New York 11722

Medical Assistant Program (1)
Bryant & Stratton Business Institute
200 Bryant & Stratton Way
Clarence, New York 14221

Medical Assistant Program (2)
The New York School for Medical and Dental Assistants
116-16 Queens Bouelvard
Forest Hills, New York 11375

Medical Assistant Program (2)
Eastern Technical School
85 5th Avenue
New York, New York 10003

Medical Assistant Program (2)
Mandle School
254 West 54th Street
New York, New York 10019

Medical Assistant Program (1)
Dutchess Community College
Pendell Road
Poughkeepsie, New York 12601

Medical Assistant Program (1)
Bryant & Stratton Business Institute
14 Franklin Street
Rochester, New York 14604

Medical Assistant Program (2)
The Stratford School
917 Main Street East
Rochester, New York 14605

Medical Assistant Program (1)
Bryant and Stratton Business Institute
400 Montgomery Street
Syracuse, New York 13202

Medical Assistant Program (2)
The Stratford School (Branch)
2301 James Street
Syracuse, New York 13206

NORTH CAROLINA

Medical Assistant Program (1)
Central Piedmont Community College
P.O. Box 35009
Charlotte, North Carolina 28235

Medical Assistant Program (1)
Kings College
322 Lamar Avenue
Charlotte, North Carolina 28204

Medical Assistant Program (1)
Gaston College
201 Highway 321 North
Dallas, North Carolina 28034-1499

Medical Assistant Program (1)
Carteret Technical College
3505 Arendell Street
Moorehead City, North Carolina 28557

Medical Assistant Program (1)
Western Piedmont Community College
1001 Burkemont Avenue
Morganton, North Carolina 28655

Medical Assistant Program (1)
Wingate College
P.O. Box 3024
Wingate, North Carolina 28174

OHIO

Medical Assistant Program (1)
Akron Institute of Medical-Dental Assistants
733 Market Street
Akron, Ohio 44303

Medical Assistant Program (1)
Southern Ohio College-Northeast
2791 Mogadore Road
Akron, Ohio 44312

Medical Assistant Program (2)
Stautzenberger College
309 South Main Street
Bowling Green, Ohio 43402

Medical Assistant Program (1)
Stark Technical College
6200 Frank Ave., N.W.
Canton, Ohio 44720

Medical Assistant Program (1)
Cincinnati Technical College
3520 Central Parkway
Cincinnati, Ohio 45223

Medical Assistant Program (2)
Institute of Medical and Dental Technology
375 Glensprings Drive, Suite 102
Cincinnati, Ohio 45246

Medical Assistant Program (2)
Ohio College of Business and Technology
415 West Court Street
Cincinnati, Ohio 45203

Medical Assistant Program (2)
Ohio College of Business and Technology
7749-53 Five Mile Road
Cincinnati, Ohio 45230

Medical Assistant Program (1)
Southern Ohio College
1055 Laidlaw Avenue
Cincinnati, Ohio 45237

Medical Assistant Program (2)
Southwestern College of Business
9910 Princeton-Glendale Road
Cincinnati, Ohio 45236

Medical Assistant Program (2)
Southwestern College of Business
717 Race Street
Cincinnati, Ohio 45202

Medical Assistant Program (2)
Cleveland Institute of Dental-Medical
Assistants, Inc.
1836 Euclid Avenue
Cleveland, Ohio 44115

Medical Assistant Program (1)
Cuyahoga Community College
700 Carnegie Avenue
Cleveland, Ohio 44115

Medical Assistant Program (1)
ICM School of Business
1375 Euclid Avenue
Cleveland, Ohio 44115

Medical Assistant Program (2)
Aristotle Institute of Medical and Dental
Technology
P.O. Box 29365
6152 Cleveland Avenue
Columbus, Ohio 43229

Medical Assistant Program (2)
Southwestern College of Business
225 West 1st Street
Dayton, Ohio 45402

Medical Assistant Program (1)
Southern Ohio College
4641 Bacher Lane
Fairfield, Ohio 45014

Medical Assistant Program (2)
Cleveland Institute of Dental-Medical Assistants,
Inc.
5564 Mayfield Road
Lyndhurst, Ohio 44124

Medical Assistant Program (2)
Cleveland Institute of Dental-Medical Assistants,
Inc. (Branch)
5733 Hopkins Road
Mentor, Ohio 44060

Medical Assistant Program (2)
Southwestern College of Business
1830 Yankee Road
Middletown, Ohio 45042

Medical Assistant Program (2)
Ohio College of Business and Technology
(Branch)
7601 Harrison Avenue
Mt. Healthy, Ohio 45231

Medical Assistant Program (1)
Hocking Technical College
Route 1
Nelsonville, Ohio 45754

Medical Assistant Program (1)
Jefferson Technical College
4000 Sunset Boulevard
Steubenville, Ohio 43952

Medical Assistant Program (1)
Davis Junior College of Business
4747 Monroe Street
Toledo, Ohio 43623

Medical Assistant Program (2)
Professional Skills Institute
1232 Flaire Drive
Toledo, Ohio 43615

Medical Assistant Program (2)
Stautzenberger College
4404 Secor Road
Toledo, Ohio 43623

Medical Assistant Program (2)
Stautzenberger College
5355 Southwyck Blvd.
Toledo, Ohio 43614

Medical Assistant Program (2)
Stautzenberger College (Branch)
4615 Woodville Road (East Campus Branch)
Toledo, Ohio 43619

Medical Assistant Program (1)
University of Toledo Comm & Tech College
2801 W. Bancroft Street
Toledo, Ohio 43606

Medical Assistant Program (1)
Muskingum Area Tech College
1555 Newark Road
Zanesville, Ohio 43701

OKLAHOMA

Medical Assistant Program (2)
Bryan Institute
2843 East 51st Street
Tulsa, Oklahoma 74105

Medical Assistant Program (2)
Oklahoma Junior College
4821 South 72 East Avenue
Tulsa, Oklahoma 74145

Medical Assistant Program (1)
Tulsa Junior College
909 S. Boston Avenue
Tulsa, Oklahoma 74119

Medical Assistant Program (2)
United Technical Institute
4233 Charter Avenue
Toledo, Ohio 43619

OREGON

Medical Assistant Program (2)
Apollo College of Medical-Dental Careers
(Branch)
2025 Lloyd Center
Portland, Oregon 97232

Medical Assistant Program (1,2)
Bradford School
921 S.W. Washington St. 200
Portland, Oregon 97205

Medical Assistant Program (1)
Portland Community College
12000 S.W. 49th Avenue
Portland, Oregon 97219

Medical Assistant Program (1)
Chemeketa Community College
P.O. Box 14007
Salem, Oregon 97309

PENNSYLVANIA

Medical Assistant Program (1)
Harcum Junior College
Montgomery Avenue
Bryn Mawr, Pennsylvania 19010

Medical Assistant Program (1)
Gannon University
University Square
Erie, Pennsylvania 16501

Medical Assistant Program (2)
Academy of Medical Arts and Business
279 Boas Street
Harrisburg, Pennsylvania 17102

Medical Assistant Program (1)
Community College of Philadelphia
1700 Spring Garden Street
Philadelphia, Pennsylvania 19130

Medical Assistant Program (2)
Delaware Valley Academy of Medical
& Dental Assistants
6539-43 Roosevelt Boulevard
Philadelphia, Pennsylvania 19149

Medical Assistant Program (2)
McCarrie School of Health Sciences & Technology
512 South Broad Street
Philadelphia, Pennsyvlania 19146

Medical Assistant Program (2)
National Schools
801 Arch Street, Fourth Floor
Philadelphia, Pennsylvania 19107

Medical Assistant Program (1,2)
Philadelphia College of Osteopathic Medicine
School of Allied Health
4190 City Avenue
Philadelphia, Pennsylvania 19131

Medical Assistant Program (1)
Community College of Allegheny City
808 Ridge Avenue
Pittsburgh, Pennsylvania 15212

Medical Assistant Program (1)
Duffs Business Institute
110 Ninth Street
Pittsburgh, Pennsylvania 15222

Medical Assistant Program (1)
ICM School of Business
10 Wood Street
Pittsburgh, Pennsylvania 15222

Medical Assistant Program (1)
Median School
121 Ninth Street
Pittsburgh, Pennsylvania 15222

Medical Assistant Program (2)
North Hills School of Health Occupations
7805 McKnight Road
Pittsburgh, Pennsylvania 15237

Medical Assistant Program (2)
The Sawyer School
717 Liberty Avenue
Pittsburgh, Pennsylvania 15222

Medical Assistant Program (2)
Western School of Health and Business
Careers, Inc.
Ruben Building, 2nd Floor
221-225 Fifth Avenue
Pittsburgh, Pennsylvania 15222

Medical Assistant Program (1)
Lehigh County Community College
2370 Main Street
Schnecksville, Pennsylvania 18078

Medical Assistant Program (1)
Central Pennsylvania Business School
Campus on College Hill
Summerdale, Pennsylvania 17093

Medical Assistant Program (2)
Lyons Technical Institute
67 Long Lane
Upper Darby, Pennsylvania 19082

PUERTO RICO

Medical Assistant Program (2)
Antilles School of Technical Careers
Calle Domenech 107
Hato Rey, Puerto Rico 00917

Medical Assistant Program (2)
Ponce Technical School, Inc.
16 Salud Street
Ponce, Puerto Rico 00731

SOUTH DAKOTA

Medical Assistant Program (1)
National College
321 Kansas City Street
Rapid City, South Dakota 57709

TENNESSEE

Medical Assistant Program (2)
Cumberland School of Medical Technology
321 North Washington Avenue
Cookeville, Tennessee 38501

Medical Assistant Program (1)
Edmondson College of Business
3635 Brainerd Road
Chattanooga, Tennessee 37411

Medical Assistant Program (1)
East Tennessee State University
1000 West E Street
Box 21190A
Elizabeth, Tennessee 37643

Medical Assistant Program (1)
Bristol College Kingsport Campus
P.O. 757
Bristol College Dr.
Kingsport, Tennessee 37655

Medical Assistant Program (2)
Excel Business College
620 Gallatin Road South
Madison, Tennessee 37115

Medical Assistant Program (2)
Nashville College
402 Plaza Professional Building
Madison, Tennessee 37115

Medical Assistant Program (1)
Trevecca Nazarene College
333 Murfreesboro Road
Nashville, Tennessee 37203

Medical Assistant Program (2)
United Technical Institute
430 Allied Drive
Nashville, Tennessee 37211

TEXAS

Medical Assistant Program (2)
Bryan Institute (Branch)
1719 West Pioneer Parkway
Arlington, Texas 76013

Medical Assistant Program (1)
El Centro College
Main & Lamar Streets
Dallas, Texas 75202

Medical Assistant Program (2)
Texas College of Medical-Dental Careers
4230 L.B.J. Freeway, Suite 150
Dallas, Texas 75244

Medical Assistant Program (1)
El Paso Community College
P.O. Box 20500
El Paso, Texas 79998

Medical Assistant Program (2)
San Antonio College of Medical & Dental
Assistants (Branch)
8375 Burnham Drive
El Paso, Texas 79907

Medical Assistant Program (2)
National Education Center
9724 Beechnut, Suite 300
Houston, Texas 77036

Medical Assistant Program (2)
Texas College of Medical-Dental Careers
1919 North Loop West
Houston, Texas 77008

Medical Assistant Program (2)
San Antonio College of Medical and Dental
Assistants (Branch)
3900 North 23rd
McAllen, Texas 78501

Medical Assistant Program (1)
San Antonio College
1300 San Pedro Avenue
San Antonio, Texas 78284

Medical Assistant Program (2)
San Antonio College of Medical and Dental
Assistants
4205 San Pedro
San Antonio, Texas 78212

Medical Assistant Program (2)
Southwest School of Medical Assistants
115 No. Broadway
San Antonio, Texas 78205

UTAH

Medical Assistant Program (2)
American Institute of Medical-Dental Technology
1675 North 200 West-Building 9A-4
Provo, Utah 84604

Medical Assistant Program (1)
LDS Business College
411 East South Temple
Salt Lake City, Utah 84111-1392

Medical Assistant Program (1)
The Bryman School
445 S. 300 East
Salt Lake City, Utah 84111

VIRGINIA

Medical Assistant Program (2)
Chesapeake Business Institute of Virginia
3823 Mount Vernon Avenue
Alexandria, Virginia 22305

Medical Assistant Program (2)
National Education Center
Temple School Campus
5832 Columbia Pike
Bailey's Crossroads, Virginia 22041

WASHINGTON

Medical Assistant Program (1)
Highline Community College
S. 240th & Pacific Hwy. S.
Des Moines, Washington 98198

Medical Assistant Program (1)
Edmonds Community College
20000 68th Avenue W.
Lynnwood, Washington 98036

Medical Assistant Program (2)
Eton Technical Institute
1516 Second Avenue, Suite 100
Seattle, Washington 98101-2884

Medical Assistant Program (1)
North Seattle Community College
9600 College Way North
Seattle, Washington 98103

Medical Assistant Program (1)
Kinman Business University
9th Floor Bon Marche Bldg.
Spokane, Washington 99201

WISCONSIN

Medical Assistant Program (1)
Lakeshore Technical Institute
1290 North Avenue
Cleveland, Wisconsin 53015

Medical Assistant Program (1)
Northeast WI Technical Institute
2740 W. Mason St., Box 19042
Green Bay, Wisconsin 54307

Medical Assistant Program (1)
Western Wisconsin Technical Institute
304 N. 6th Street
P.O. Box 908
La Crosse, Wisconsin 54602

Medical Assistant Program (1)
Madison Area Technical College
3550 Anderson Street
Madison, Wisconsin 53704

Medical Assistant Program (1)
Mid State Voc Tech Institute
110 W. Third Street
Marshfield, Wisconsin 54449

Medical Assistant Program (1)
Milwaukee Area Technical College
1015 N. 6th Street
Milwaukee, Wisconsin 53203

Medical Assistant Program (1)
WI Indianhead Technical Institute
1019 S. Knowles Avenue
New Richmond, Wisconsin 54017

Medical Assistant Program (1)
Waukesha County Technical Institute
800 Main Street
Pewaukee, Wisconsin 53072

Medical Assistant Program (1)
Gateway Technical Institute
1001 S. Main Street
Racine, Wisconsin 53403

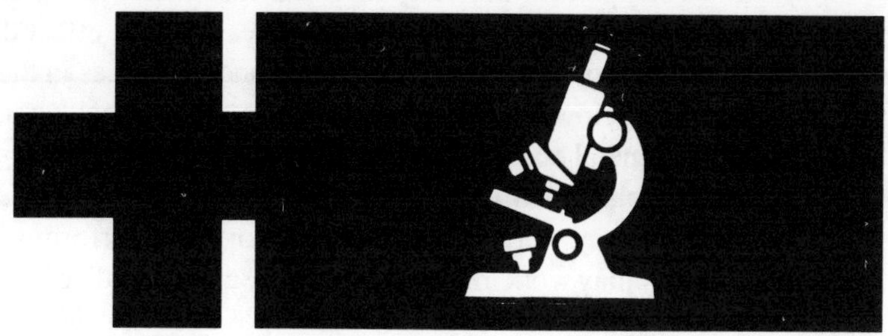

MEDICAL LABORATORY

The medical or clinical laboratory is essential to the modern practice of medicine. Tests and studies are carried out in the medical laboratory with the use of precision instruments and automated and electronic equipment to determine causes and patterns of disease, to develop better diagnostic procedures, and to innovate new methodologies in preventive medicine. The tests are specifically designed to both assist medical staff in making or confirming diagnoses and also to evaluate the effectiveness of medical treatment.

Laboratories are located in hospitals of all sizes; clinics; physicians' offices; independent laboratory companies; public health agencies; pharmaceutical and industrial companies; medical, dental, and veterinary schools; and research institutions.

In medical laboratories tests are generally performed in six fields of basic science, all oriented to provide data on the cause, cure, and prevention of disease. They are as follows: *bacteriology (microbiology)* is the study of microorganisms in the human body; *cytology* is the study of human cells; *histology* is the study of human tissue; *biochemistry* is the study of chemical processes within the human body and of the effects of chemical compounds upon the body's physiological and biochemical functions; *immunology* is the study of the mechanisms that fight infection; and *hematology* tests blood specimens. In a large hospital each of these six fields is usually established as a specialized laboratory unit. Also in large hospitals blood banks are usually part of the hematology unit. The bank receives, stores, and preserves blood and tests it to determine its suitability for transfusion.

Career opportunities are found at every level in the medical laboratory. The pathologist (a physician who specializes in the causes and nature of disease) is the director of the medical laboratory, and he or she directly supervises laboratory specialists, or scientists, including the biochemist (a scientist who studies the chemical components of living things) and the microbiologist (a scientist who studies the relationship between bacteria and disease or the effect that antibodies have on bacteria), both of whom have earned advanced degrees in their respective fields.

Discussed below are the other careers in the medical laboratory, all of which fall under the general occupational heading of medical technology. Medical technology personnel include *medical technologists,* and *medical technicians.* Personnel in these occupations may work in a small laboratory and perform a wide range of clinical tests, or they may work in a large laboratory and specialize in one of the six previously discussed scientific fields. Certain positions in *blood banking technology, cytotechnology,* and *histologic technology* are also discussed in detail below.

In addition to all these laboratory personnel there are two occupations that provide essential services to the laboratory but require only minimal training. They are the *laboratory aide* and the *morgue attendant.*

Medical Technologist

As a top-level laboratory worker the *medical technologist* is supervised by, and works in conjunction with, the pathologist and also with other physicians and scientists. The medical technologist exercises independent judgment in carrying out a broad range of complex chemical, microscopic, and bacteriological laboratory procedures that help to identify and control disease. The technologist supervises laboratory technicians and assists in their training. She or he may also calibrate equipment and evaluate the accuracy and utility of new laboratory tests.

In a small laboratory the worker performs many types of tests and is known as a medical technologist. In a larger laboratory setting, where the technologist usually specializes in a field and has had more specialized training, he or she is referred to as a *microbiology technologist, histologic technologist, chemistry technologist, immunology technologist, hematology technologist, blood bank technologist*, or as a *cytotechnologist*, or even with more training, as a *specialist in blood bank technology, specialist in chemistry, specialist in immunology*, or *specialist in microbiology.*

The minimum educational requirement for the medical technologist is completion of a bachelor's degree program, which includes three-to-four years of course work plus a twelve-month clinical experience in an accredited hospital laboratory educational program in medical technology.

Educational programs are offered in colleges, universities and hospitals throughout the country. Accredited hospital programs affiliated with universities and colleges offer bachelor's degrees upon completion. Graduate degrees in medical technology are also available for those who wish to become highly specialized in a certain area of laboratory work or obtain upper echelon positions in teaching, administration, or research.

After graduation from an accredited bachelor's degree program which includes the twelve-month hospital course in medical technology, the candidate may take the registry examinations, and become certified as a Medical Technologist, MT(ASCP), by the Board of Registry of the American Society of Clinical Pathologists; or as a Medical Technologist,

MT, by the American Medical Technologists; or as a Registered Medical Technologist, RMT, by the International Society of Clinical Laboratory Technology, or as a Certified Medical Technologist by the National Certification Agency for Medical Laboratory Personnel. Certification is also available by the Board of Registry of the American Society of Clinical Pathologists for categorical technologists, including the Technologist in Blood Banking, BB(ASCP); Technologist in Chemistry, C(ASCP); Technologist in Hematology, H(ASCP); Technologist in Immunology, I(ASCP); Technologist in Microbiology, M(ASCP); Cytotechnologist, CT(ASCP); and Histotechnologist, HTL(ASCP). To qualify for certification, these categorical technologists must have a bachelor's degree plus one-to-two years of full-time acceptable laboratory experience in their respective fields, and successful completion of the categorical certification examination.

To date, a license to practice as a medical technologist is required in the following states: California, Florida, Hawaii, Nevada, and Tennessee. Georgia requires certification for practicing medical technologists. Write to the State Board of Occupational Licensing for specifics on state requirements.

Scholarships are available for qualified high school seniors who are entering a medical technology career. Interested students should contact the Scholarship Committee, American Medical Technologists, 710 Higgins Road, Park Ridge, Illinois 60068. For information on other types of financial assistance, write directly to the colleges and universities listed at the end of this chapter.

Based on a 1987 salary survey conducted by the University of Texas Medical Branch, starting salaries for medical technologists working in hospitals, medical schools, and medical centers averaged $19,800 annually, while those medical technologists with several years experience average $27,000.

For more details on a career in medical technology, write to the American Medical Technologists, 710 Higgins Road, Park Ridge, Illinois 60068, and the American Society of Clinical Pathologists, 2100 W. Harrison Street, Chicago, Illinois 60612.

Certification information can be obtained from any of the following agencies: American Society of Clinical Pathologists, Board of Registry, 2100 West Harrison St., Chicago, Illinois 60612; American Medical Technologists, 710 Higgins Road, Park Ridge, Illinois 60068; International Society for Clinical Laboratory Technology, 818 Olive Street, St. Louis, Missouri 63101; or the National Certification Agency for Medical Laboratory Personnel, P.O. Box 705, Ben Franklin Station, Washington, D.C. 20044.

Below is a list of educational programs in medical technology accredited by the American Medical Association's Committee on Allied Health Education and Accreditation. These programs are usually twelve-to-eighteen months in length, require two-to-four years of college as their entrance requirement, and award bachelor's degrees and/or certificates.

SOURCES:

American Medical Technologists
American Society of Clinical Pathologists
Occupational Outlook Handbook

Medical Technologist Programs

ALABAMA

Medical Technologist Program
Baptist Medical Centers
3201 Fourth Avenue, S.
Birmingham, Alabama 35222

Medical Technologist Program
St. Vincent's Hospital
2701 9th Court, S.
P.O. Box 915
Birmingham, Alabama 35201

Medical Technologist Program
The University of Alabama at Birmingham
University Station
Birmingham, Alabama 35294

Medical Technologist Program
Lloyd Noland Hospital
701 Ridgeway Road
Birmingham, Alabama 35064

Medical Technologist Program
Holy Name of Jesus Hospital
Moragne Park
Gadsden, Alabama 35901

Medical Technologist Program
Huntsville Cooperative School of Med. Tech
101 Sivley Road
Huntsville, Alabama 35801

Medical Technologist Program
Mobile Infirmary Medical Center
N. End of Louiselle St.
Mobile, Alabama 36652

Medical Technologist Program
University of South Alabama
307 University Boulevard
Mobile, Alabama 36688

Medical Technologist Program
Auburn University of Montgomery
Montgomery, Alabama 36193

Medical Technologist Program
Baptist Medical Center
2105 E. South Boulevard
Montgomery, Alabama 36198

Medical Technologist Program
St. Margaret's Hospital
301 S. Ripley Street
P.O. Drawer 311
Montgomery, Alabama 36195-4701

Medical Technologist Program
DCH Regional Medical Center
809 University Blvd. E.
Tuscaloosa, Alabama 35403

Medical Technologist Program
Tuskegee University
Kresge Center
Tuskegee Institute, Alabama 36088

ARIZONA

Medical Technologist Program
Arizona State University
Tempe, Arizona 85287

Medical Technologist Program
University of Arizona
Tucson, Arizona 85721

ARKANSAS

Medical Technologist Program
Arkansas College
2300 Highland Road
Batesville, Arkansas 72501

Medical Technologist Program
Antaeus Lineal Research Associates
2470 N. Gregg, Box 817
Fayetteville, Arkansas 72701

Medical Technologist Program
Sparks Regional Medical Center
1311 South "I" Street
Fort Smith, Arkansas 72901

Medical Technologist Program
St. Edward Mercy Medical Center
7301 Rogers Avenue
Fort Smith, Arkansas 72903

Medical Technologist Program
Baptist Medical Center
9601 Interstate 630 Exit 7
Little Rock, Arkansas 72205-7299

Medical Technologist Program
University of Arkansas for Medical Sciences
4301 W. Markham
Little Rock, Arkansas 72205

Medical Technologist Program
Arkansas State University
P.O. Box 10
State University, Arkansas 72467

CALIFORNIA

Medical Technologist Program
California State College
9001 Stockdale Hwy.
Bakersfield, California 93309

Medical Technologist Program
Kern Medical Center
1830 Flower Street
Bakersfield, California 93305-4197

Medical Technologist Program
St. Joseph Medical Center
Buena Vista & Alameda Sts.
Burbank, California 91505

Medical Technologist Program
Peninsula Hospital & Medical Center
1783 El Camino Real
Burlingame, California 94010

Medical Technologist Program
California State University
1000 E. Victoria Street
Carson, California 90747

Medical Technologist Program
Fresno Community Hospital & Medical Center
P.O. Box 1232
Fresno, California 93715

Medical Technologist Program
Valley Childrens Hospital
3151 N. Millbrook Avenue
Fresno, California 93703

Medical Technologist Program
Valley Medical Center at Fresno
445 S. Cedar Avenue
Fresno, California 93702

Medical Technologist Program
Centinela Hospital Medical Center
555 E. Hardy Street, Box 720
Inglewood, California 90307

Medical Technologist Program
Daniel Freeman Memorial Hospital
333 N. Prairie Ave.
Inglewood, California 90301

Medical Technologist Program
The Green Hospital of Scripps Clinic
10666 North Torrey Pines Rd.
La Jolla, California 92037

Medical Technologist Program
Scripps Memorial Hospital
9888 Genesee Avenue
La Jolla, California 92037

Medical Technologist Program
Grossmont District Hospital
5555 Grossmont Center Dr.
La Mesa, California 92041

Medical Technologist Program
Loma Linda University
School of Allied Health Professions
Loma Linda, California 92350

Medical Technologist Program
Memorial Medical Center
2801 Atlantic Avenue
Long Beach, California 90801-1428

Medical Technologist Program
St. Mary Medical Center-Bauer Hospital
1050 Linden Avenue
Long Beach, California 90813

Medical Technologist Program
VA Medical Center
5901 East 7th Street
Long Beach, California 90822

Medical Technologist Program
Cedars-Sinai Medical Center
8700 Beverly Boulevard
Los Angeles, California 90048

Medical Technologist Program
Childrens Hospital of Los Angeles
4650 Sunset Boulevard
Los Angeles, California 90027

Medical Technologist Program
Clinical Lab Med Group & Affiliated Labs
2222 Ocean View Avenue
Los Angeles, California 90057

Medical Technologist Program
Hollywood Presbyterian Medical Center
1300 North Vermont Avenue
Los Angeles, California 90027

Medical Technologist Program
King Drew Medical Center
1621 E. 120th Street
Los Angeles, California 90059

Medical Technologist Program
Los Angeles County-USC Medical Center
1200 N. State Street
Los Angeles, California 90033

Medical Technologist Program
UCLA Center for Health Sciences-Clinical Labs
10833 Le Conte Avenue
Los Angeles, California 90024

Medical Technologist Program
VA-Wadsworth Medical Center
Wilshire & Sawtelle Boulevards
Los Angeles, California 90073

Medical Technologist Program
White Memorial Medical Center
1720 Brooklyn Avenue
Los Angeles, California 90033

Medical Technologist Program
Veterans Administration Medical Center
150 Muir Road
Martinez, California 94553

Medical Technologist Program
El Camino Hospital
2500 Grant Road
Mountain View, California 94040

Medical Technologist Program
St. Joseph Hospital
1100 Stewart Drive
Orange, California 92668

Medical Technologist Program
Univ. of CA Irvine Medical Center & Blood Bank
101 City Drive South
Orange, California 92668

Medical Technologist Program
Huntington Memorial Hospital
100 Congress Street
Pasadena, California 91105

Medical Technologist Program
St. Luke Hospital
2632 E. Washington Blvd.
Pasadena, California 91109-7021

Medical Technologist Program
Eisenhower Medical Center
39000 Bob Hope Drive
Rancho Mirage, California 92270

Medical Technologist Program
Sutter Community Hospitals
1111 Howe Ave., Suite 600
Sacramento, California 95825

Medical Technologist Program
University of CA Davis Medical Center
2315 Stockton Boulevard
Sacramento, California 95817

Medical Technologist Program
Natividad Medical Center
1330 Natividad Road
P.O. Box 1611
Salinas, California 93902

Medical Technologist Program
San Bernardino County Medical Center
780 E. Gilbert Street
San Bernardino, California 92415-0935

Medical Technologist Program
Mercy Hospital & Medical Center
4077 Fifth Avenue
San Diego, California 92103

Medical Technologist Program
Sharp Memorial Hospital
7901 Frost Street
San Diego, California 92123

Medical Technologist Program
Children's Hospital of San Francisco
3700 California Street
San Francisco, California 94118

Medical Technologist Program
Mt. Zion Hospital & Medical Center
1600 Divisadero Street
San Francisco, California 94115

Medical Technologist Program
San Francisco State University
1600 Holloway
San Francisco, California 94132

Medical Technologist Program
San Jose Hospital & Health Center, Inc.
675 E. Santa Clara Street
San Jose, California 95112

Medical Technologist Program
Santa Clara Valley Medical Center
751 S. Bascom Avenue
San Jose, California 95128

Medical Technologist Program
Santa Barbara Cottage Hospital
P.O. Box 689, Pueblo at Bath
Santa Barbara, California 93102

Medical Technologist Program
St. John's Hospital and Health Center
1328 22nd Street
Santa Monica, California 90404

Medical Technologist Program
Sepulveda VA Medical Center
16111 Plummer Street
Sepulveda, California 91343

Medical Technologist Program
Little Company of Mary Hospital
4101 Torrance Boulevard
Torrance, California 90503

Medical Technologist Program
LAC Harbor-UCLA Medical Center
1000 W. Carson Street
Torrance, California 90509

COLORADO

Medical Technologist Program
Memorial Hospital
1400 E. Boulder Street
P.O. Box 1326
Colorado Springs, Colorado 80901

Medical Technologist Program
Penrose Hospitals
2215 N. Cascade Avenue
P.O. Box 7021
Colorado Springs, Colorado 80933

Medical Technologist Program
Presbyterian St. Luke's Medical Center
1719 E. 19th Avenue
Denver, Colorado 80218

Medical Technologist Program
St. Anthony Hospital
4231 West 16th
Denver, Colorado 80204

Medical Technologist Program
Univ. of Colorado Health Science Center
4200 E. 9th Avenue
Denver, Colorado 80262

Medical Technologist Program
North Colorado Medical Center
1801 16th Street
Greeley, Colorado 80631-5199

Medical Technologist Program
Parkview Episcopal Medical Center
400 W. 16th Street
Pueblo, Colorado 81003

CONNECTICUT

Medical Technologist Program
Bridgeport Hospital
267 Grant Street
Bridgeport, Connecticut 06610

Medical Technologist Program
St. Vincent's Medical Center
2800 Main Street
Bridgeport, Connecticut 06606

Medical Technologist Program
Danbury Hospital
24 Hospital Avenue
Danbury, Connecticut 06810

Medical Technologist Program
Quinnipiac College
Mt. Carmel Avenue
Hamden, Connecticut 06518

Medical Technologist Program
Hartford Hospital
80 Seymour Street
Hartford, Connecticut 06115

Medical Technologist Program
St. Joseph Hospital
128 Strawberry Hill Ave.
Stamford, Connecticut 06904-1222

Medical Technologist Program
St. Mary's Hospital
56 Franklin Street
Waterbury, Connecticut 06702

Medical Technologist Program
Waterbury Hospital Health Center
64 Robbins Street
Waterbury, Connecticut 06721

Medical Technologist Program
The University of Hartford
200 Bloomfield Avenue
West Hartford, Connecticut 06117

DELAWARE

Medical Technologist Program
Wesley College
College Square
Dover, Delaware 19901

Medical Technologist Program
University of Delaware
Hullihen Hall
Newark, Delaware 19716

DISTRICT OF COLUMBIA

Medical Technologist Program
George Washington University Medical Center
2121 Eye Street, N.W., Suite. 800
Washington, D.C. 20037

Medical Technologist Program
Howard University
2400 6th Street, N.W.
Washington, D.C. 20059

Medical Technologist Program
The Catholic University of America
103 Executive Bldg.
Washington, D.C. 20064

Medical Technologist Program
Walter Reed Army Medical Center
Washington, D.C. 20307-5001

Medical Technologist Program
Washington Hospital Center
110 Irving Street, N.W.
Washington, D.C. 20010

FLORIDA

Medical Technologist Program
Florida Atlantic University
Boca Raton, Florida 33431

Medical Technologist Program
Bethune-Cookman College
640 Second Avenue
Daytona Beach, Florida 32015

Medical Technologist Program
University of Florida
226 Tigert Hall
Gainesville, Florida 32611

Medical Technologist Program
Baptist Medical Center
800 Prudential Drive
Jacksonville, Florida 32207

Medical Technologist Program
St. Vincent's Medical Center
1800 Barrs Street
P.O. Box 2982
Jacksonville, Florida 32203

Medical Technologist Program
University Hospital of Jacksonville
655 West 8th Street
Jacksonville, Florida 32209

Medical Technologist Program
Florida International University
Tamiami Trail
Miami, Florida 33199

Medical Technologist Program
Mt. Sinai Medical Center
4300 Alton Road
Miami Beach, Florida 33140

Medical Technologist Program
Florida Hospital
601 E. Rollins Street
Orlando, Florida 32803

Medical Technologist Program
University of Central Florida
P.O. Box 25000
Orlando, Florida 32816

Medical Technologist Program
Baptist Hospital
1000 W. Moreno Street
Pensacola, Florida 32501

Medical Technologist Program
Sacred Heart Hospital
5151 N. 9th Avenue
Pensacola, Florida 32504

Medical Technologist Program
Bayfront Medical Center, Inc.
701 6th Street, South
St. Petersburg, Florida 33701

Medical Technologist Program
Tallahassee Memorial Regional Medical Center
Magnolia Road
Tallahassee, Florida 32308

Medical Technologist Program
The Tampa General Hospital
Davis Island
Tampa, Florida 33606

GEORGIA

Medical Technologist Program
Crawford W. Long Memorial Hospital
35 Linden Avenue
Atlanta, Georgia 30365

Medical Technologist Program
Emory University Hospital
1364 Clifton Rd., N.E.
Atlanta, Georgia 30322

Medical Technologist Program
Georgia Baptist Medical Center
300 Boulevard, N.E.
Atlanta, Georgia 30312

Medical Technologist Program
Georgia State University
University Plaza
Atlanta, Georgia 30303-3090

Medical Technologist Program
Grady Memorial Hospital
80 Butler Street, S.E.
Atlanta, Georgia 30335

Medical Technologist Program
Piedmont Hospital
1968 Peachtree Rd., NW
Atlanta, Georgia 30309

Medical Technologist Program
Medical College of Georgia
Office of the President, AA-31
Augusta, Georgia 30912-0450

Medical Technologist Program
Columbus College
Algonquin Drive
Columbus, Georgia 31993

Medical Technologist Program
Armstrong State College
11935 Abercorn Street
Savannah, Georgia 31419-1997

HAWAII

Medical Technologist Program
Kaiser Foundation Hospital
3288 Moanalua
Honolulu, Hawaii 96819

Medical Technologist Program
St. Francis Hospital
2230 Liliha Street
Honolulu, Hawaii 96817

Medical Technologist Program
The Queen's Medical Center
1301 Punchbowl Street
Honolulu, Hawaii 96813

Medical Technologist Program
University of Hawaii at Manoa
2538 The Mall
Honolulu, Hawaii 96822

IDAHO

Medical Technologist Program
St. Alphonsus Regional Medical Center
1055 N. Curtis Road
Boise, Idaho 83706

Medical Technologist Program
St. Luke's Regional Medical Center
190 E. Bannock
Boise, Idaho 83712

Medical Technologist Program
Bannock Regional Medical Center
Memorial Drive
Pocatello, Idaho 83201

ILLINOIS

Medical Technologist Program
St. Elizabeth Hospital
211 S. Third Street
Belleville, Illinois 62221

Medical Technologist Program
St. Francis Hospital
12935 S. Gregory Street
Blue Island, Illinois 60406

Medical Technologist Program
Burnham Hospital
407 S. Fourth Street
Champaign, Illinois 61820

Medical Technologist Program
Holy Cross Hospital
2701 W. 68th Street
Chicago, Illinois 60629

Medical Technologist Program
Illinois Masonic Medical Center
836 W. Wellington Avenue
Chicago, Illinois 60657

Medical Technologist Program
Louis A. Weiss Memorial Hospital
4646 N. Marine Drive
Chicago, Illinois 60640

Medical Technologist Program
Michael Reese Hospital & Medical Center
29th South Ellis
Chicago, Illinois 60616

Medical Technologist Program
Rush Presbyterian-St. Luke's Medical Center
1653 West Congress Parkway
Chicago, Illinois 60612

Medical Technologist Program
St. Joseph Hospital
2900 N. Lake Shore Drive
Chicago, Illinois 60657

Medical Technologist Program
St. Mary of Nazareth Hospital Center
2233 West Division Street
Chicago, Illinois 60622

Medical Technologist Program
University of Illinois at Chicago
1737 W. Polk Street
Chicago, Illinois 60680

Medical Technologist Program
Lake View Medical Center
812 N. Logan Avenue
Danville, Illinois 61832

Medical Technologist Program
Decatur Memorial Hospital
2300 N. Edward Street
Decatur, Illinois 62526

Medical Technologist Program
St. Mary's Hospital
1800 E. Lake Shore Drive
Decatur, Illinois 62521-3883

Medical Technologist Program
Evanston Hospital
2650 Ridge Avenue
Evanston, Illinois 60201

Medical Technologist Program
Freeport Memorial Hospital
1045 W. Stephenson Street
Freeport, Illinois 61032

Medical Technologist Program
Edward Hines Jr. VA Hospital
Fifth Ave. & Roosevelt Rd.
Hines, Illinois 60141

Medical Technologist Program
Hinsdale Hospital
120 N. Oak Street
Hinsdale, Illinois 60521

Medical Technologist Program
St. Joseph Hospital
333 N. Madison Street
Joliet, Illinois 60435

Medical Technologist Program
Foster G. McGaw Hospital of Loyola Univ.
2160 S. First Avenue
Maywood, Illinois 60153

Medical Technologist Program
Univ. of Health Sciences/Chicago Medical School
3333 Greenbay Road
North Chicago, Illinois 60064

Medical Technologist Program
Christ Hospital
4440 W. 95th Street
Oak Lawn, Illinois 60453

Medical Technologist Program
West Suburban Hospital Medical Center
Erie at Austin Boulevard
Oak Park, Illinois 60302

Medical Technologist Program
Lutheran General Hospital
1775 Dempster Street
Park Ridge, Illinois 60068

Medical Technologist Program
Methodist Medical Center of Illinois
221 N.E. Glen Oak
Peoria, Illinois 61636

Medical Technologist Program
St. Francis Medical Center
530 N.E. Glen Oak Avenue
Peoria, Illinois 61637

Medical Technologist Program
St. Mary Hospital
1415 Vermont Street
Quincy, Illinois 62301

Medical Technologist Program
Augustana College-Quad-City Hospital
Rock Island, Illinois 61201

Medical Technologist Program
Rockford Memorial Hospital
2400 N. Rockton Avenue
Rockford, Illinois 61103

Medical Technologist Program
St. Anthony Hospital Medical Center
5666 E. State Street
Rockford, Illinois 61108

Medical Technologist Program
Swedish American Hospital
1400 Charles Street
Rockford, Illinois 61108

Medical Technologist Program
Sangamon State University
Shepherd Road
Springfield, Illinois 62708

Medical Technologist Program
St. John's Hospital
800 E. Carpenter
Springfield, Illinois 62769

Medical Technologist Program
Governors State University
Route 54 & Stuenkel Road
University Park, Illinois 60466

Medical Technologist Program
Carle Foundation Hospital
611 W. Park Street
Urbana, Illinois 61801

Medical Technologist Program
St. Therese Hospital
2615 W. Washington Street
Waukegan, Illinois 60085

INDIANA

Medical Technologist Program
St. John's Medical Center
2015 Jackson Street
Anderson, Indiana 46014

Medical Technologist Program
St. Francis Hospital Center
1600 Albany Street
Beech Grove, Indiana 46107

Medical Technologist Program
Deaconess Hospital, Inc.
600 Mary Street
Evansville, Indiana 47747

Medical Technologist Program
St. Mary's Medical Center
3700 Washington Avenue
Evansville, Indiana 47750

Medical Technologist Program
Lutheran Hospital
3024 Fairfield Avenue
Fort Wayne, Indiana 46807

Medical Technologist Program
Parkview Memorial Hospital
2200 Randallia Drive
Fort Wayne, Indiana 46805

Medical Technologist Program
St. Joseph's Hospital of Fort Wayne, Inc.
700 Broadway
Fort Wayne, Indiana 46802

Medical Technologist Program
St. Mary Medical Center
640 Tyler Street
Gary, Indiana 46402

Medical Technologist Program
St. Margaret Hospital
5454 Hohman Avenue
Hammond, Indiana 46320

Medical Technologist Program
Community Hospital of Indianapolis, Inc.
1500 N. Ritter Avenue
Indianapolis, Indiana 46219

Medical Technologist Program
Indiana University School of Medicine
1120 South Drive
Indianapolis, Indiana 46223

Medical Technologist Program
Methodist Hospital of Indiana, Inc.
1604 N. Capitol Ave., Box 1367
Indianapolis, Indiana 46206

Medical Technologist Program
St. Vincent Hospital & Health Care Center
2001 W. 88th Street
Box 40970
Indianapolis, Indiana 46240-0970

Medical Technologist Program
St. Joseph Memorial Hospital
1907 W. Sycamore Street
Kokomo, Indiana 46901

Medical Technologist Program
Ball Memorial Hospital Association, Inc.
2401 University Avenue
Muncie, Indiana 47302

Medical Technologist Program
Indiana State University
Terre Haute, Indiana 47809

Medical Technologist Program
Good Samaritan Hospital
520 South 7th Street
Vincennes, Indiana 47591

IOWA

Medical Technologist Program
St. Luke's Methodist Hospital
1026 "A" Avenue N.E.
Cedar Rapids, Iowa 52402

Medical Technologist Program
Mercy Hospital
P.O. Box 1C
Council Bluffs, Iowa 51502

Medical Technologist Program
Iowa Methodist Medical Center
1200 Pleasant Street
Des Moines, Iowa 50308

Medical Technologist Program
Mercy Hospital Medical Center
6th & University
Des Moines, Iowa 50314

Medical Technologist Program
The University of Iowa
101 Jessup Hall
Iowa City, Iowa 52242

Medical Technologist Program
Marian Health Center
801 5th Street
Sioux City, Iowa 51101

Medical Technologist Program
St. Luke's Medical Center
2720 Stone Park Boulevard
Sioux City, Iowa 51104

Medical Technologist Program
Allen Memorial Hospital
1825 Logan Ave-Administration
Waterloo, Iowa 50613

Medical Technologist Program
Consolidated Regional Labs
Kimball & Ridgeway
Waterloo, Iowa 50702

KANSAS

Medical Technologist Program
Providence-St. Margaret Health Center
8929 Parallel Parkway
Kansas City, Kansas 66112

Medical Technologist Program
University of Kansas Medical Center
39th & Rainbow Boulevard
Kansas City, Kansas 66103

Medical Technologist Program
Topeka School of Medical Technology
1505 W. 8th Street
Topeka, Kansas 66606

Medical Technologist Program
St. Francis Regional Medical Center
929 N. St. Francis Avenue
Wichita, Kansas 67214

Medical Technologist Program
Wichita State University
P.O. Box 1
Wichita, Kansas 67208

KENTUCKY

Medical Technologist Program
St. Elizabeth Medical Center
401 E. 20th Street
Covington, Kentucky 41014

Medical Technologist Program
University of Kentucky
103 Administration Bldg.
Lexington, Kentucky 40506-0032

Medical Technologist Program
Sts Mary & Elizabeth Hospital
4400 Churchman Avenue
Louisville, Kentucky 40215

Medical Technologist Program
University of Louisville
Administration Bldg.
Louisville, Kentucky 40292

Medical Technologist Program
Owensboro-Daviess County Hospital
Box 2799
12th & Triplett Streets
Owensboro, Kentucky 42302-2799

Medical Technologist Program
Lourdes Hospital
1530 Lone Oak Road
Paducah, Kentucky 42001

Medical Technologist Program
Methodist Hospital of Kentucky
US 23 By-Pass; H. Branch Rd.
Pikeville, Kentucky 41501

Medical Technologist Program
Eastern Kentucky University
Coates Admin. Bldg.
Richmond, Kentucky 40475

LOUISIANA

Medical Technologist Program
Rapides General Hospital
Box 30101
211 Fourth Street
Alexandria, Louisiana 71301

Medical Technologist Program
St. Frances Cabrini Hospital
3330 Masonic Drive
Alexandria, Louisiana 71301

Medical Technologist Program
Earl K. Long Memorial Hospital
5825 Airline Hwy.
Baton Rouge, Louisiana 70805

Medical Technologist Program
Our Lady of the Lake Regional Medical Center
500 Hennessy Boulevard
Baton Rouge, Louisiana 70809

Medical Technologist Program
Southeastern Louisiana University
P.O. Box 784
Hammond, Louisiana 70402

Medical Technologist Program
South Louisiana Medical Center
1978 Industrial Boulevard
Houma, Louisiana 70363

Medical Technologist Program
University Medical Center
2390 W. Congress
P.O. Box 4016-C
Lafayette, Louisiana 70502

Medical Technologist Program
Lake Charles Memorial Hospital
1701 Oak Park Boulevard
Lake Charles, Louisiana 70601

Medical Technologist Program
St. Patrick Hospital
524 S. Ryan Street
Lake Charles, Louisiana 70601

Medical Technologist Program
St. Francis Medical Center
309 Jackson Street
Monroe, Louisiana 71201

Medical Technologist Program
Alton Ochsner Medical Foundation
1516 Jefferson Hwy.
New Orleans, Louisiana 70121

Medical Technologist Program
Charity Hospital of LA at New Orleans
1532 Tulane Avenue
New Orleans, Louisiana 70140

Medical Technologist Program
L.S.U. Medical Center
1440 Canal Street
New Orleans, Louisiana 70112

Medical Technologist Program
Southern Baptist Hospital
2700 Napoleon Avenue
New Orleans, Louisiana 70175

Medical Technologist Program
Touro Infirmary
1401 Foucher Street
New Orleans, Louisiana 70115

Medical Technologist Program
Veterans Administration Hospital
1601 Perdido Street
New Orleans, Louisiana 70146

Medical Technologist Program
Schumpert Medical Center
915 Margaret Place
Shreveport, Louisiana 71101

Medical Technologist Program
Veterans Administration Medical Center
510 East Stoner Avenue
Shreveport, Louisiana 71130

MAINE

Medical Technologist Program
Eastern Maine Medical Center
489 State Street
Bangor, Maine 04401-6674

Medical Technologist Program
Central Maine Medical Center
300 Main Street
Lewiston, Maine 04240-0305

Medical Technologist Program
Maine Medical Center
22 Bramhall Street
Portland, Maine 04102

MARYLAND

Medical Technologist Program
Mercy Hospital, Inc.
301 St. Paul Place
Baltimore, Maryland 21202

Medical Technologist Program
The Union Memorial Hospital
201 E. University Pkwy.
Baltimore, Maryland 21218

Medical Technologist Program
University of Maryland School of Medicine
522 W. Lombard Street
Baltimore, Maryland 21201

Medical Technologist Program
Oscar B. Hunter Memorial Laboratory
8218 Wisconsin Ave., Suite 201
Bethesda, Maryland 20014

Medical Technologist Program
Malcolm Grow USAF Medical Center
Andrews AFB, DC
Camp Springs, Maryland 20331

Medical Technologist Program
Salisbury State College
Holloway Hall
Salisbury, Maryland 21801

Medical Technologist Program
Columbia Union College
7600 Flower Avenue
Takoma Park, Maryland 20912

MASSACHUSETTS

Medical Technologist Program
Carney Hospital
2100 Dorchester Avenue
Boston, Massachusetts 02124

Medical Technologist Program
New England Deaconess Hospital
110 Francis Street
Boston, Massachusetts 02215

Medical Technologist Program
Northeastern University
360 Huntington Avenue
Boston, Massachusetts 02115

Medical Technologist Program
Veterans Administration Medical Center
150 S. Huntington Avenue
Boston, Massachusetts 02130

Medical Technologist Program
The Cambridge Hospital
1493 Cambridge Street
Cambridge, Massachusetts 02139

Medical Technologist Program
Burbank Hospital School of Medical Technology
42 Nichols Road
Fitchburg, Massachusetts 01420

Medical Technologist Program
Framingham Union Hospital
115 Lincoln Street
Framingham, Massachusetts 01701

Medical Technologist Program
Lawrence General Hospital
1 General Street
Lawrence, Massachusetts 01842

Medical Technologist Program
University of Lowell
1 University Avenue
Lowell, Massachusetts 01854

Medical Technologist Program
Newton-Wellesley Hospital
2014 Washington Street
Newton, Massachusetts 02162

Medical Technologist Program
Southeastern Massachusetts University
North Dartmouth, Massachusetts 02747

Medical Technologist Program
Berkshire Medical Center
725 North Street
Pittsfield, Massachusetts 01201

Medical Technologist Program
Salem Hospital
81 Highland Avenue
Salem, Massachusetts 01970

Medical Technologist Program
Baystate Medical Center
759 Chestnut Street
Springfield, Massachusetts 01199

Medical Technologist Program
Mercy Hospital
271 Carew Street
P.O. Box 9012
Springfield, Massachusetts 01102-9012

Medical Technologist Program
Worcester City Hospital
26 Queen Street
Worcester, Massachusetts 01610

MICHIGAN

Medical Technologist Program
University of Michigan
Fleming Admin. Bldg.
Ann Arbor, Michigan 48109

Medical Technologist Program
Ferris State College
901 S. State Street, Starr 304
Big Rapids, Michigan 49307

Medical Technologist Program
Oakwood Hospital
18101 Oakwood Boulevard
Dearborn, Michigan 48124

Medical Technologist Program
Detroit Receiving Hospital-University Health Center
4201 St. Antoine
Detroit, Michigan 48201

Medical Technologist Program
Harper-Grace Hospitals
3990 John R Street
Detroit, Michigan 48201-2097

Medical Technologist Program
Henry Ford Hospital
2799 W. Grand Boulevard
Detroit, Michigan 48202

Medical Technologist Program
Hutzel Hospital
4707 St. Antoine
Detroit, Michigan 48201

Medical Technologist Program
Mercy College of Detroit
8200 W. Outer Drive, Box 99
Detroit, Michigan 48219

Medical Technologist Program
St. John Hospital
22101 Moross Road
Detroit, Michigan 48236

Medical Technologist Program
Wayne State University
1142 Mackenzie Hall
Detroit, Michigan 48202

Medical Technologist Program
Michigan State University
438 Administration Bldg.
East Lansing, Michigan 48824

Medical Technologist Program
Flint Osteopathic Hospital
3921 Beecher Road
Flint, Michigan 48502

Medical Technologist Program
Hurley Medical Center
Number One Hurley Plaza
Flint, Michigan 48502

Medical Technologist Program
Mc Laren General Hospital
401 S. Ballenger Hwy.
Flint, Michigan 48502

Medical Technologist Program
St. Joseph Hospital
302 Kensington Avenue
Flint, Michigan 48502

Medical Technologist Program
Garden City Hospital, Osteopathic
6245 N. Inkster Road
Garden City, Michigan 48135

Medical Technologist Program
Blodgett Memorial Medical Center
1840 Wealthy Street, S.E.
Grand Rapids, Michigan 49506

Medical Technologist Program
Butterworth Hospital
100 Michigan, N.E.
Grand Rapids, Michigan 49503

Medical Technologist Program
St. Mary's Hospital
200 Jefferson Avenue, S.E.
Grand Rapids, Michigan 49503

Medical Technologist Program
W.A. Foote Memorial Hospital, Inc.
205 N. East Avenue
Jackson, Michigan 49201

Medical Technologist Program
Borgess Medical Center
1521 Gull Road
Kalamazoo, Michigan 49001

Medical Technologist Program
Bronson Methodist Hospital
252 E. Lovell Street
Kalamazoo, Michigan 49007

Medical Technologist Program
Edward W. Sparrow Hospital
1215 E. Michigan
P.O. Box 30480
Lansing, Michigan 48909

Medical Technologist Program
St. Lawrence Hospital
1210 W. Saginaw
Lansing, Michigan 48915

Medical Technologist Program
Northern Michigan Hospitals, Inc.
416 Connable Avenue
Petoskey, Michigan 49770

Medical Technologist Program
Pontiac General Hospital
Pontiac, Michigan 48053

Medical Technologist Program
Port Huron Hospital
1001 Kearney Street
Port Huron, Michigan 48060

Medical Technologist Program
William Beaumont Hospital
3601 W. 13 Miles Road
Royal Oak, Michigan 48072

Medical Technologist Program
Saginaw Medical Center School of Clinical
Laboratory Science
100 Houghton Avenue
Saginaw, Michigan 48602

Medical Technologist Program
St. Mary's Hospital
830 S. Jefferson
Saginaw, Michigan 48601

Medical Technologist Program
Providence Hospital
16001 W. Nine Mile Road
Southfield, Michigan 48037

Medical Technologist Program
Munson Medical Center
6th & Madison Streets
Traverse City, Michigan 49684

Medical Technologist Program
Westland Medical Center
2345 Merriman Road
Westland, Michigan 48185

Medical Technologist Program
Eastern Michigan University
143 Pierce Hall
Ypsilanti, Michigan 48197

MINNESOTA

Medical Technologist Program
College of St. Scholastica
1200 Kenwood Avenue
Duluth, Minnesota 55811

Medical Technologist Program
St. Luke's Hospital
915 E. 1st Street
Duluth, Minnesota 55805

Medical Technologist Program
Abbott-Northwestern Hospital, Inc.
800 E. 28th Street
Minneapolis, Minnesota 55407

Medical Technologist Program
Hennepin County Medical Center
701 Park Avenue S.
Minneapolis, Minnesota 55415

Medical Technologist Program
Metropolitan Medical Center
900 S. 8th Street
Minneapolis, Minnesota 55404

Medical Technologist Program
University of Minnesota Health Science Center
213 Morrill Hall
Minneapolis, Minnesota 55455

Medical Technologist Program
St. Cloud Hospital
1406 6th Avenue N.
St. Cloud, Minnesota 56301

Medical Technologist Program
St. Joseph's Hospital
69 W. Exchange Street
St. Paul, Minnesota 55102

Medical Technologist Program
St. Paul-Ramsey Medical Center
640 Jackson Street
St. Paul, Minnesota 55101

Medical Technologist Program
United Hospitals, Inc.
333 N. Smith Avenue
St. Paul, Minnesota 55102

MISSISSIPPI

Medical Technologist Program
University of Southern Mississippi
Southern Station
Hattiesburg, Mississippi 39406

Medical Technologist Program
William Carey College
Tuscan Avenue
Hattiesburg, Mississippi 39401

Medical Technologist Program
Mississippi Baptist Medical Center
1225 N. State Street
Jackson, Mississippi 39202

Medical Technologist Program
University of Mississippi Medical Center
2500 N. State Street
Jackson, Mississippi 39216-4505

Medical Technologist Program
North Mississippi Medical Center
830 S. Gloster
Tupelo, Mississippi 38801

MISSOURI

Medical Technologist Program
St. Francis Medical Center
211 St. Francis Drive
Cape Giradeau, Missouri 63701

Medical Technologist Program
University of Missouri-Columbia
105 Jesse Hall
Columbia, Missouri 65211

Medical Technologist Program
St. John's Regional Medical Center
2727 McClelland Boulevard
Joplin, Missouri 64801

Medical Technologist Program
Avila College
11901 Wornall Road
Kansas City, Missouri 64145-9990

Medical Technologist Program
Baptist Medical Center
6601 Rockhill Road
Kansas City, Missouri 64131

Medical Technologist Program
Menorah Medical Center
4949 Rockhill Road
Kansas City, Missouri 64110

Medical Technologist Program
Research Medical Center
2316 E. Meyer Boulevard
Kansas City, Missouri 64132

Medical Technologist Program
St. Luke's Hospital of Kansas City
Wornall Road at 44th
Kansas City, Missouri 64111

Medical Technologist Program
St. Mary's Hospital
101 Memorial Drive
Kansas City, Missouri 64108

Medical Technologist Program
Trinity Lutheran Hospital
3030 Baltimore Street
Kansas City, Missouri 64108

Medical Technologist Program
North Kansas City Memorial Hospital
2800 Hospital Drive
North Kansas City, Missouri 64116

Medical Technologist Program
Lester E. Cox Medical Center
1423 N. Jefferson Street
Springfield, Missouri 65802

Medical Technologist Program
St. John's Regional Health Center
1235 E. Cherokee
Springfield, Missouri 65802

Medical Technologist Program
St. John's Mercy Medical Center
615 S. New Ballas Road
St. Louis, Missouri 63141

Medical Technologist Program
St. Louis University
3556 Caroline
St. Louis, Missouri 63104

Medical Technologist Program
The Jewish Hospital of St. Louis
216 S. Kingshighway Boulevard
P.O. Box 14
St. Louis, Missouri 63178

MONTANA

Medical Technologist Program
St. James Community Hospital
400 S. Clark Street
Butte, Montana 59701

Medical Technologist Program
Columbus Hospital
500 15th Avenue S.
P.O. Box 5013
Great Falls, Montana 59403

NEBRASKA

Medical Technologist Program
Nebraska Wesleyen University
50th & St. Paul Streets
Lincoln, Nebraska 68504

Medical Technologist Program
Bergan Mercy Hospital
7500 Mercy Road
Omaha, Nebraska 68124

Medical Technologist Program
Bishop Clarkson Memorial Hospital
44th & Dewey Avenue
Omaha, Nebraska 68105

Medical Technologist Program
Creighton University
California at 24th Street
Omaha, Nebraska 68178

Medical Technologist Program
Nebraska Methodist Hospital
8303 Dodge Street
Omaha, Nebraska 68114

Medical Technologist Program
University of Nebraska Medical Center
42nd & Dewey Avenue
Omaha, Nebraska 68105

NEVADA

Medical Technologist Program
University of Nevada
Reno, Nevada 89557

NEW HAMPSHIRE

Medical Technologist Program
Dartmouth Hitchcock Medical Center
Hanover, New Hampshire 03755

Medical Technologist Program
Notre Dame College
2321 Elm Street
Manchester, New Hampshire 03104

NEW JERSEY

Medical Technologist Program
Cooper Hospital-Univ. Medical Center
One Cooper Plaza
Camden, New Jersey 08103

Medical Technologist Program
Monmouth Medical Center
300 Second Avenue
Long Branch, New Jersey 07740

Medical Technologist Program
The Mountainside Hospital
Bay & Highland Avenue
Montclaire, New Jersey 07042

Medical Technologist Program
Morristown Memorial Hospital
100 Madison Avenue
Morristown, New Jersey 07960

Medical Technologist Program
Jersey Shore Medical Center-Fitkin Hospital
1945 Corlies Avenue
Neptune, New Jersey 07753

Medical Technologist Program
St. Peter's Medical Center
254 Easton Avenue
New Brunswick, New Jersey 08903

Medical Technologist Program
University of Med. & Dental of NJ-Rutgers Med School
100 Bergen Street
Newark, New Jersey 07103

Medical Technologist Program
The Hospital Center at Orange
188 S. Essex Avenue
Orange, New Jersey 07051

Medical Technologist Program
Bergen Pines County Hospital
E. Ridgewood Avenue
Paramus, New Jersey 07652

Medical Technologist Program
St. Mary's Hospital, Passaic
211 Pennington Avenue
Passaic, New Jersey 07055

Medical Technologist Program
Barnert Memorial Hospital Center
680 Broadway
Paterson, New Jersey 07514

Medical Technologist Program
St. Joseph's Hospital Medical Center
703 Main Street
Paterson, New Jersey 07503

Medical Technologist Program
Muhlenberg Hospital
Park Ave. & Randolph Road
Plainfield, New Jersey 07061

Medical Technologist Program
The Valley Hospital
Linwood & N. Van Dien Ave.
Ridgewood, New Jersey 07451

Medical Technologist Program
Somerset Medical Center
110 Rehill Avenue
Somerville, New Jersey 08876

NEW MEXICO

Medical Technologist Program
Univ. of New Mexico School of Medicine
Basic Medical Sciences Bldg.
Albuquerque, New Mexico 87131

Medical Technologist Program
Memorial General Hospital
Telshor Blvd. & University Ave.
Las Cruces, New Mexico 88001

NEW YORK

Medical Technologist Program
Albany Medical Center Hospital
New Scotland Avenue
Albany, New York 12208

Medical Technologist Program
College of Saint Rose
432 Western Avenue
Albany, New York 12203

Medical Technologist Program
St. Peter's Hospital
315 S. Manning Boulevard
Albany, New York 12208

Medical Technologist Program
Daemen College
Box 584
Amherst, New York 14226

Medical Technologist Program
United Health Services, Inc.
Box 540
Binghamton, New York 13790

Medical Technologist Program
Methodist Hospital of Brooklyn
506 6th Street
Brooklyn, New York 11215

Medical Technologist Program
Mercy Hospital
565 Abbott Road
Buffalo, New York 14220

Medical Technologist Program
Millard Fillmore Hospital
3 Gates Circle
Buffalo, New York 14209

Medical Technologist Program
SUNY at Buffalo
501 Capen Hall
Buffalo, New York 14260

Medical Technologist Program
The Buffalo General Hospital
100 High Street
Buffalo, New York 14203

Medical Technologist Program
Long Island University C.W. Post Campus
Northern Boulevard
Greenvale, New York 11548

Medical Technologist Program
Catholic Medical Center
38-25 153rd Street
Jamaica, New York 11432

Medical Technologist Program
Women's Christian Association Hospital
207 Foote Avenue
Jamestown, New York 14701

Medical Technologist Program
Northern Westchester Hospital Center
Mt. Kisco, New York 10549

Medical Technologist Program
Cabrini Health Care Center
227 E. 19th Street
New York, New York 10003

Medical Technologist Program
St. Vincent's Hospital & Medical Center of NY
153 West 11th Street
New York, New York 10011

Medical Technologist Program
Mount Saint Mary College
Powell Avenue
Newburgh, New York 12550

Medical Technologist Program
Rochester General Hospital
1425 Portland Avenue
Rochester, New York 14621

Medical Technologist Program
St. Mary's Hospital of Rochester
89 Genesee Street
Rochester, New York 14611

Medical Technologist Program
State University of New York at Stony Brook
Stony Brook, New York 11794-0701

Medical Technologist Program
SUNY Upstate Medical Center
155 Elizabeth Blackwell Street
Syracuse, New York 13210

Medical Technologist Program
Utica College of Syracuse U
Burrstone Road
Utica, New York 13502

NORTH CAROLINA

Medical Technologist Program
University of North Carolina
103-C South Bldg. 005A
Chapel Hill, North Carolina 27514

Medical Technologist Program
Charlotte Memorial Hosp & Medical Center
P.O. Box 32861
Charlotte, North Carolina 28232

Medical Technologist Program
Mercy Hospital, Inc.
2001 Vail Avenue
Charlotte, North Carolina 28207

Medical Technologist Program
Presbyterian Hospital
Box 33549, 200 Hawthorne Lane
Charlotte, North Carolina 28233

Medical Technologist Program
Western Carolina University
511 HF Robinson Admin. Bldg.
Cullowhee, North Carolina 28723

Medical Technologist Program
Duke University Medical Center
P.O. Box 3701
M106A Davison Bldg.
Durham, North Carolina 27710

Medical Technologist Program
Moses H. Cone Memorial Hospital
1200 North Elm Street
Greensboro, North Carolina 27401-1020

Medical Technologist Program
East Carolina University
Greenville, North Carolina 27834

Medical Technologist Program
New Hanover Memorial Hospital
2131 S. 17th Street
Wilmington, North Carolina 28402

Medical Technologist Program
Atlantic Christian College
West Lee Street
Wilson, North Carolina 27893

Medical Technologist Program
Bowman Gray School of Med. of Wake Forest U.
300 S. Hawthorne Road
Winston-Salem, North Carolina 27103

Medical Technologist Program
Forsyth City Hospital Authority, Inc.
3333 Silas Creek Pkwy.
Winston-Salem, North Carolina 27103

Medical Technologist Program
Winston-Salem State University
Office of the Chancellor
Winston-Salem, North Carolina 27110

NORTH DAKOTA

Medical Technologist Program
St. Alexius Medical Center
900 E. Broadway, Box 1658
Bismarck, North Dakota 58501

Medical Technologist Program
University of North Dakota
University Station
Grand Forks, North Dakota 58202

Medical Technologist Program
St. Joseph's Hospital
3rd Street, S.E. & Burdick Expressway
Minot, North Dakota 58701

Medical Technologist Program
Trinity Medical Center
Burdick Expressway at Main Street
Minot, North Dakota 58701

OHIO

Medical Technologist Program
Akron City Hospital
525 E. Market Street
Akron, Ohio 44309

Medical Technologist Program
Akron General Medical Center
400 Wabash Avenue
Akron, Ohio 44307

Medical Technologist Program
Children's Hospital Medical Center of Akron
281 Locust Street
Akron, Ohio 44308

Medical Technologist Program
St. Thomas Hospital Med. Center
444 N. Main Street
Akron, Ohio 44310

Medical Technologist Program
Bowling Green State University
220 McFall Center
Bowling Green, Ohio 43403

Medical Technologist Program
Aultman Hospital
2600 Sixth Street, S.W.
Canton, Ohio 44710

Medical Technologist Program
Providence Hospital
2446 Kipling Avenue
Cincinnati, Ohio 45239

Medical Technologist Program
The Christ Hospital
2139 Auburn Avenue
Cincinnati, Ohio 45219

Medical Technologist Program
University of Cincinnati
Mail Location 63
Cincinnati, Ohio 45221-0063

Medical Technologist Program
Cleveland Clinic Foundation
9500 Euclid Avenue
Cleveland, Ohio 44106

Medical Technologist Program
Cleveland Metropolitan General Hospital
3395 Scranton Road
Cleveland, Ohio 44109

Medical Technologist Program
Fairview General Hospital
18101 Lorain Avenue
Cleveland, Ohio 44111

Medical Technologist Program
Mt. Sinai Medical Center
University Circle
Cleveland, Ohio 44106

Medical Technologist Program
St. Alexis Hospital
5163 Broadway Avenue
Cleveland, Ohio 44127

Medical Technologist Program
St. Vincent Charity Hospital
2351 E. 22nd Street
Cleveland, Ohio 44115

Medical Technologist Program
University Hospitals of Cleveland
2074 Abington Road
Cleveland, Ohio 44106

Medical Technologist Program
The Ohio State University
190 N. Oval Mall
Columbus, Ohio 43210-1234

Medical Technologist Program
Good Samaritan Hospital & Health Center
2222 Philadelphia Drive
Dayton, Ohio 45406

Medical Technologist Program
Miami Valley Hospital
1 Wyoming Street
Dayton, Ohio 45409

Medical Technologist Program
St. Elizabeth Medical Center
601 Edwin C. Moses Boulevard
Dayton, Ohio 45408

Medical Technologist Program
Wright State University
Administrative Wing
Dayton, Ohio 45435

Medical Technologist Program
Mercy Hospital
P.O. Box 418
Hamilton, Ohio 45012

Medical Technologist Program
Kettering College of Medical Arts
3535 Southern Boulevard
Kettering, Ohio 45429

Medical Technologist Program
Southwest General Hospital
18697 E. Bagley Road
Middleburg Heights, Ohio 44130

Medical Technologist Program
St. Charles Hospital
2600 Navarre Avenue
Oregon, Ohio 43616

Medical Technologist Program
Salem Community Hospital
1995 E. State Street
Salem, Ohio 44460

Medical Technologist Program
Ohio Valley Hospital
1 Ross Park
Steubenville, Ohio 43952

Medical Technologist Program
Mercy Hospital
2200 Jefferson Avenue
Toledo, Ohio 43624

Medical Technologist Program
Riverside Hospital
1600 N. Superior Street
Toledo, Ohio 43604

Medical Technologist Program
Trumbull Memorial Hospital
1350 E. Market Street
Warren, Ohio 44482

Medical Technologist Program
St. Elizabeth Hospital Medical Center
1044 Belmont Avenue
Youngstown, Ohio 44504

Medical Technologist Program
The Youngstown Hosp. Assoc-North Unit
345 Oak Hill Avenue
Youngstown, Ohio 44502

OKLAHOMA

Medical Technologist Program
Valley View Hospital
1300 E. Sixth Street
Ada, Oklahoma 74820

Medical Technologist Program
Jane Phillips Episcopal-Memorial Medical Center
3500 E.F. Phillips Boulevard
Bartlesville, Oklahoma 74006

Medical Technologist Program
St. Mary's Hospital
305 S. Fifth Street
Enid, Oklahoma 73701

Medical Technologist Program
Comanche County Memorial Hospital
P.O. Box 129
Lawton, Oklahoma 73502

Medical Technologist Program
Muskogee Regional Medical Center
300 Rockefeller Drive
Muskogee, Oklahoma 74401

Medical Technologist Program
Norman Regional Hospital
P.O. Box 1308
Norman, Oklahoma 73070

Medical Technologist Program
Baptist Medical Center of Oklahoma
3300 N.W. Expressway
Oklahoma City, Oklahoma 73112

Medical Technologist Program
Mercy Health Center
4300 W. Memorial Road
Oklahoma City, Oklahoma 73120

Medical Technologist Program
St. Anthony Hospital
1000 N. Lee Street
Oklahoma City, Oklahoma 73102

Medical Technologist Program
University of Oklahoma at Oklahoma City
P.O. Box 26901
Oklahoma City, Oklahoma 73190

Medical Technologist Program
Hillcrest Medical Center
1120 S. Utica
Tulsa, Oklahoma 74104

Medical Technologist Program
St. Francis Hospital
6161 S. Yale Avenue
Tulsa, Oklahoma 74136

Medical Technologist Program
St. John Medical Center
1923 S. Utica Avenue
Tulsa, Oklahoma 74104

OREGON

Medical Technologist Program
Sacred Heart General Hospital
1255 Hilyard Street
P.O. Box 10905
Eugene, Oregon 97440

Medical Technologist Program
Oregon Institute of Technology
Oretech Branch Post Office
Klamath Falls, Oregon 97601

Medical Technologist Program
Oregon Health Sciences University
3181 S.W. Sam Jackson Park Road
Portland, Oregon 97201

Medical Technologist Program
St. Vincent Hospital & Medical Center
9205 S.W. Barnes Road
Portland, Oregon 97225

PENNSYLVANIA

Medical Technologist Program
Abington Memorial Hospital
1200 Old York Road
Abington, Pennsylvania 19001

Medical Technologist Program
Allentown Hospital Association
17th & Chew Streets
Allentown, Pennsylvania 18102

Medical Technologist Program
Sacred Heart Hospital
421 Chew Street
Allentown, Pennsylvania 18102

Medical Technologist Program
Altoona Hospital
7th & Howard Avenue
Altoona, Pennsylvania 16603

Medical Technologist Program
Neumann College
Convent Road
Aston, Pennsylvania 19014

Medical Technologist Program
St. Luke's Hospital
801 Ostrum Street
Bethlehem, Pennsylvania 18015

Medical Technologist Program
Lower Bucks Hospital
Bath Road at Orchard Ave.
Bristol, Pennsylvania 19007

Medical Technologist Program
Bryn Mawr Hospital
Bryn Mawr Avenue
Bryn Mawr, Pennsylvania 19010

Medical Technologist Program
Geisinger Medical Center
North Academy Avenue
Danville, Pennsylvania 17822

Medical Technologist Program
Rolling Hill Hospital
60 E. Township Line Road
Elkins Park, Pennsylvania 19117

Medical Technologist Program
Saint Vincent Health Center
232 W. 25th Street
Erie, Pennsylvania 16544

Medical Technologist Program
Harrisburg Hospital
South Front Street
Harrisburg, Pennsylvania 17101

Medical Technologist Program
Polyclinic Medical Center
2601 N. Third Street
Harrisburg, Pennsylvania 17110

Medical Technologist Program
Conemaugh Valley Memorial Hospital
1086 Franklin Street
Johnstown, Pennsylvania 15905

Medical Technologist Program
Lancaster General Hospital
555 N. Duke Street
P.O. Box 3555
Lancaster, Pennsylvania 17603

Medical Technologist Program
St. Joseph Hospital & Health Care Center
250 College Avenue
P.O. Box 3509
Lancaster, Pennsylvania 17604

Medical Technologist Program
Latrobe Area Hospital
West 2nd Avenue
Latrobe, Pennsylvania 15650

Medical Technologist Program
McKeesport Hospital
1500 Fifth Avenue
McKeesport, Pennsylvania 15132

Medical Technologist Program
Hahnemann University
Broad & Vine Streets
Philadelphia, Pennsylvania 19102

Medical Technologist Program
Lankenau Hospital
Lancaster & City Line Avenues
Philadelphia, Pennsylvania 19151

Medical Technologist Program
Medical College of Pennsylvania
3300 Henry Avenue
Philadelphia, Pennsylvania 19129

Medical Technologist Program
Nazareth Hospital
2601 Holme Avenue
Philadelphia, Pennsylvania 19152

Medical Technologist Program
Pennsylvania Hospital
8th & Spruce Streets
Philadelphia, Pennsylvania 19107

Medical Technologist Program
Temple University Hospital
Broad Street & Montgomery Avenue
Philadelphia, Pennsylvania 19122

Medical Technologist Program
Thomas Jefferson University
Scott Bldg., 1020 Walnut Street
Philadelphia, Pennsylvania 19107

Medical Technologist Program
Allegheny General Hospital
320 E. North Avenue
Pittsburgh, Pennsylvania 15212-9986

Medical Technologist Program
Mercy Hospital of Pittsburgh
1400 Locust Street
Pittsburgh, Pennsylvania 15219

Medical Technologist Program
University of Pittsburgh
4200 Fifth Avenue
Pittsburgh, Pennsylvania 15260

Medical Technologist Program
Western Pennsylvania Hospital
4800 Friendship Avenue
Pittsburgh, Pennsylvania 15224

Medical Technologist Program
Reading Hospital and Medical Center
Reading, Pennsylvania 19603

Medical Technologist Program
Saint Joseph Hospital
12th & Walnut Streets, Box 316
Reading, Pennsylvania 19603

Medical Technologist Program
Robert Packer Hospital
Guthrie Square
Sayre, Pennsylvania 18840

Medical Technologist Program
Scranton Medical Technology Consortium
700 Quincy Avenue
Scranton, Pennsylvania 18510

Medical Technologist Program
Washington Hospital
155 Wilson Avenue
Washington, Pennsylvania 15301

Medical Technologist Program
Wilkes-Barre General Hospital
N. River & Auburn Streets
Wilkes-Barre, Pennsylvania 18764

Medical Technologist Program
Divine Providence Hospital
1100 Grampian Boulevard
Williamsport, Pennsylvania 17701

Medical Technologist Program
Williamsport Hospital
777 Rural Avenue
Williamsport, Pennsylvania 17701-3198

Medical Technologist Program
York Hospital
1001 S. George Street
York, Pennsylvania 17405

PUERTO RICO

Medical Technologist Program
Catholic University of Puerto Rico
Ponce, Puerto Rico 00731

Medical Technologist Program
Inter American Univ. of Puerto Rico
G.P.O. Box 3255
San German, Puerto Rico 00753

Medical Technologist Program
University of Puerto Rico
G.P.O. Box 5067
San Juan, Puerto Rico 00936

RHODE ISLAND

Medical Technologist Program
General Hospital, RI Medical Center
P.O. Box 8269
Cranston, Rhode Island 02920

Medical Technologist Program
Newport Hospital
19 Friendship Street
Newport, Rhode Island 02840

Medical Technologist Program
Memorial Hospital
Prospect & Pond Streets
Pawtucket, Rhode Island 02860

Medical Technologist Program
Rhode Island Hospital
593 Eddy Street
Providence, Rhode Island 02902

Medical Technologist Program
St. Joseph Hospital-OLP Unit
200 High Service Avenue
North Providence, Rhode Island 02904

Medical Technologist Program
The Miriam Hospital
164 Summit Avenue
Providence, Rhode Island 02906

SOUTH CAROLINA

Medical Technologist Program
Anderson Memorial Hospital
800 N. Fant Street
Anderson, South Carolina 29621

Medical Technologist Program
Medical University of South Carolina
171 Ashley Avenue
Charleston, South Carolina 29425

Medical Technologist Program
Baptist Medical Center at Columbia
Taylor at Marion Street
Columbia, South Carolina 29220

Medical Technologist Program
McLeod Regional Medical Center
555 E. Cheves Street
Florence, South Carolina 29501

Medical Technologist Program
Self Memorial Hospital
1325 Spring Street
Greenwood, South Carolina 29646

SOUTH DAKOTA

Medical Technologist Program
St. Luke's Hospital
305 S. State Street
Aberdeen, South Dakota 57401

Medical Technologist Program
Rapid City Regional Hospital, Inc.
353 Fairmont Boulevard
Rapid City, South Dakota 57709

Medical Technologist Program
Sioux Valley Hospital
1100 S. Euclid Ave., PO 5039
Sioux Falls, South Dakota 5717-5039

Medical Technologist Program
Sacred Heart Hospital
501 Summit Street
Yankton, South Dakota 57078

TENNESSEE

Medical Technologist Program
Erlanger Medical Center
975 E. Third Street
Chattanooga, Tennessee 37403

Medical Technologist Program
Cumberland School of Med. Tech.
321 N. Washington
Cookeville, Tennessee 38501

Medical Technologist Program
Holston Valley Hospital & Med Center
West Ravine Street
Kingsport, Tennessee 37662

Medical Technologist Program
East Tennessee Baptist Hospital
P.O. Box 1788
Knoxville, Tennessee 37901

Medical Technologist Program
UTN Memorial Hosp. & Research Center
1924 Alcoa Highway
Knoxville, Tennessee 37920

Medical Technologist Program
Baptist Memorial Hospital
899 Madison Avenue
Memphis, Tennessee 38146

Medical Technologist Program
Methodist Hospital of Memphis
1265 Union Avenue
Memphis, Tennessee 38104

Medical Technologist Program
St. Francis Hospital
P.O. Box 171808
Memphis, Tennessee 38187-1808

Medical Technologist Program
University of Tennessee
800 Madison Avenue
Memphis, Tennessee 38163

Medical Technologist Program
Baptist Hospital, Inc.
2000 Church Street
Nashville, Tennessee 37236

Medical Technologist Program
St. Thomas Hospital
P.O. Box 380
4220 Harding Road
Nashville, Tennessee 37202

Medical Technologist Program
Tennessee State University, Meharry Med Coll.
3500 John A. Merritt Boulevard
Nashville, Tennessee 37203

Medical Technologist Program
Vanderbilt University Medical Center
21st & Garland
Nashville, Tennessee 37232

TEXAS

Medical Technologist Program
Hendrick Medical Center
19th & Hickory Streets
Abilene, Texas 79601

Medical Technologist Program
Northwest Texas Hospital
1501 Coulter
Amarillo, Texas 79106

Medical Technologist Program
St. Anthony's Hospital
P.O. Box 950
Amarillo, Texas 79176

Medical Technologist Program
Austin State Hospital
4110 Guadalupe Street
Austin, Texas 78751

Medical Technologist Program
Brackenridge Hospital
601 E. 15th Street
Austin, Texas 78701

Medical Technologist Program
St. Elizabeth Hospital
P.O. Box 5405
Beaumont, Texas 77706

Medical Technologist Program
The Baptist Hospital of SE Texas, Inc.
P.O. Drawer 1591
Beaumont, Texas 77704

Medical Technologist Program
Corpus Christi State University
6300 Ocean Drive
Corpus Christi, Texas 78412

Medical Technologist Program
Baylor University Medical Center
3500 Gaston Avenue
Dallas, Texas 75246

Medical Technologist Program
St. Paul Medical Center
5909 Harry Hines Boulevard
Dallas, Texas 75235

Medical Technologist Program
University of Texas
5323 Harry Hines Boulevard
Dallas, Texas 75235

Medical Technologist Program
Pan American University
1201 W. University Drive
Edinburg, Texas 78539

Medical Technologist Program
University of Texas at El Paso
Administration Building 500
El Paso, Texas 79968

Medical Technologist Program
Brooke Army Medical Center
Fort Sam Houston, Texas 78234-6200

Medical Technologist Program
Harris Hospital-Methodist
1301 Pennsylvania
Fort Worth, Texas 76104

Medical Technologist Program
Tarleton State University
Tarleton Station
Steohenville, Texas 76402

Medical Technologist Program
USAF Regional Hospital Carswell
Carswell AFB, Texas 76127-5300

Medical Technologist Program
The University of Texas Medical Branch
Galveston, Texas 77550

Medical Technologist Program
Harris City Hosp. Dist-Ben Taub Hospital
726 Gillette Street
Houston, Texas 77019

Medical Technologist Program
Methodist Hospital
6565 Fannin, Mail Station 101
Houston, Texas 77030

Medical Technologist Program
St. Luke's Episcopal Hospital
6720 Bertner
Houston, Texas 77030

Medical Technologist Program
University of Texas School of Allied Health Sciences
P.O. Box 20036
Houston, Texas 77225

Medical Technologist Program
Wilford Hall USAF Medical Center
Lackland AFB, Texas 78236-5300

Medical Technologist Program
Lubbock General Hospital
602 Indiana Avenue, Box 5980
Lubbock, Texas 79417

Medical Technologist Program
Methodist Hospital
3615 19th Street
Lubbock, Texas 79410

Medical Technologist Program
Texas Tech University Health Sciences Center
Office of the President, 2B158
Lubbock, Texas 79430

Medical Technologist Program
Midland Memorial Hospital
2200 W. Illinois Street
Midland, Texas 79701

Medical Technologist Program
Shannon West Texas Memorial Hospital
120 East Harris
P.O. Box 1879
San Angelo, Texas 76902

Medical Technologist Program
Baptist Memorial Hospital System
111 Dallas Street
San Antonio, Texas 78286

Medical Technologist Program
SW Texas Methodist Hospital
7700 Floyd Curl Drive
San Antonio, Texas 78229

Medical Technologist Program
University of Texas Health Science Center at San Antonio
7703 Floyd Curl Drive
San Antonio, Texas 78284

Medical Technologist Program
Southwest Texas State University
JC Kellam Building
San Marcos, Texas 78666

WASHINGTON

Medical Technologist Program
Deaconess Hospital
800 West 5th
Spokane, Washington 99210

Medical Technologist Program
Sacred Heart Medical Center
W. 101 Eighth Avenue, TAF-C9
Spokane, Washington 99220

Medical Technologist Program
Tacoma General Hospital
315 South "K" Street
Tacoma, Washington 98405

WEST VIRGINIA

Medical Technologist Program
Cabell Huntington Hospital
1340 Hal Greer Boulevard
Huntington, West Virginia 25701

Medical Technologist Program
West Virginia University
Stewart Hall
Morgantown, West Virginia 26506

Medical Technologist Program
West Liberty State College
West Liberty, West Virginia 26074

Medical Technologist Program
Wheeling College
316 Washington Avenue
Wheeling, West Virginia 26003

WISCONSIN

Medical Technologist Program
St. Elizabeth Hospital
1506 S. Oneida Street
Appleton, Wisconsin 54915

Medical Technologist Program
Sacred Heart Hospital
900 W. Clairemont Avenue
Eau Claire, Wisconsin 54701

Medical Technologist Program
St. Vincent Hospital
P.O. Box 13508
Green Bay, Wisconsin 54307-3508

Medical Technologist Program
Kenosha Memorial Hospital
6308 8th Avenue
Kenosha, Wisconsin 53140

Medical Technologist Program
St. Catherine's Hospital
3556 7th Avenue
Kenosha, Wisconsin 53140

Medical Technologist Program
St. Francis Medical Center
700 West Avenue South
La Crosse, Wisconsin 54601

Medical Technologist Program
University of Wisconsin-Madison
Bascom Hall
Madison, Wisconsin 53706

Medical Technologist Program
St. Joseph's Hospital
611 St. Joseph's Avenue
Marshfield, Wisconsin 54449

Medical Technologist Program
Clement J. Zablocki VA Medical Center
5000 W. National Avenue
Milwaukee, Wisconsin 53193

Medical Technologist Program
Family Hospital
2711 W. Wells Street
Milwaukee, Wisconsin 53208

Medical Technologist Program
Milwaukee Children's Hospital
1700 W. Wisconsin Avenue
Milwaukee, Wisconsin 53233

Medical Technologist Program
Milwaukee County Medical Complex
8700 West Wisconsin Avenue
Milwaukee, Wisconsin 53226

Medical Technologist Program
Mount Sinai Medical Center
950 N. 12th Street
P.O. Box 342
Milwaukee, Wisconsin 53201

Medical Technologist Program
St. Joseph's Hospital
5000 W. Chambers Street
Milwaukee, Wisconsin 53210

Medical Technologist Program
St. Mary's Hospital
2323 N. Lake Drive
P.O.Box 503
Milwaukee, Wisconsin 53201

Medical Technologist Program
St. Michael Hospital
2400 W. Villard Avenue
Milwaukee, Wisconsin 53209

Medical Technologist Program
Theda Clark Regional Medical Center
130 Second Street
Neehan, Wisconsin 54956

Medical Technologist Program
St. Luke's Memorial Hospital
1320 S. Wisconsin Avenue
Racine, Wisconsin 53403

Medical Technologist Program
St. Mary's Medical Center
3801 Spring Street
Racine, Wisconsin 53405

Medical Technologist Program
St. Michael's Hospital
900 Illinois Avenue
Stevens Point, Wisconsin 54481

Medical Technologist Program
Waukesha Memorial Hospital
725 American Avenue
Waukesha, Wisconsin 53186

Medical Technologist Program
Wausau Hospital Center
333 Pine Ridge Boulevard
Wausau, Wisconsin 54401

Medical Technologist Program
West Allis Memorial Hospital
8901 W. Lincoln Avenue
West Allis, Wisconsin 53227

WYOMING

Medical Technologist Program
University of Wyoming
Box 3434, University Station
Laramie, Wyoming 82071

Medical Laboratory Technician

The *medical laboratory technician* is an intermediate-level worker on the laboratory career ladder. Requiring only a limited amount of supervision by the pathologist or the medical technologist, the medical laboratory technician does not possess the same level of knowledge as the medical technologist and performs less complicated tests. However, the technician still uses a high degree of skill and some independent judgment in carrying out a wide range of tests and procedures that provides data for diagnosis and treatment of disease.

Like the medical technologist, the technician may work in all fields of laboratory testing or specialize in one, such as immunology, hematology, cytology, and so on. The position of histologic technician is described in detail later in this section.

The medical laboratory technician must graduate from an accredited two-years community college, junior college, vocational-technical, hospital or armed forces program that includes supervised clinical experience in an approved laboratory. Many programs lead to an associate degree. The technician may advance to become a medical technologist with additional training and work experience.

The societies that certify medical technologists also certify medical laboratory technicians and the same states require licensure to practice.

Recommended high school courses are chemistry, biology, and mathematics.

According to a recent survey conducted by the University of Texas Medical Branch, starting annual salaries for medical laboratory technicians employed in hospitals, medical centers, and medical schools, averaged $15,500, while those with experience averaged $20,600.

Below is a list of schools that offer accredited two-year and certificate programs for the medical laboratory technician.

KEY:

(1) Accredited by the American Medical Association Committee on Allied Health Education and Accreditation

(2) Accredited by the Accrediting Bureau of Medical Laboratory Schools

SOURCES:

Accrediting Bureau of Medical Laboratory Schools
American Medical Technologists
American Society of Clinical Pathologists
Occupational Outlook Handbook

Medical Laboratory Technician Program

ALABAMA

Medical Laboratory Technician Program (1)
Jefferson State Junior College
Pinson Valley Pky-2601 Carson
Birmingham, Alabama 35215-3098

Medical Laboratory Technician Program (1)
The University of AL at Birmingham
University Station
Birmingham, Alabama 35294

Medical Laboratory Technician Program (1)
George C. Wallace State Community College
Administration
Dothan, Alabama 36303

Medical Laboratory Technician Program (1)
Gadsden State Community College
Number One State College Boulevard
Gadsden, Alabama 35999

Medical Laboratory Technician Program (1)
Wallace State Community College
P.O. Box 250
Hanceville, Alabama 35077-9080

ALASKA

Medical Laboratory Technician Program (1)
Anchorage Community College
2533 Providence Drive
Anchorage, Alaska 99508-4670

ARIZONA

Medical Laboratory Technician Program (2)
Health Careers Institute
3320 W. Flower
Phoenix, Arizona 85017

Medical Laboratory Technician Program (1)
Phoenix College
1202 W. Thomas Road
Phoenix, Arizona 85013

Medical Laboratory Technician Program (2)
Health Careers Institute (Branch)
4444 East Grant Road, Suite 120
Tucson, Arizona 85712

Medical Laboratory Technician Program (2)
Pima Medical Institute
1010 North Alvernon Way
P.O. Box 30622
Tucson, Arizona 85711

ARKANSAS

Medical Laboratory Technician Program (1)
Southern AR University-Eldorado Branch
300 South West Avenue
El Dorado, Arkansas 71730

Medical Laboratory Technician Program (1)
Phillips County Community College
P.O. Box 785
Helena, Arkansas 72342

Medical Laboratory Technician Program (1)
Garland County Community College
No. 1 College Drive
Hot Springs, Arkansas 71913

CALIFORNIA

Medical Laboratory Technician Program (2)
Oakland College of Dental-Medical Assistants
388 17th Street
Oakland, California 94612

Medical Laboratory Technician Program (2)
Technical Health Careers School, Inc.
1843 West Imperial Highway
Los Angeles, California 90047

Medical Laboratory Technician Program (1)
Naval School of Health Sciences
San Diego, California 92134-6000

Medical Laboratory Technician Program (2)
Bay City College of Dental-Medical Assistants
211 Sutter Street, 10th Floor
San Francisco, California 94108

COLORADO

Medical Laboratory Technician Program (1)
T.H. Pickens Technical Center
500 Buckley Road
Aurora, Colorado 80011

Medical Laboratory Technician Program (2)
Pikes Peak Institute of Medical Technology
820 Arcturus Drive
Colorado Springs, Colorado 80906

Medical Laboratory Technician Program (1)
Arapahoe Community College
5900 South Santa Fe Drive
Littleton, Colorado 80120

CONNECTICUT

Medical Laboratory Technician Program (1)
Housatonic Community College
510 Barnum Avenue
Bridgeport, Connecticut 06608

Medical Laboratory Technician Program (1)
Manchester Community College
60 Bidwell Street
Mail Station 1
Manchester, Connecticut 06040

DELAWARE

Medical Laboratory Technician Program (1)
Delaware Technical and Community College
P.O. Box 610
Georgetown, Delaware 19947

DISTRICT OF COLUMBIA

Medical Laboratory Technician Program (2)
Georgetown School of Science and Arts, Ltd.
2461 Wisconsin Avenue, N.W.
Washington, D.C. 20007

FLORIDA

Medical Laboratory Technician Program (1)
Brevard Community College
1519 Clearlake Road
Cocoa, Florida 32922

Medical Laboratory Technician Program (1)
Broward Community College
225 East Las Olas Boulevard
Fort Lauderdale, Florida 33301

Medical Laboratory Technician Program (2)
Keiser Institute of Technology School of Allied Health
4861 N. Dixie Highway 200
Ft. Lauderdale, Florida 33334

Medical Laboratory Technician Program (1)
Indian River Community College
3209 Virginia Avenue
Fort Pierce, Florida 33450-9003

Medical Laboratory Technician Program (1)
Sheridan Vocational Technical Center
5400 Sheridan Street
Hollywood, Florida 33021

Medical Laboratory Technician Program (1)
Florida Junior College at Jacksonville
501 West State Street
Jacksonville, Florida 32202

Medical Laboratory Technician Program (1)
Florida Institute of Techology
1707 N.E. Indian River Drive
Jensen Beach, Florida 33457

Medical Laboratory Technician Program (2)
American Medical Training Institute
10700 Caribbean Boulevard
Miami, Florida 33189

Medical Laboratory Technician Program (1)
Miami-Dade Community College
11011 S.W. 104th Street
Miami, Florida 33176

Medical Laboratory Technician Program (1)
Valencia Community College
190 S. Orange Ave., POB 3028
Orlando, Florida 32802

Medical Laboratory Technician Program (1)
Manatee Community College-Sarasota Vocational Center
4748 Beneva Road
Sarasota, Florida 34233

Medical Laboratory Technician Program (1)
St. Petersburg Junior College
P.O. Box 13489
St. Petersburg, Florida 33733

Medical Laboratory Technician Program (1)
Erwin Area Vocational Technical Center
2010 E. Hillsborough Avenue
Tampa, Florida 33610

GEORGIA

Medical Laboratory Technician Program (1)
Albany Junior College
2400 Gillionville Road
Albany, Georgia 31707

Medical Laboratory Technician Program (1)
Atlanta Area Technical School
1560 Stewart Ave., S.W.
Atlanta, Georgia 30310

Medical Laboratory Technician Program (2)
Atlanta College of Medical and Dental Careers
1240 West Peachtree Street, N.W.
Atlanta, Georgia 30309

Medical Laboratory Technician Program (1)
Augusta Area Technical School
3116 Deans Bridge Road
Augusta, Georgia 30906

Medical Laboratory Technician Program (1)
Brunswick Junior College
Altama at Fourth Street
Brunswick, Georgia 31523

Medical Laboratory Technician Program (1)
De Kalb Community College
495 N. Indian Creek Dr.
Clarkston, Georgia 30021

Medical Laboratory Technician Program (1)
North Georgia Technical & Vocational School
Highway 197 North
P.O. Box 65
Clarkesville, Georgia 30523

Medical Laboratory Technician Program (1)
Dalton Junior College
College Drive
Dalton, Georgia 30720

Medical Laboratory Technician Program (1)
Macon Area Vocational-Technical School
3300 Macon Tech Drive
Macon, Georgia 31206

Medical Laboratory Technician Program (1)
Lanier Area Technical School
P.O. Box 58
Oakwood, Georgia 30566

Medical Laboratory Technician Program (1)
Floyd Junior College
P.O. Box 1864
Rome, Georgia 30163

Medical Laboratory Technician Program (1)
Valdosta Area Vocational Technical School
Route 1, Box 202
Valdosta, Georgia 31602

Medical Laboratory Technician Program (1)
Waycross-Ware County Area Vocational-Technical School
1701 Carswell Avenue
Waycross, Georgia 31501

HAWAII

Medical Laboratory Technician Program (1)
Kapiolani Community College
620 Pensacola Street
Honolulu, Hawaii 96814

ILLINOIS

Medical Laboratory Technician Program (1)
Belleville Area College
2500 Carlyle Road
Belleville, Illinois 62221-9989

Medical Laboratory Technician Program (1)
Oakton Community College
1600 E. Golf Road
Des Plaines, Illinois 60016

Medical Laboratory Technician Program (1)
Sauk Valley College
RR-5
Dixon, Illinois 61021

Medical Laboratory Technician Program (1)
Illinois Central College
East Peoria, Illinois 61635

Medical Laboratory Technician Program (1)
Lewis & Clark Community College
5800 Godfrey Road
Godfrey, Illinois 62035

Medical Laboratory Technician Program (1)
College of Lake County
19351 W. Washington Street
Grayslake, Illinois 60030

Medical Laboratory Technician Program (1)
Kankakee Community College
P.O. Box 888
Kankakee, Illinois 60901

Medical Laboratory Technician Program (1)
Moraine Valley Community College
10900 S. 88th Avenue
Palos Hills, Illinois 60465

Medical Laboratory Technician Program (1)
Blessing Hospital
1005 Broadway Street
Quincy, Illinois 62301

Medical Laboratory Technician Program (1)
Triton College
2000 Fifth Avenue
River Grove, Illinois 60171

INDIANA

Medical Laboratory Technician Program (1)
Caylor-Nickel Hospital, Inc.
One Caylor-Nickel Square
Bluffton, Indiana 46714

Medical Laboratory Technician Program (2)
Elkhart Institute of Technology
516 South Main Street
Elkhart, Indiana 46516

Medical Laboratory Technician Program (1)
Indiana Vocational Technical College
One W. 26th Street
P.O. Box 1763
Indianapolis, Indiana 46206-1763

Medical Laboratory Technician Program (1)
Marion College
4201 S. Washington Street
Marion, Indiana 46953

Medical Laboratory Technician Program (1)
Lakeshore Med.-Lab Training Program, Inc.
422 Franklin Street
P.O. Box 341
Michigan City, Indiana 46360

Medical Laboratory Technician Program (1)
Indiana Vocational Technical College
One W. 26th Street
Richmond, Indiana 46206

Medical Laboratory Technician Program (1)
Indiana Vocational Technical College-Northcentral
1534 W. Sample Street
South Bend, Indiana 46619

Medical Laboratory Technician Program (1)
Indiana State University
Terra Haute, Indiana 47809

Medical Laboratory Technician Program (1)
Indiana Vocational Technical College
7377 S. Dixie Bee Road
Terre Haute, Indiana 47802

IOWA

Medical Laboratory Technician Program (1)
Des Moines Area Community College
2006 Ankeny Boulevard
Ankeny, Iowa 50021

Medical Laboratory Technician Program (1)
Scott Community College of EICCD
Belmont Road
Bettendorf, Iowa 52722

Medical Laboratory Technician Program (1)
Hawkeye Institute of Technology
P.O. Box 8015
Waterloo, Iowa 50704

KANSAS

Medical Laboratory Technician Program (1)
Coffeyville Community Junior College
304 Centennial
Coffeyville, Kansas 67337

Medical Laboratory Technician Program (1)
Barton City Community College
RR-3
Great Bend, Kansas 67530-9803

Medical Laboratory Technician Program (1)
Seward County Community College
Box 1137
Liberal, Kansas 67901

Medical Laboratory Technician Program (1)
Wichita Area Vocational Technical School
301 S. Grove
Wichita, Kansas 67211

LOUISIANA

Medical Laboratory Technician Program (1)
Baton Rouge Reg'l Vocational Technical Institute
4350 N. Acadian Thruway
Baton Rouge, Louisiana 70805

Medical Laboratory Technician Program (1)
Lafayette Reg'l Vocational Technical Institute
1101 Bertrand Drive
Lafayette, Louisiana 70506

KENTUCKY

Medical Laboratory Technician Program (1)
Henderson Community College
2660 South Green Street
Henderson, Kentucky 42420

Medical Laboratory Technician Program (1)
Jefferson Community College-University of Kentucky
109 East Broadway
Louisville, Kentucky 40202

Medical Laboratory Technician Program (2)
Louisville College of Medical and Dental Careers
1512 Crums Lane
Louisville, Kentucky 40216

Medical Laboratory Technician Program (2)
Watterson College
4400 Breckinridge Lane
Louisville, Kentucky 40218

Medical Laboratory Technician Program (1)
Madisonville Area Vocational School
P.O. Box 608
Madisonville, Kentucky 42431

Medical Laboratory Technician Program (1)
Midway College
Midway, Kentucky 40347

Medical Laboratory Technician Program (1)
Murray State University
Murray, Kentucky 42071

Medical Laboratory Technician Program (1)
Eastern Kentucky University
Coates Admin. Bldg.
Richmond, Kentucky 40475

Medical Laboratory Technician Program (1)
Somerset Community College
Somerset, Kentucky 42501

MAINE

Medical Laboratory Technician Program (1)
University of Maine at Augusta
University Height's
Augusta, Maine 04330

Medical Laboratory Technician Program (1)
Eastern Maine Vocational Technical Institute
354 Hogan Road
Bangor, Maine 04401

Medical Laboratory Technician Program (1)
University of Maine at Presque Isle
181 Maine Street, 22 Preble Hall
Presque Isle, Maine 04769

MARYLAND

Medical Laboratory Technician Program (1)
Essex Community College-Johns Hopkins Hosp.
7201 Rossville Boulevard
Baltimore, Maryland 21237

Medical Laboratory Technician Program (1)
Naval School of Health Sciences
Building 141
Bethesda, Maryland 20814-5033

Medical Laboratory Technician Program (1)
Allegany Community College
Willow Brook Road
Cumberland, Maryland 21502

Medical Laboratory Technician Program (1)
Prince George's Community College
301 Largo Road
Largo, Maryland 20772

Medical Laboratory Technician Program (2)
Temple School of Maryland
8635 Colesville Road
Silver Spring, Maryland 20910

Medical Laboratory Technician Program (1)
Villa Julie College
Greenspring Valley Road
Stevenson, Maryland 21153

Medical Laboratory Technician Program (1)
Columbia Union College
7600 Flower Avenue
Takoma Park, Maryland 20912

Medical Laboratory Technician Program (1)
Montgomery College
Takoma Avenue & Fenton Street
Takoma Park, Maryland 20912

Medical Laboratory Technician Program (1)
Chesapeake College
P.O. Box 8
Wye Mills, Maryland 21679

MASSACHUSETTS

Medical Laboratory Technician Program (1)
Middlesex Community College
Springs Road
Bedford, Massachusetts 01730

Medical Laboratory Technician Program (1)
Northeastern University
360 Huntington Avenue
Boston, Massachusetts 02115

Medical Laboratory Technician Program (1)
Massasoit Community College
One Massasoit Boulevard
Brockton, Massachusetts 02402

Medical Laboratory Technician Program (1)
Bristol Community College
777 Elsbree Street
Fall River, Massachusetts 02720

Medical Laboratory Technician Program (1)
Mt. Wachusett Community College
444 Green Street
Gardner, Massachusetts 01440

Medical Laboratory Technician Program (1)
Anna Maria College
Sunset Lane
Paxton, Massachusetts 01612-1198

Medical Laboratory Technician Program (1)
Springfield Tech. Community College
1 Armory Square
Springfield, Massachusetts 01105

Medical Laboratory Technician Program (1)
Massachusetts Bay Community College
50 Oakland Street
Wellesley Hills, Massachusetts 02181

MICHIGAN

Medical Laboratory Technician Program (1)
Kellogg Community College
Battle Creek, Michigan 49016

Medical Laboratory Technician Program (1)
Lake Michigan College
2755 E. Napler Avenue
Benton Harbor, Michigan 49022

Medical Laboratory Technician Program (1)
Ferris State College
901 S. State Street, Starr 304
Big Rapids, Michigan 49307

Medical Laboratory Technician Program (1)
Oakland Community College
2480 Opdyke Road
Bloomfield Hills, Michigan 48085

Medical Laboratory Technician Program (2)
Krainz Woods Academy of Medical Laboratory
Technology
4327 East Seven Mile Road
Detroit, Michigan 48234

Medical Laboratory Technician Program (1)
Mercy College of Detroit
8200 W. Outer Drive, Box 99
Detroit, Michigan 48219

Medical Laboratory Technician Program (1)
Mid Michigan Community College
1375 S. Clare Avenue
Harrison, Michigan 48625

Medical Laboratory Technician Program (1)
Highland Park Community College
Glendale at Third
Highland Park, Michigan 48203

Medical Laboratory Technician Program (1)
Schoolcraft College
18600 Haggerty Road
Livonia, Michigan 49152

Medical Laboratory Technician Program (1)
Northern Michigan University
602 Cohodas Administration Center
Marquette, Michigan 49855

Medical Laboratory Technician Program (2)
Michigan Para-Professional Training Institute
21800 Greenfield Road
Oak Park, Michigan 48237

Medical Laboratory Technician Program (2)
Michigan Para-Professional Training Institute
(Branch)
29814 Smith ROad
Romulus, Michigan 48174

MINNESOTA

Medical Laboratory Technician Program (1)
Alexandria Area Vocational Technical Institute
1601 Jefferson Street
Alexandria, Minnesota 56308

Medical Laboratory Technician Program (1)
Duluth Area Vocational Technical Institute
2101 Trinity Road
Duluth, Minnesota 55811

Medical Laboratory Technician Program (1)
East Grand Forks Area Vocational Technical Institute
Highway 220 North
East Grand Forks, Minnesota 56721

Medical Laboratory Technician Program (1)
Fairbault Area Vocational Technical Institute
1225 S.W. 3rd Street
Faribault, Minnesota 55021

Medical Laboratory Technician Program (1)
Fergus Falls Community College
1414 College Way
Fergus Falls, Minnesota 56537

Medical Laboratory Technician Program (1)
Hibbing Area Vocational Technical Institute
2900 E. Beltline
Hibbing, Minnesota 55746

Medical Laboratory Technician Program (1)
Lakeland Medical-Dental Academy
1402 W. Lake Street
Minneapolis, Minnesota 55408

Medical Laboratory Technician Program (1,2)
Medical Institute of Minnesota
2309 Nicollet Avenue
Minneapolis, Minnesota 55404

Medical Laboratory Technician Program (1)
St. Mary's Junior College
2500 S. 6th Street
Minneapolis, Minnesota 55454

Medical Laboratory Technician Program (1)
St. Paul Technical Vocational Institute
235 Marshall Avenue
St. Paul, Minnesota 55102

MISSISSIPPI

Medical Laboratory Technician Program (1)
Northeast Mississippi Junior College
Cunningham Boulevard
Booneville, Mississippi 38829

Medical Laboratory Technician Program (1)
Mississippi Gulf Coast Junior College
Perkinston, Mississippi 39573

Medical Laboratory Technician Program (1)
Meridian Junior College
5500 Hwy 19 North
Meridian, Mississippi 39305

Medical Laboratory Technician Program (1)
Mississippi Delta Junior College
Olive Street, P.O. Box 668
Moorhead, Mississippi 38761

Medical Laboratory Technician Program (1)
Hinds Junior College
Raymond, Mississippi 39154

Medical Laboratory Technician Program (1)
Copiah-Lincoln Junior College
P.O. Box 457
Wesson, Mississippi 39191

MISSOURI

Medical Laboratory Technician Program (1)
Three Rivers Community College
Three Rivers Boulevard
Poplar Bluff, Missouri 63901

Medical Laboratory Technician Program (1)
St. Louis Community College at Forest Park
5600 Oakland Avenue
St. Louis, Missouri 63110

NEBRASKA

Medical Laboratory Technician Program (1)
Southeast Community College
800 "O" Street
Lincoln, Nebraska 68520

Medical Laboratory Technician Program (1)
Mid-Plains Community College
I-80 & Hwy. 83
North Platte, Nebraska 69101

NEW HAMPSHIRE

Medical Laboratory Technician Program (1)
New Hampshire Vocational Technical College
Hanover Street Extension
Claremont, New Hampshire 03743

Medical Laboratory Technician Program (1)
Rivier College
429 Main Street
Nashua, New Hampshire 03060

NEW JERSEY

Medical Laboratory Technician Program (1)
Camden County College
Little Gloucester Road
Blackwood, New Jersey 08012

Medical Laboratory Technician Program (2)
Lyons Institute
16 Springdale Road
Cherry Hill, New Jersey 08003

Medical Laboratory Technician Program (2)
Lyons Institute
10 Commerce Place
Clark, New Jersey 07066

Medical Laboratory Technician Program (1)
Union County College
1033 Springfield Avenue
Cranford, New Jersey 07016

Medical Laboratory Technician Program (1)
Middlesex County College
155 Mill Road
P.O. Box 3050
Edison, New Jersey 08818-3050

Medical Laboratory Technician Program (2)
Lyons Institute
320 Main Street
Hackensack, New Jersey 07601

Medical Laboratory Technician Program (1)
Brookdale Community College
765 Newman Springs Road
Lincroft, New Jersey 07738

Medical Laboratory Technician Program (1)
Felician College
South Main Street
Lodi, New Jersey 07644

Medical Laboratory Technician Program (1)
Atlantic Community College
Black Horse Pike
Mays Landing, New Jersey 08330

Medical Laboratory Technician Program (1)
Bergen Community College
400 Paramus Road
Paramus, New Jersey 07652

Medical Laboratory Technician Program (1)
Burlington County College
Pemberton, New Jersey 08068

Medical Laboratory Technician Program (1)
County College of Morris
Route 10 & Center Grove Road
Randolph, New Jersey 07869

Medical Laboratory Technician Program (1)
Community Memorial Hospital
99 Route 37
Toms River, New Jersey 08753

Medical Laboratory Technician Program (1)
Mercer County Community College
1200 Old Trenton Road
Trenton, New Jersey 08690

NEW MEXICO

Medical Laboratory Technician Program (1)
New Mexico State University at Alamogordo
Box 477
Alamogordo, New Mexico 88310

Medical Laboratory Technician PRogram (2)
Pima Medical Institute (Branch)
5509 Menaul Boulevard, N.E.
Albuquerque, New Mexico 87110

Medical Laboratory Technician Program (1)
University of New Mexico
200 College Road
Gallup, New Mexico 87301

Medical Laboratory Technician Program (1)
New Mexico Junior College
Lovington Highway
Hobbs, New Mexico 88240

NEW YORK

Medical Laboratory Technician Program (1)
SUNY, Agricultural & Technical College
Administration Bldg.-ASC
Alfred, New York 14802

Medical Laboratory Technician Program (1)
Broome Community College
P.O. Box 10017
Binghamton, New York 13902

Medical Laboratory Technician Program (1)
Erie Community College
121 Ellicott Street
Buffalo, New York 14202

Medical Laboratory Technician Program (1)
State Univeristy of NY Agric. & Tech. College
Cornell Drive
Canton, New York 13617

Medical Laboratory Technician Program (2)
The New York School for Medical and Dental Assistants
116-16 Queens Boulevard
Forest Hills, New York 11375

Medical Laboratory Technician Program (1)
Orange County Community College
115 South Street
Middletown, New York 10940

Medical Laboratory Technician Program (2)
Eastern Technical School
85 5th Avenue
New York, New York 10003

Medical Laboratory Technician Program (1)
Clinton Community College
Bluff Point
Plattsburgh, New York 12901

Medical Laboratory Technician Program (1)
Dutchess Community College
Pendell Road
Poughkeepsie, New York 12601

Medical Laboratory Technician Program (1)
Monroe Community College
1000 E. Henrietta Road
Rochester, New York 14623

Medical Laboratory Technician Program (1)
North Country Community College
Saranac Lake, New York 12983

Medical Laboratory Technician Program (1)
The College of Staten Island
130 Stuyvesant Place
Staten Island, New York 10301

Medical Laboratory Technician Program (1)
Rockland Community College
145 College Road
Suffern, New York 10901

NORTH CAROLINA

Medical Laboratory Technician Program (1)
Asheville-Buncombe Technical College
340 Victoria Road
Asheville, North Carolina 28801

Medical Laboratory Technician Program (1)
Sandhills Community College
Rt. 3, Box 182-C
Carthage, North Carolina 28327

Medical Laboratory Technician Program (1)
Bladen Technical College
P.O. Box 266
Dublin, North Carolina 28332

Medical Laboratory Technician Program (1)
Elon College
Box 2185
Elon College, North Carolina 27244

Medical Laboratory Technician Program (1)
Coastal Carolina Community College
444 Western Boulevard
Jacksonville, North Carolina 28540

Medical Laboratory Technician Program (1)
Western Piedmont Community College
1001 Burkemont Avenue
Morganton, North Carolina 28655

Medical Laboratoary Technician Program (2)
Northern Hospital of Surry County
School of Medical Technology
P.O. Box 1101
830 Rockford Street
Mt. Airy, North Carolina 27030

Medical Laboratory Technician Program (1)
Southwestern Technical College
275 Webster Road
Sylva, North Carolina 28779

Medical Laboratory Technician Program (1)
Beaufort County Community College
P.O. Box 1069
Washington, North Carolina 27889

Medical Laboratory Technician Program (1)
Halifax Community College
Box 809
Weldon, North Carolina 27890

NORTH DAKOTA

Medical Laboratory Technician Program (1)
Bismark Junior College
Schaffer Heights
Bismarck, North Dakota 58501

Medical Laboratory Technician Program (2)
Turtle Mountain School of Paramedical Technique
Box 203
Bottineau, North Dakota 58318

OHIO

Medical Laboratory Technician Program (1)
Stark Technical College
6200 Frank Avenue, N.W.
Canton, Ohio 44720

Medical Laboratory Technician Program (1)
Cincinnati Technical College
3520 Central Parkway
Cincinnati, Ohio 45223

Medical Laboratory Technician Program (1)
Quyahoga Community College
700 Carnegie Avenue
Cleveland, Ohio 44115

Medical Laboratory Technnician Program (20
Cleveland Institute of Dental-Medical
Assistants, Inc.
183 Euclid Avenue
Cleveland, Ohio 44115

Medical Laboratory Technician Program (1)
Columbus Technical Institute
550 E. Spring Street
Columbus, Ohio 43215

Medical Laboratory Technician Program (1)
Lorain County Community College
1005 N. Abbe Road
Elyria, Ohio 44035

Medical Laboratory Technician Program (1)
Kettering College of Medical Arts
3535 Southern Boulevard
Kettering, Ohio 45429

Medical Laboratory Technician Program (1)
Lima Memorial Hospital
1001 Bellefontaine Avenue
Lima, Ohio 45804

Medical Laboratory Technician Program (1)
Washington Technical College
Rt. 2, State Rt. 676
Marietta, Ohio 45750

Medical Laboratory Technician Program (1)
Marion Technical College
1465 Mt. Vernon Avenue
Marion, Ohio 43302

Medical Laboratory Technician Program (1)
Lakeland Community College
Mentor, Ohio 44060

Medical Laboratory Technician Program (1)
Middletown Regional Hospital
105 McKnight Drive
Middletown, Ohio 45044

Medical Laboratory Technician Program (1)
College of Mount St. Joseph
5701 Delhi Road
Mt. St. Joseph, Ohio 45051

Medical Laboratory Technician Program (1)
Shawnee State Community College
940 Second Street
Portsmouth, Ohio 45662

Medical Laboratory Technician Program (1)
Rio Grande College & Community College
Rio Grande, Ohio 45674

Medical Laboratory Technician Program (1)
Clark Technical College
1343 N. Fountain Boulevard
Springfield, Ohio 45501

Medical Laboratory Technician Program (1)
Mercy Medical Center
1343 N. Fountain Boulevard
Springfield, Ohio 45501

Medical Laboratory Technician Program (1)
Jefferson Technical College
4000 Sunset Boulevard
Steubenville, Ohio 43952

Medical Laboratory Technician Program (2)
Stautzenberger College
4404 Secor Road
Toledo, Ohio 43623

Medical Laboratory Technician Program (1)
Youngstown State University
410 Wick Avenue
Youngstown, Ohio 44555

Medical Laboratory Technician Program (1)
Muskingum Area Technical College
1555 Newark Road
Zanesville, Ohio 43701

OKLAHOMA

Medical Laboratory Technician Program (1)
Northeaster OK A & M College
2nd and 1 Streets, N.E.
Miami, Oklahoma 74354

Medical Laboratory Technician Program (1)
Rose State College
6420 S.E. 15th
Midwest City, Oklahoma 73110

Medical Laboratory Technician Program (2)
United Technical Institute
4533 Enterprise Drive
Oklahoma City, Oklahoma 73128

Medical Laboratory Technician Program (2)
Sayre Junior College
716 N.E. 66 Highway
Sayre, Oklahoma 73662

Medical Laboratory Technician Program (1)
Seminole Junior College
P.O. Box 351
Seminole, Oklahoma 74868

Medical Laboratory Technician Program (1)
Tulsa Junior College
6111 E. Skelly Drive
Tulsa, Oklahoma 74135-6101

OREGON

Medical Laboratory Technician Program (1)
Portland Community College
12000 S.W. 49th Avenue
Portland, Oregon 97219

PENNSYLVANIA

Medical Laboratory Technician Program (1)
Ashland State General Hospital
Route 61
Ashland, Pennsylvania 17921

Medical Laboratory Technician Program (1)
Northampton County Area Community College
3835 Green Pond Road
Bethlehem, Pennsylvania 18017

Medical Laboratory Technician Program (1)
Montgomery County Community College
340 DeKalb Pike
Blue Bell, Pennsylvania 19422

Medical Laboratory Technician Program (1)
Harcum Junior College
Bryn Mawr, Pennsylvania 19010

Medical Laboratory Technician Program (1)
Mt. Aloysius Junior College
William Penn Hwy.
Cresson, Pennsylvania 16630

Medical Laboratory Technician Program (1)
Chambersburg Hospital
112 N. Seventh Street
Chambersburg, Pennsylvania 17201

Medical Laboratory Technician Program (1)
Hamot Medical Center
201 State Street
Erie, Pennsylvania 16550

Medical Laboratory Technician Program (1)
Westmoreland Hospital Association
532 W. Pittsburgh Street
Greensburg, Pennsylvania 15601

Medical Laboratory Technician Program (1)
Gwynedd-Mercy College
Sumneytown Pike
Gwynedd Valley, Pennsylvania 19437

Medical Laboratory Technician Program (1)
Harrisburg Area Community College
3300 Cameron St. Road
Harrisburg, Pennsylvania 17110-2999

Medical Laboratory Technician Program (1)
PA State University-Hazleton Campus
Hazelton Campus
Hazelton, Pennsylvania 18201

Medical Laboratory Technician Program (1)
Manor Junior College
Fox Chase Road
Jenkintown, Pennsylvania 19046

Medical Laboratory Technician Program (1)
Conemaugh Valley Memorial Hospital
1086 Franklin Street
Johnstown, Pennsylvania 15905

Medical Laboratory Technician Program (1)
Community College of Beaver County
College Drive
Monaca, Pennsylvania 15061

Medical Laboratory Technician Program (1)
The Pennsylvania State University
3550 Seventh St. Road
New Kensington, Pennsylvania 15068

Medical Laboratory Technician Program (1)
Community College of Philadelphia
1700 Spring Garden Street
Philadelphia, Pennsylvania 19130

Medical Laboratory Technician Program (1)
Hahnemann University
Broad & Vine Streets
Philadelphia, Pennsylvania 19102

Medical Laboratory Technician Program (2)
James Martin School
Adult Vocational Training Center
Richmond and Ontario Streets
Philadelphia, Pennsylvania 19134

Medical Laboratory Technician Program (2)
McCarrie School of Health Sciences and Technology
132 North 12 Street
Philadelphia, Pennsylvania 19107

Medical Laboratory Technician Program (1)
Spring Garden College
7500 Germantown Avenue
Philadelphia, Pennsylvania 19118

Medical Laboratory Technician Program (1)
Community College of Allegheny Cty-Allegheny Campus
808 Ridge Avenue
Pittsburgh, Pennsylvania 15212

Medical Laboratory Technician Program (1)
Reading Area Community College
P.O. Box 1706
10 S. Second Street
Reading, Pennsylvania 19606

Medical Laboratory Technician Program (1)
Community College of Allegheny Cty
1750 Clairton Road
West Mifflin, Pennsylvania 15122

RHODE ISLAND

Medical Laboratory Technician Program (1)
Community College of Rhode Island
400 East Avenue
Warwick, Rhode Island 02886

SOUTH CAROLINA

Medical Laboratory Technician Program (1)
Trident Technical College
P.O. Box 10367
Charleston, South Carolina 29411

Medical Laboratory Technician Program (1)
Midlands Technical College
P.O. Box 2408
Columbia, South Carolina 29202

Medical Laboratory Technician Program (1)
Florence-Darlington Technical College
P.O. Drawer F-8000
Florence, South Carolina 29501

Medical Laboratory Technician Program (1)
Greenville Technical College
P.O. Box 5616-Station B
Greenville, South Carolina 29606-5616

Medical Laboratory Technician Program (1)
Orangeburg-Calhoun Technical College
3250 St. Matthews Road
Orangeburg, South Carolina 29115

Medical Laboratory Technician Program (1)
Tri-County Technical College
P.O. Box 587
Pendleton, South Carolina 29670

Medical Laboratory Technician Program (1)
York Technical College
US Hwy 21 A By-Pass
Rock Hill, South Carolina 29730

Medical Laboratory Technician Program (1)
Spartanburg Technical College
P.O. Drawer 4386
Spartanburg, South Carolina 29305

SOUTH DAKOTA

Medical Laboratory Technician Program (1)
Presentation College
1500 N. Main Street
Aberdeen, South Dakota 57401-1299

Medical Laboratory Technician Program (1)
Mitchell Area Vocational Technical School
821 N. Capital Street
Mitchell, South Carolina 57301

Medical Laboratory Technician Program (1)
Lake Area Vocational Technical School
200 N.E. 9th
Watertown, South Dakota 57201

TENNESSEE

Medical Laboratory Technician Program (1)
Cleveland State Community College
P.O. Box 3750
Cleveland, Tennessee 37320-3570

Medical Laboratory Technician Program (1)
Columbia State Community College
P.O. Box 1315
Columbia, Tennessee 38401

Medical Laboratory Technician Program (1,2)
Cumberland School of Medical Technology
321 N. Washington
Cookeville, Tennessee 38501

Medical Laboratory Technician Program (1)
Volunteer State Community College
Nashville Pike
Gallatin, Tennessee 37066

Medical Laboratory Technician Program (1)
Roane State Community College
Patton Lane
Harriman, Tennessee 37748

Medical Laboratory Technician Program (1)
Jackson State Community College
P.O. Box 2487
Jackson, Tennessee 38302

Medical Laboratory Technician Program (1)
East Tennessee State University
Box 24, 520A
Johnson City, Tennessee 37614

Medical Laboratory Technician Program (1)
Knoxville City Board of Education
101 E. 5th Avenue
Knoxville, Tennessee 37917

Medical Laboratory Technician Program (1)
Sea Isle Vocational Technical Center
5250 Sea Isle Road
Memphis, Tennessee 38117

Medical Laboratory Technician Program (1)
Shelby State Community College
1256 Union Ave. POB 40568
Memphis, Tennessee 38174-0568

Medical Laboratory Technician Program (1)
Nashville State Technical Institute
120 White Bridge Road
Nashville, Tennessee 37209

TEXAS

Medical Laboratory Technician Program (1)
Alvin Community College
3110 Mustang Road
Alvin, Texas 77511

Medical Laboratory Technician Program (1)
Amarillo College
P.O. Box 447
Amarillo, Texas 79178

Medical Laboratory Technician Program (1)
Austin Community College
P.O. Box 2285
Austin, Texas 78768

Medical Laboratory Technician Program (1)
Texas Southmost College
80 Fort Brown
Brownsville, Texas 78520

Medical Laboratory Technician Program (2)
Navarro College
P.O. Box 1170
West Seventh Avenue
Corsicana, Texas 75110

Medical Laboratory Technician Program (1)
Del Mar College
Baldwin & Ayers
Corpus Christi, Texas 78404

Medical Laboratory Technician Program (1)
El Centro College
Main & Lamar
Dallas, Texas 75202-3604

Medical Laboratory Technician Program (1)
Grayson County College
6101 Grayson Drive
Denison, Texas 75020

Medical Laboratory Technician Program (1)
El Paso Community College
P.O. Box 20500
El Paso, Texas 79998

Medical Laboratory Technician Program (1)
Houston Community College System
22 Waugh Drive
P.O. Box 7849
Houston, Texas 77270-7849

Medical Laboratory Technician Program (1)
Tarrant County Junior College
828 Harwood Road
Hurst, Texas 76054

Medical Laboratory Technician Program (1)
Kilgore College
1100 Broadway
Kilgore, Texas 75662

Medical Laboratory Technician Program (1)
Laredo Junior College
West End Washington Street
Laredo, Texas 78040

Medical Laboratory Technician Program (1)
Odessa College
201 W. University
Odessa, Texas 79764

Medical Laboratory Technician Program (1)
Orange Memorial Hospital
P.O. Box 37
Orange, Texas 77630

Medical Laboratory Technician Program (1)
San Antonio State Chest Hospital
P.O. 23340 Highland Hills Station
San Antonio, Texas 78223

Medical Laboratory Technician Program (1)
St. Philip's College
2111 Nevada Street
San Antonio, Texas 78203

Medical Laboratory Technician Program (2)
Southwest School of Medical Assistants
115 North Braodway
San Antonio, Texas 78205

Medical Laboratory Technician Program (1)
School of Health Care Sciences, USAF
Sheppard AFB, Texas 76311-5465

Medical Laboratory Technician Program (1)
Temple Junior College
2600 S 1
Temple, Texas 76501

Medical Laboratory Technician Program (1)
Tyler Junior College
E. 5th Street, Box 9020
Tyler, Texas 75711

Medical Laboratory Technician Program (1)
Victoria College
2200 E. Red River
Victoria, Texas 77901

Medical Laboratory Technician Program (1)
McLennan Community College
1400 College Drive
Waco, Texas 76708

Medical Laboratory Technician Program (1)
Midwestern State University
3400 Taft Boulevard
Wichita Falls, Texas 76308

UTAH

Medical Laboratory Technician Program (1)
Weber State College
M S 1001
Ogden, Utah 88408

VERMONT

Medical Laboratory Technician Program (1)
Vermont College of Norwich University
Office of the President
Northfield, Vermont 05764

VIRGINIA

Medical Laboratory Technician Program (1)
Northern Virginia Community College
8333 Little River Turnpike
Annandale, Virginia 22003

Medical Laboratory Technician Program (2)
Temple School (Branch)
5832 Columbia Pike
Bailey's Crossroads, Virginia 22041

Medical Laboratory Technician Program (1)
Thomas Nelson Community College
P.O. Box 9407
Hampton, Virginia 23670

Medical Laboratory Technician Program (1)
Norfolk General Hospital
600 Gresham Drive
Norfolk, Virginia 23507

Medical Laboratory Technician Program (1)
Central Virginia Community College
3506 Wards Road
Lynchburg, Virginia 24502

Medical Laboratory Technician Program (1)
Maryview Hospital
3636 High Street
Portsmouth, Virginia 23707-3274

Medical Laboratory Technician Program (1)
J. Sargeant Reynolds Community College
P.O. Box C-32040
Richmond, Virginia 23261-2040

Medical Laboratory Technician Program (1)
Wytheville Community College
1000 E. Main Street
Wytheville, Virginia 24382

WASHINGTON

Medical Laboratory Technician Program (1)
Shoreline Community College
16101 Greenwood Ave. N.
Seattle, Washington 98133

Medical Laboratory Technician Program (1)
Clover Park School District-400 Ed. Center
4500 Steilacoom Blvd., S.W.
Tacoma, Washington 98499

Medical Laboratory Technician Program (1)
Wenatchee Valley College
1300 Fifth Street
Wenatchee, Washington 98801

WEST VIRGINIA

Medical Laboratory Technician Program (1)
Veterans Administration Medical Center
200 Veterans Avenue
Beckley, West Virginia 25801

Medical Laboratory Technician Program (1)
Bluefield Community Hospital, School of MT
500 Cherry Street
Bluefield, West Virginia 24701-3306

Medical Laboratory Technician Program (2)
Boone County Career Center
Box 50 B
Danville, West Virginia 25053

Medical Laboratory Technician Program (1)
Fairmont State College
Locust Avenue
Fairmont, West Virginia 26554

Medical Laboratory Technician Program (1)
Marshall University
Huntington, West Virginia 25701

Medical Laboratory Technician Program (1)
West Virginia Northern Community College
College Square
Wheeling, West Virginia 26003

WISCONSIN

Medical Laboratory Technician Program (1)
VTAE District One Technical Institute
620 W. Clairemont Avenue
Eau Claire, Wisconsin 54701

Medical Laboratory Technician Program (1)
Western Wisconsin Technical Institute
304 North 6th Street
P.O. Box 908
La Crosse, Wisconsin 54602-0908

Medical Laboratory Technician Program (1)
Madison Area Technical College
211 N. Carroll Street
Madison, Wisconsin 53703

Medical Laboratory Technician Program (1)
Milwaukee Area Technical College
1015 N. Sixth Street
Milwaukee, Wisconsin 53203

WYOMING

Medical Laboratory Technician Program (1,2)
Northwest Community College
231 W. Sixth Street
Powell, Wyoming 82435

Medical Laboratory Technician Program (1)
Western Wyoming College
2500 College Drive
P.O. Box 428
Rock Springs, Wyoming 82901

Specialist in Blood Bank Technology

Under the direction of a pathologist or other physician, the *specialist in blood bank technology* specializes in typing, crossmatching, and testing of blood for life-giving transfusions. In collecting. classifying, storing, and processing blood, the specialist detects and identifies antibodies in patient and donor bloods and selects suitable blood for transfusion.

Although medical technologists and medical laboratory technicians may all perform various tests in blood bank technology, the specialist is a more highly trained individual who interprets technical work and who performs specialized tests such as *immunohematology* (the study of blood and its immunities). The specialist may also be a blood bank supervisor, an educator, a consultant, or a researcher.

Certification in medical technology, MT(ASCP), or blood bank technology, BB(ASCP), or a bachelor's degree in biological or physical sciences, or medical technology, plus work experience, are prerequisites for entrance into an accredited twelve-month advanced training program in blood bank technology.

After completion of this program certification as a specialist in blood bank technology, SBB(ASCP) is available from the Board of Registry of the American Society of Clinical Pathologists.

For further career information, write to the American Association of Blood Banks, 1117 North 19th Street, Arlington, Virginia 22209.

Following is a list of educational programs for the specialist in blood bank technology, accredited by the American Association of Blood Banks, in conjunction with the Committee on Allied Health Education and Accreditation of the American Medical Association.

SOURCES:

American Association of Blood Banks
American Society of Clinical Pathologists

Specialist in Blood Bank Technology Programs

ALABAMA

Specialist in Blood Bank Technology Program
University of Alabama Hospitals Blood Bank and American Red Cross Services
Alabama Region
619 19th Street, South
Birmingham, Alabama 35233

CALIFORNIA

Specialist in Blood Bank Technology Program
American Red Cross Blood Services
Central California Region
333 McKendrie Street
San Jose, California 95110-9990

Specialist in Blood Bank Technology Program
Sacramento Medical Foundation Blood Bank
1625 Stockton Boulevard
Sacramento, California 95816-7089

Specialist in Blood Bank Technology Program
San Diego Blood Bank
440 Upas Street
P.O. Box 3757
San Diego, California 92103

CONNECTICUT

Specialist in Blood Bank Technology Program
American Red Cross Blood Services
Connecticut Region
209 Farmington Avenue
Farmington, Connecticut 06032

DISTRICT OF COLUMBIA

Specialist in Blood Bank Technology Program
Walter Reed Army Medical Center Blood Bank
Building 2
6825 16th Street, N.W.
Washington, D.C. 20307-5001

FLORIDA

Specialist in Blood Bank Technology Program
Central Florida Blood Bank, Inc.
1300 South Kuhl Avenue
Orlando, Florida 32806

Specialist in Blood Bank Technology Program
Southwest Florida Blood Bank, Inc.
P.O. Box 2125
Tampa, Florida 33601

GEORGIA

The Atlanta Specialist in Blood Bank Technology Program
1925 Monroe Drive, N.E.
Atlanta, Georgia 30324

ILLINOIS

Specialist in Blood Bank Technology Program
LifeSource Blood Center
43 East Ohio Street
Chicago, Illinois 60611

Specialist in Blood Bank Technology Program
Michael Reese Hospital & Medical Center
School of Health Sciences
29th & Ellis Avenue
Chicago, Illinois 60616

Specialist in Blood Bank Technology Program
University of Illinois at Chicago
Medical Laboratory Sciences Department
808 S. Wood Street
Box 6998
Chicago, Illinois 60612

INDIANA

Specialist in Blood Bank Technology Program
Central Indiana Regional Blood Center
3450 North Meridian
Indianapolis, Indiana 46208

LOUISIANA

Specialist in Blood Bank Technology Program
Alton Ochsner Foundation
Hospital Blood Bank
1516 Jefferson Highway
New Orleans, Louisiana 70121

Specialist in Blood Bank Technology Program
Charity Hospital of Louisiana at New Orleans
Blood Bank Program
1532 Tulane Avenue
New Orleans, Louisiana 70140

Specialist in Blood Bank Technology Program
Southern Baptist Hospital Blood Bank
2700 Napoleon Avenue
New Orleans, Louisiana 70175

MARYLAND

Specialist in Blood Bank Technology Program
Johns Hopkins Hospital Blood Bank
600 North Wolfe
Baltimore, Maryland 21205

Specialist in Blood Bank Technology Program
National Institute of Health
Department of Transfusion Medicine
9000 Rockville Pike, Bldg. 10-A
Bethesda, Maryland 20014

MASSACHUSETTS

Specialist in Blood Bank Technology Program
New England Deaconess Hospital Blood Bank
185 Pilgrim Road
Boston, Massachusetts 02215

MICHIGAN

Specialist in Blood Bank Technology Program
American Red Cross Blood Services
Southeastern Michigan Region
P.O. Box 33351
Detroit, Michigan 48232

Specialist in Blood Bank Technology Program
William Beaumont Hospital
School of Specialist in Blood Banking
3601 West Thirteen Mile Road
Royal Oak, Michigan 48072

MINNESOTA

Specialist in Blood Bank Technology Program
Memorial Blood Center of Minneapolis
2304 Park Avenue
Minneapolis, Minnesota 55404

MISSOURI

Specialist in Blood Bank Technology Program
Barnes Hospital
School of Blood Banking
4949 Barnes Hospital Plaza
St. Louis, Missouri 63110

NEW YORK

Specialist in Blood Bank Technology Program
State University of New York
Upstate Medical Center
750 East Adams Street
Syracuse, New York 13210

NORTH CAROLINA

Specialist in Blood Bank Technology Program
Duke University Medical Center Blood Bank
Box 2929
Durham, North Carolina 27710

OHIO

Specialist in Blood Bank Technology Program
American Red Cross Blood Services
Northern Ohio Region
3950 Chester Avenue
Cleveland, Ohio 44114-4690

Specialist in Blood Bank Technology Program
Hoxworth Blood Center of the University of
Cincinnati
3231 Burnet Avenue
Cincinnati, Ohio 45267-1127

Specialist in Blood Bank Technology Program
Ohio State University Hospitals-Central
Ohio Red Cross Transfusion Service
410 W. 10th Avenue
Columbus, Ohio 43210-1228

OKLAHOMA

Specialist in Blood Bank Technology Program
Oklahoma Blood Institute
Sylvan N. Goldman Center
1001 N. Lincoln Boulevard
Oklahoma City, Oklahoma 73104

OREGON

Specialist in Blood Bank Technology Program
Pacific Northwest Regional Red Cross Blood
Services
3131 North Vancouver
P.O. Box 3200
Portland, Oregon 97208

SOUTH CAROLINA

Specialist in Blood Bank Technology Program
Medical University of South Carolina & American Red Cross Bood Services
Department of Laboratory Medicine
171 Ashley Avenue
Charleston, South Carolina 29425-1097

TENNESSEE

Specialist in Blood Bank Technology Program
Baptist Memorial Hospital Blood Bank
899 Madison Avenue
Memphis, Tennessee 38146

TEXAS

Specialist in Blood Bank Technology Program
St. Luke's Episcopal Hospital
School of Blood Bank Technology
6720 Bertner Avenue
Houston, Texas 77030

Specialist in Blood Bank Technology Program
University of Texas
Health Science Center
5323 Harry Hines Boulevard
Dallas, Texas 75235

Specialist in Blood Bank Technology Program
University of Texas Blood Bank of the Medical Branch Hospitals
8th and Mechanic Streets
Galveston, Texas 77550-2780

Specialist in Blood Bank Technology Program
University of Texas HSC
Medical Center Hospital
7703 Floyd Curl Drive
San Antonio, Texas 78284

UTAH

Specialist in Blood Bank Technology Program
LDS Hospital Hospital Bank
325 Eighth Avenue
Salt Lake City, Utah 84143

WISCONSIN

Specialist in Blood Bank Technology Program
American Red Cross Blood Services
Badger Region, School of Blood Bank Tech.
4860 Sheboygan Ave., P.O. Box 5905
Madison, Wisconsin 53701

Cytotechnologist

The *cytotechnologist* is a medical technologist who specializes in cytology, the medical science that detects early evidence of cancerous cells and usually allows for effective treatment of lung, stomach, mouth, cervical, and other cancers. With minimal supervision from the pathologist, the cytotechnologist screens specially stained slides of human cells under the microscope. In the delicate patterns of the cell's cytoplasm and nucleus, the technologist looks for minute abnormalities in cell structure that might be the first warning signs of cancer. The most familiar cytologic test is the Pap smear, which tests cervical cancer in the female reproductive tract. Most cytotechnologists do their work in hospitals and private laboratories.

The minimum educational requirement for the cytotechnologist is an associate degree or two-to-three years of college with emphasis on courses in biological sciences, both followed by completion of a twelve-month accredited certificate program in cytotechnology. A bachelor's degree in cytotechnology is available and there is a trend to require a bachelor's degree for certification.

Certification as a cytotechnologist, CT(ASCP), is available and recommended upon successful completion of an accredited program and the American Society of Clinical Pathologist's certification examination.

Average starting salaries for the cytotechnologist equalled $19,000, while experienced technologists earned $24,800, according to a University of Texas Medical Branch survey.

Below is a list supplied by the American Society of Cytology of accredited programs in cytotechnology. For more information on a career as a cytotechnologist, write to the American Society of Cytology, 130 South 9th Street, Philadelphia, Pennsylvania 19107.

KEY:

(1) Bachelor's degree program

(2) Certificate program

SOURCES:

American Society of Clinical Pathologists
American Society of Cytology

Cytotechnologist Programs

ALABAMA

Cytotechnologist Program (1)
University of Alabama
School of Community and Allied Health
University Station
Birmingham, Alabama 35294

Cytotechnologist Program (1,2)
University of South Alabama Medical Center
Moorer Clinical Sciences Building
2451 Fillingim Street
Mobile, Alabama 36617

ARKANSAS

Cytotechnologist Program (2)
University of Arkansas for Medical Sciences
College of Health Related Professions
4301 West Markham, Slot 620
Little Rock, Arkansas 72205

CALIFORNIA

Cytotechnologist Program (1,2)
Loma Linda University
School of Allied Health Professions
Dept. of Clinical Laboratory Science
Loma Linda, California 92350

Cytotechnologist Program (2)
Los Angeles County-University of Southern California
School of Cytotechnology
1200 North Street Street
Los Angeles, California 90033

Cytotechnologist Program (2)
The Hospital of the Good Samaritan
616 South Witmer Street
Los Angeles, California 90017

Cytotechnologist Program (2)
M.S. Hippen School of Cytotechnology
D.N. Sharp Memorial Hospital
7901 Frost Street
San Diego, California 92123

Cytotechnologist Program (2)
University of California
Curriculum in Exfoliative Cytology
Third and Parnassus, HSW 595
San Francisco, California 94143

CONNECTICUT

Cytotechnologist Program (1,2)
University of Connecticut Health Center
Department of Pathology
263 Farmington Avenue
Farmington, Connecticut 06032

FLORIDA

Cytotechnologist Program (1,2)
University of Miami
Department of Pathology
Box 016960 (R-1)
Miami, Florida 33101

GEORGIA

Cytotechnologist Program (2)
Grady Memorial Hospital
80 Butler Street, S.E.
Atlanta, Georgia 30335

ILLINOIS

Cytotechnologist Program (1,2)
Michael Reese Hospital and Medical Center
Lake Shore Drive at 31st Street
Chicago, Illinois 60616

Cytotechnologist Program (1,2)
University of Chicago
Chicago Lying-In-Hospital
5841 South Maryland Ave., HM 449
Chicago, Illinois 60637

INDIANA

Cytotechnologist Program (1)
Indiana University School of Medicine
Fesler Hall 409
1120 South Drive
Indianapolis, Indiana 46223

KANSAS

Cytotechnologist Program (1,2)
University of Kansas Medical Center
1600 Bell Memorial
39th and Rainbow Boulevard
Kansas City, Kansas 66103

KENTUCKY

Cytotechnologist Program (1,2)
University of Louisville
Health Sciences Center
Division of Allied Health
Louisville, Kentucky 40292

LOUISIANA

Cytotechnologist Program (1)
Louisiana State University Medical Center
Department of Medical Technology
1900 Gravier Street
New Orleans, Louisiana 70112

MARYLAND

Cytotechnologist Program (2)
The Johns Hopkins Hospital
610 Pathology Building
Baltimore, Maryland 21205

Cytotechnologist Program (2)
Naval School of Health Sciences
Cytology Technician School
Bethesda, Maryland 20814-5033

MASSACHUSETTS

Cytotechnologist Program (1,2)
Berkshire Medical Center
725 North Street
Pittsfield, Massachusetts 01201

MICHIGAN

Cytotechnologist Program (1,2)
Harper-Grace Hospitals
Department of Pathology
3990 John R Street
Detroit, Michigan 48201-2097

Cytotechnologist Program (2)
Wayne State University
Department of Pathology
540 East Canfield Avenue
Detroit, Michigan 48201

Cytotechnologist Program (1)
William Beaumont Hospital
Department of Anatomic Pathology
3601 West 13 Mile Road
Royal Oak, Michigan 48072

MINNESOTA

Cytotechnologist Program (2)
Mayo School of Health-Related Sciences
200 First Street, S.W.
Rochester, Minnesota 55905

MISSISSIPPI

Cytotechnologist Program (1)
University of Mississippi Medical Center
School of Health-Related Professions
2500 North State Street
Jackson, Mississippi 39216

MISSOURI

Cytotechnologist Program (1)
University of Missouri-Columbia
Department of Pathology - M646
1 Hospital Drive
Columbia, Missouri 65211

NEW JERSEY

Cytotechnologist Program (2)
University of Medicine and Dentistry of New Jersey (UMD-NJ)
School of Health-Related Professions
100 Bergen Street
Newark, New Jersey 07103

Cytotechnologist Program (2)
Muhlenberg Hospital
Park Avenue and Randolph Road
Plainfield, New Jersey 07061

NEW YORK

Cytotechnologist Program (1,2)
Albany School of Cytotechnology
College of St. Rose
432 Western Avenue, Box 189
Albany, New York 12203

Cytotechnologist Program (2)
Memorial Sloan-Kettering Cancer Center
1275 York Avenue
New York, New York 10021

Cytotechnologist Program (2)
Papanicolaou School of Cytotechnology
The New York Hospital
525 East 68th Street
New York, New York 10021

Cytotechnologist Program (1)
State University of New York
S.U.N.Y.-Upstate Medical Center
766 Irving Avenue
Syracuse, New York 13210

NORTH CAROLINA

Cytotechnologist Program (2)
University of North Carolina
North Carolina Memorial Hospital
Medical School Wing E
Chapel Hill, North Carolina 27514

Cytotechnologist Program (1,2)
Elon College
Campus Box 2213
Elon College, North Carolina 27244

NORTH DAKOTA

Cytotechnologist Program (1,2)
University of North Dakota
Department of Pathology
University Station
Grand Forks, North Dakota 58202

OHIO

Cytotechnologist Program (1,2)
Akron General Medical Center
400 Wabash Avenue
Akron, Ohio 44307

Cytotechnologist Program (1,2)
St. Luke's Hospital
11311 Shaker Boulevard
Cleveland, Ohio 44104

Cytotechnologist Program (1,2)
St. Elizabeth Hospital Medical Center
1044 Belmont Avenue
Youngstown, Ohio 44501

OKLAHOMA

Cytotechnologist Program (1)
University of Oklahoma
Dept. of Clinical Laboratory Sciences
P.O. Box 26901, 801 N.E. 13th St.
Oklahoma City, Oklahoma 73190

PENNSYLVANIA

Cytotechnologist Program (1)
Thomas Jefferson University
Department of Cytotechnology
Philadelphia, Pennsylvania 19107

Cytotechnologist Program (2)
Hospital of the University of Pennsylvania
School of Cytotechnology
3400 Spruce Street
Philadelphia, Pennsylvania 19104

Cytotechnologist Program (2)
University Health Center of Pittsburgh
Magee-Women's Hospital
Forbes Avenue & Halket Street
Pittsburgh, Pennsylvania 15213

RHODE ISLAND

Cytotechnologist Program (1,2)
St. Joseph Hospital
Our Lady of Fatima Unit
200 High Service Avenue
North Providence, Rhode Island 02904

SOUTH CAROLINA

Cytotechnologist Program (1)
Medical University of South Carolina
Cytotechnology-Histotechnology Education Department
171 Ashley Avenue
Charleston, South Carolina 29425

TENNESSEE

Cytotechnologist Program (2)
University of Tennessee
Memorial Hospital & Research Center
1924 Alcoa Highway
Knoxville, Tennessee 37920

Cytotechnologist Program (1)
University of Tennessee
Center for the Health Sciences
858 Madison Avenue
Memphis, Tennessee 38163

TEXAS

Cytotechnologist Program (2)
Brooke Army Medical Center
U.S. Army School of Cytotechnology
Department of Pathology & ALS
Fort Sam Houston, Texas 78234-6200

Cytotechnologist Program (2)
University of Texas
Health Science Center at Houston
P.O. Box 20708
Houston, Texas 77225

Cytotechnologist Program (2)
Medical Center Hospital at San Antonio
Pathology Department
7703 Floyd Curl Drive
San Antonio, Texas 78284

UTAH

Cytotechnologist Program (1)
University of Utah Medical Center
Department of Pathology
50 North Medical Drive
Salt Lake City, Utah 84132

VERMONT

Cytotechnologist Program (2)
Medical Center Hospital of Vermont
DeGoesbriand Unit
1 South Prospect Street
Burlington, Vermont 05401

WASHINGTON

Cytotechnologist Program (2)
Harborview Medical Center
University of Washington
325 Ninth Avenue
Seattle, Washington 98104

WEST VIRGINIA

Cytotechnologist Program (2)
Charleston Area Medical Center
3200 MacCorkle Avenue, S.E.
Charleston, West Virginia 25304

Cytotechnologist Program (1,2)
Cabell Huntington Hospital
1340 Hal Greer Boulevard
Huntington, West Virginia 25701

WISCONSIN

Cytotechnologist Program (2)
University of Wisconsin-Madison
Center for Health Sciences
465 Henry Mall
Madison, Wisconsin 53706

Cytotechnologist Program (2)
Marshfield Clinic
School of Cytotechnology
1000 North Oak Avenue
Marshfield, Wisconsin 54449

Cytotechnologist Program (2)
Milwaukee County Medical Complex
Cytotechnology Training Program
8700 West Wisconsin Avenue
Milwaukee, Wisconsin 53226

Histologic Technician

The *histologic technician* or *histology technician* is a medical laboratory technician who specializes in preparing sections of body tissues for microscopic examination by the pathologist. Often while the patient lies in the operating room, the histologic technician, under supervision of the pathologist, freezes and sections tissue samples taken from the patient, mounts them on slides, and stains them with special dyes to make details visible under the microscope. The pathologist then looks for malignant or questionable cells and makes his final diagnosis, allowing the surgeons to proceed with the operation in the appropriate manner.

High school graduation or the equivalent is the prerequisite for entrance into a twelve-month accredited clinical pathology program in histologic techniques. Community college programs that offer associate degrees in histologic techniques are recommended after they have received accreditation.

Certification as a histologic technician, HT(ASCP), is available for graduates of an American Medical Association — accredited program who pass the American Society of Clinical Pathologists' examination.

Recent starting salaries for the histologic technician average $16,000 and experienced technicians average $20,700.

Below is a list of educational programs accredited by the American Medical Association's Committee on Allied Health Education and Accreditation for the histologic technician. Contact the program directly for details on entrance prerequisites and length of program.

SOURCE:

American Society of Clinical Pathologists

Histologic Technician Programs

ARKANSAS

Histologic Technician Program
Baptist Medical Center
9601 Interstate 630 Exit 7
Little Rock, Arkansas 72205-7299

CALIFORNIA

Histologic Technician Program
Cedars-Sinai Medical Center
8700 Beverly Boulevard
Los Angeles, California 90048

COLORADO

Histologic Technician Program
Penrose Hospitals
2215 N. Cascade Avenue
P.O. Box 7021
Colorado Springs, Colorado 80933

CONNECTICUT

Histologic Technician Program
Hartford Hospital
80 Seymour Street
Hartford, Connecticut 06115

GEORGIA

Histologic Technician Program
Georgia Baptist Medical Center
300 Boulevard, N.E.
Atlanta, Georgia 30312

Histologic Technician Program
St. Joseph Hospital
5665 Peachtree-Dunwoody Road, N.E.
Atlanta,Georgia, 30342

ILLINOIS

Histologic Technician Program
Holy Cross Hospital
2701 W. 68th Street
Chicago, Illinois 60629

Histologic Technician Program
St. Joseph Hospital
2900 N. Lake Shore Drive
Chicago, Illinois 60657

Histologic Technician Program
University of Chicago
5841 S. Maryland, Box 417
Chicago, Illinois 60637

Histologic Technician Program
Methodist Medical Center of Illinois
221 N.E. Glen Oak
Peoria, Illinois 61636

Histologic Technician Program
St. Francis Medical Center
530 N.E. Glen Oak Avenue
Peoria, Illinois 61637

Histologic Technician Program
Memorial Medical Center
800 N. Rutledge Street
Springfield, Illinois 62781

Histologic Technician Program
St. John's Hospital
800 E. Carpenter
Springfield, Illinois 62769

KANSAS

Histologic Technician Program
St. Francis Regional Medical Center
929 N. St. Francis Avenue
Wichita, Kansas 67214

MARYLAND

Histologic Technician Program
Harford Community College
401 Thomas Run Road
Bel Air, Maryland 21014

MICHIGAN

Histologic Technician Program
Hurley Medical Center
Number One Hurley Plaza
Flint, Michigan 48502

Histologic Technician Program
Blodgett Memorial Medical Center
1840 Wealthy Street, S.E.
Grand Rapids, Michigan 49506

Histologic Technician Program
William Beaumont Hospital
3601 W. 13 Mile Road
Royal Oak, Michigan 48072

Histologic Technician Program
St. Mary's Hospital
830 South Jefferson
Saginaw, Michigan 48601

MINNESOTA

Histologic Technician Program
Fergus Falls Community College
1414 College Way
Fergus Falls, Minnesota 56537

MISSOURI

Histologic Technician Program
University of Missouri-Columbia
105 Jesse Hall
Columbia, Missouri 65211

Histologic Technician Program
St. Mary's Hospital
101 Memorial Drive
Kansas City, Missouri 64108

NEW JERSEY

Histologic Technician Program
The Mountainside Hospital
Bay & Highland Avenue
Montclair, New Jersey 07042

Histologic Technician Program
Muhlenberg Hospital
Park Avenue & Randolph Road
Plainfield, New Jersey 07061

NEW YORK

Histologic Technician Program
SUNY Agricultural & Technical College
Cobleskill, New York 12043

NORTH DAKOTA

Histologic Technician Program
University of North Dakota
University Station
Grand Forks, North Dakota 58202

OHIO

Histologic Technician Program
Aultman Hospital
2600 Sixth Street S.W.
Canton, Ohio 44710

OKLAHOMA

Histologic Technician Program
Rose State College
6420 S.E 15th
Midwest City, Oklahoma 73110

PENNSYLVANIA

Histologic Technician Program
Geisinger Medical Center
North Academy Avenue
Danville, Pennsylvania 17822

Histologic Technician Program
Conemaugh Valley Memorial Hospital
1086 Franklin Street
Johnstown, Pennsylvania 15905

Histologic Technician Program
Hospital of the University of PA
3400 Spruce Street
Philadelphia, Pennsylvania 19104

SOUTH CAROLINA

Histologic Technician Program
Medical University of South Carolina
171 Ashley Avenue
Charleston, South Carolina 29425

TENNESSEE

Histologic Technician Program
Methodist Hospital of Memphis
1265 Union Avenue
Memphis, Tennessee 38104

Histologic Technician Program
University of Tennessee
800 Madison Avenue
Memphis, Tennessee 38163

TEXAS

Histologic Technician Program
St. Paul Medical Center
5909 Harry Hines Boulevard
Dallas, Texas 75235

Histologic Technician Program
St. Luke's Episcopal Hospital
6720 Bertner
Houston, Texas 77030

Histologic Technician Program
University of Texas School of Allied Health Sciences
P.O. Box 20036
Houston, Texas 77225

Histologic Technician Program
Medical Center Hospital
4502 Medical Drive
San Antonio, Texas 78284

WASHINGTON

Histologic Technician Program
Shoreline Community College
16101 Greenwood Avenue, N.
Seattle, Washington 98133

WISCONSIN

Histologic Technician Program
VTAE District One Tech Institute
620 W. Clairemont Avenue
Eau Claire, Wisconsin 54701

Histologic Technician Program
Madison General Hospital School of Rad. Tech.
202 South Park Street
Madison, Wisconsin 53715

Histologic Technician Program
St. Joseph's Hospital
611 St. Josephs Avenue
Marshfield, Wisconsin 54449

Histologic Technician Program
Clement J. Zablocki VA Medical Center
5000 W. National Avenue
Milwaukee, Wisconsin 53193

Laboratory Aide

Under direct supervision of the medical technologist, the *laboratory aide* requires minimal training to carry out routine responsibilities in the laboratory. The aide cleans and sterilizes instruments and equipment, maintains records of specimens, keeps an inventory of supplies, and assembles and repairs laboratory equipment. He or she may also perform simple tests such as determining the quantity of sugar and albumen in urine and preparing simple stains, solutions, and culture media. The laboratory aide is also responsible for keeping the laboratory clean, which means scrubbing walls, floors, tables, sinks, and shelves.

In a small hospital the laboratory aide may also be in charge of caring for the animals kept in the laboratory for research purposes. (Refer to the section on Animal Technology).

High school education, usually including courses in biology and chemistry, is the prerequisite for on-the-job training in a hospital laboratory. Training usually lasts about two months.

Individuals interested in career opportunities and salaries for this job, should contact the Personnel Director of their local hospital.

Morgue Attendant

Directly responsible to, and supervised by the pathologist, the *morgue attendant* maintains the hospital morgue room and equipment in a clean, well stocked, and orderly condition. Besides performing janitorial duties, the morgue attendant also assists the pathologist in autopsy procedures. Before the autopsy the attendant prepares the body for examination, during which he or she hands the pathologist surgical instruments, prepares specimens for microscopic examination, and may perform minor prosections. Afterwards the morgue attendant closes the incisions in the body cavities and prepares the body for the undertaker.

High school graduation, or the equivalent, and three months on-the-job training is required to work as a morgue attendant.

For persons interested in this position, information on job opportunities and salaries may be obtained from the Personnel Director of their local hospital.

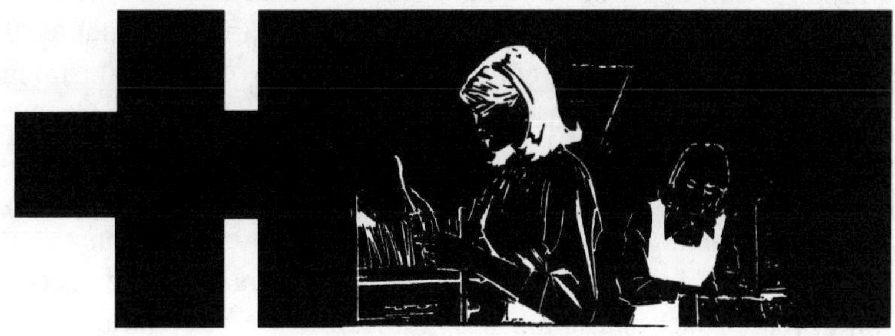

MEDICAL RECORDS

A medical record is a complete and permanent documentation of a patient's history of illnesses and injuries, and of all related medical treatments. Among other data, the record includes all medical observations and findings, laboratory and X-ray reports, diets, and medications. Compiled from the records of each healthcare facility the patient has attended, the comprehensive medical record is used by a physician to aid in the diagnosis and treatment of illness, and to ensure continuity of care in the future. The record may also be used by healthcare researchers, hospital administrators and planners, community public health officials, insurance companies, and legal professionals in their planning and research. There are three levels of careers for medical record personnel: *medical record administrator, medical record technician* and *medical record clerk.*

Medical Record Administrator

The *medical record administrator* is a professional member of a medical health team, and is responsible for the innovation and management of health information systems. In administering the medical record department of a hospital, clinic, or other healthcare facility, the medical record administrator plans and directs a system of medical record retention and retrieval systems, and compiles statistical data from medical records. Medical record administrators often manage the medical record department and train and supervise medical record technicians and clerks. Although the medical record administrator interacts with other members of the facility staff, the position does not provide any patient contact.

As a specialist in information management, the medical record administrator is often relied upon to provide information to members of the facility staff for research projects utilizing healthcare information, and for cost-saving studies. The medical record administrator may also assist administrative staff in evaluating the performance of the healthcare facility, provide consultant services to other healthcare facilities and health data systems, and provide statistical facts to government agencies. Although most work in a healthcare facility, the medical record administrator may also find employment with insurance companies, and state and federal health agencies.

Training for high school graduates involves completion of an accredited four year bachelor's degree program in medical record administration or completion of the third and fourth year of such a program after graduating from a community college. Individuals who have already earned a bachelor's degree in a related field, with required courses in liberal arts and biological sciences, may also be trained by completing a one to two year post-graduate certificate program in medical record administration. Both classroom and clinical experience are incorporated in the accredited training programs for medical record administration. The student completes courses in anatomy and physiology, computer science and information systems management, medical terminology, financial and administrative management, and statistics. Recommended high school subjects include mathematics, biology, chemistry, English, typing, and computer science.

The graduate of an accredited program is eligible to complete a national registration examination, sponsored by the American Medical Record Association, and if successful, become designated as a professional Registered Record Administrator (RRA).

Salaries vary as a result of degree earned, credentials awarded, experience level, size of facility and geographic location. According to a recent survey by the University of Texas Medical Branch, average annual starting salaries for Registered Record Administrators equalled $26,000, while those with experience average $33,500, with some administrators earning salaries in the mid-$50's.

For more information on a career as a medical record administrator, contact the American Medical Record Association, 875 North Michigan Avenue, Suite 1850, Chicago, Illinois 60611.

Below is a list of university and college educational programs accredited by the Committee on Allied Health Education and Accreditation of the American Medical Association, in cooperation with the Council on Education of the American Medical Record Association, and offering bachelor degrees and/or certificate programs in medical record administration.

KEY:

(1) Four year program with a high school education as entrance prerequisite.
(2) Two year program with two years college as entrance prerequisite.
(3) One year program with three years college as entrance prerequisite.
(4) One year program with three years college or degree as entrance prerequisite.
(5) Two year program with bachelor's degree as entrance prerequisite.
Program offers post-graduate certificate program.

* Program provides progression training for Accredited Record Technicians who wish to become Registered Record Administrators.

Medical Record Administration Programs

ALABAMA

Medical Record Administration Program (2,#)
University of Alabama at Birmingham
1629 University Blvd.
Birmingham, Alabama 35294

ARKANSAS

Medical Record Administration Program (2)
Arkansas Tech University
Russellville, Arkansas 72801

CALIFORNIA

Medical Record Administration Program (2,#)
Loma Linda University
1934 Nichol Hall
Loma Linda, California 92350

COLORADO

Medical Record Administration Program (2,#)
Regis College
50th Avenue and Lowell Blvd.
Denver, Colorado 80221

FLORIDA

Medical Record Administration Program (2,#)
Florida International University
NE 151st Street and Biscayne Blvd.
North Miami, Florida 33181

Medical Record Administration Program (2,#)
University of Central Florida
P.O. Box 25000
Orlando, Florida 32816

Medical Record Administration Program (2)
Florida A & M University
Tallahassee, Florida 32307

GEORGIA

Medical Record Administration Program (2)
Medical College of Georgia
15th Street and Laney Walker Blvd.
Augusta, Georgia 30912

ILLINOIS

Medical Record Administration Program (1,#)
Chicago State University
College of Allied Health
95th at King Drive
Chicago, Illinois 60628

Medical Record Administration Program (2)
University of Illinois at Chicago
808 South Wood Street
Chicago, Illinois 60612

Medical Record Administration Program (2,#)
Illinois State University
Dept. of Health Science
Normal, Illinois 61761

INDIANA

Medical Record Administration Program (3,#)
Indiana University School of Medicine
1140 W. Michigan Street
Indianapolis, Indiana 46223

KANSAS

Medical Record Administration Program (4,#)
University of Kansas Medical Center
School of Allied Health
39th & Rainbow Blvd.
Kansas City, Kansas 66103

KENTUCKY

Medical Record Administration Program (1,#)
Eastern Kentucky University
608 Begley
Richmond, Kentucky 40475

LOUISANA

Medical Record Administration Program (1,#)
University of Southwestern Louisiana
P.O. Box 41007, USL Station
Lafayette, Louisiana 70504

Medical Record Administration Program (1,#)
Louisiana Tech University
P.O. Box 3171
Ruston, Louisiana 71272

MASSACHUSETTS

Medical Record Administration Program (1,#,*)
Northeastern University
College of Pharmacy & Allied Health Prof.
Boston, Massachusetts 02115

MICHIGAN

Medical Record Administration Program (2)
Ferris State College
Big Rapids, Michigan 49307

Medical Record Administration Program (1,#)
Mercy College of Detroit
8200 West Outer Drive, Box 8
Detroit, Michigan 48219

MINNESOTA

Medical Record Administration Program (1,#)
College of St.Scholastica
1200 Kenwood Avenue
Duluth, Minnesota 55811

MISSISSIPPI

Medical Record Administration Program (2)
University of Mississippi Medical Center
School of Health Related Professions
2500 North State Street
Jackson, Mississippi 39216-4505

MISSOURI

Medical Record Administration Program (1,#,*)
Stephens College
Box 2083
Columbia, Missouri 65215

Medical Record Administration Program (1)
St. Louis University
School of Allied Health Professions
1504 South Grand Blvd.
St. Louis, Missouri 63104

MONTANA

Medical Record Administration Program (1)
Carroll College
Helena, Montana 59625

NEBRASKA

Medical Record Administration Program (2,#,*)
College of Saint Mary
1901 South 72nd Street
Omaha, Nebraska 68124

NEW JERSEY

Medical Record Administration Program (2,#,*)
Kean College of New Jersey
Morris Avenue
Union, New Jersey 07083

NEW YORK

Medical Record Administration Program (2,*)
State University of New York
Health Science Center at Brooklyn
College of Health Related Professions
450 Clarkson Avenue
Box 105
Brooklyn, New York 11203

Medical Record Administration Program (2,#,*)
Daemen College
4380 Main Street
Buffalo, New York 14226

Medical Record Administration Program (1,#)
Ithaca College
Danby Road
Ithaca, New York 14850

Medical Record Administration Program (2,#)
Touro College
30 West 44th Street
New York, New York 10036

Medical Record Administration Program (2,#)
SUNY College of Technology
P.O. Box 3050
Utica, New York 13504-3050

NORTH CAROLINA

Medical Record Administration Program (2,#)
Western Carolina University
School of Nursing and Health Sciences
Cullowhee, North Carolina 28723

Medical Record Administration Program (2)
East Carolina University
Greenville, North Carolina 27834

OHIO

Medical Record Administration Program (2)
Bowling Green State University
114 Health Center
Bowling Green, Ohio 43403-0287

Medical Record Administration Program (2,#,*)
The Ohio State University
School of Allied Medical Professions
1583 Perry Street
Columbus, Ohio 43210

OKLAHOMA

Medical Record Administration Program (2)
East Central University
Ada, Oklahoma 74820

Medical Record Administration Program (2,#)
Southwestern Oklahoma State University
100 Campus Drive
Weatherford, Oklahoma 73096

PENNSYLVANIA

Medical Record Administration Program (2,#)
Temple University
College of Allied Health Professions
3307 North Broad Street
Philadelphia, Pennsylvania 19140

Medical Record Administration Program (2,#,*)
University of Pittsburgh
School of Health Related Professions
308 Pennsylvania Hall
Pittsburgh, Pennsylvania 15261

Medical Record Administration Program (2,#)
York College of Pennsylvania
Country Club Road
York, Pennsylvania 17405-9987

SOUTH CAROLINA

Medical Record Administration Program (2)
Medical University of South Carolina
College of Allied Health Sciences
171 Ashley Avenue
Charleston, South Carolina 29425

SOUTH DAKOTA

Medical Record Administration Program (1,#)
Dakota State College
Madison, South Dakota 57042

TENNESSEE

Medical Record Administration Program (3,*)
University of Tennessee, Memphis
The Health Science Center
956 Court
Memphis, Tennessee 38163

Medical Record Administration Program (2,#)
Tennessee State University
3500 John A. Merritt Blvd.
Nashville, Tennessee 37203

TEXAS

Medical Record Administration Program (2,#)
Texas Woman's University
1810 Inwood Road
Dallas, Texas 75235-7299

Medical Record Administration Program (2,#)
University of Texas Medical Branch
School of Allied Health Sciences J28
Galveston, Texas 77550

Medical Record Administration Program (2,#)
Southwest Texas State University
Dept. of Health Administration
San Marcos, Texas 78666

VIRGINIA

Medical Record Administration Program (1)
Norfolk State University
Health Related Professions & Natural Sciences
2401 Corprew Avenue
Norfolk, Virginia 23504

Medical Record Administration Program (2)
Medical College of Virginia
School of Allied Health Professions
MCV Station - Box 203
Richmond, Virginia 23298-0001

WASHINGTON

Medical Record Administration Program (4,#,*)
Seattle University
12th & East Columbia
Seattle, Washington 98122

WISCONSIN

Medical Record Administration Program (2,#)
University of Wisconsin-Milwaukee
School of Allied Health Professions
Box 413
Milwaukee, Wisconsin 53201

PUERTO RICO

Medical Record Administration Program (5,#)
University of Puerto Rico
College of Health Related Professions
Medical Science Campus, GPO Box 5067
San Juan, Puerto Rico 00936

Medical Record Technician

As a specially trained and skilled assistant to the medical record administrator, the *medical record technician* performs the many technical activities in a medical record department. In general, the technician compiles codes, analyzes, prepares, and maintains health information. Specifically, the technician reviews medical records for completeness and accuracy, codes symptoms, diseases, operations and therapies, indexes and classifies diagnoses and treatments, prepares special studies for medical and administrative staff, and supervises medical records clerks. The medical record technician has no direct patient contact.

In addition to being employed in a large hospital, the medical record technician may be employed as a director of a medical record department in a small hospital, nursing home, outpatient clinic, or community health center, and have full responsibility for the medical record department. He or she may also be employed as a consultant to several small health facilities, or even work for insurance companies or manufacturers of medical record systems and equipment.

Those interested in becoming a medical record technician should enroll in an accredited two year community college, junior college, or vocational/technical institute associate degree program.

For those individuals interested in entering the medical record field, or for medical record clerks who wish to advance to the technician level, the American Medical Record Association offers a home-study, independent study program in medical record technology. Requirements for enrollment include a high school degree or equivalent, and a minimum recommended typing speed of 45 words per minute. The program is self-paced and must be completed within 36 months. A certificate of completion is granted after successfully completing the program. For additional information on the home study program write to the American Medical Record Association, Independent Study Division, 875 N. Michigan Avenue, Suite 1850, Chicago, Illinois 60611.

Upon completion of an approved academic program, the graduate is qualified to take the accreditation examination sponsored by the American Medical Record Association, and if successful, can apply to become an Accredited Record Technician (ART). Graduates of the independent study program who also have completed 30 semester credits of approved college work, may also apply to take the accreditation examination.

Recommended high school subjects include science, English, typing, mathematics, office procedures and computer science.

According to a recent survey by the University of Texas Medical Branch, starting salaries for medical record technicians averaged $15,700, while experienced technicians averaged $20,200. For further career information in medical record technology, contact the American Medical Record Association, 875 North Michigan Avenue, Suite 1850, Chicago, Illinois 60611.

Below is a list of academic programs accredited by the Committee on Allied Health Education and Accreditation of the American Medical Association in cooperation with the Council on Education of the American Medical Record Association.

SOURCES:

American Medical Record Association
Occupational Outlook Handbook

Medical Record Technician Programs

ALABAMA

Medical Record Technician Program
University of Alabama at Birmingham
Regional Technical Institute
1629 University Blvd.
Birmingham, Alabama 35294

Medical Record Technician Program
Wallace State Community College
P.O. Box 180
Hanceville, Alabama 35077

ARIZONA

Medical Record Technician Program
Phoenix College
1202 West Thomas Road
Phoenix, Arizona 85013

CALIFORNIA

Medical Record Technician Program
Cypress College
9200 Valley View
Cypress, California 90630

Medical Record Technician Program
Chabot College
25555 Hesperian Blvd.
Hayward, California 94545

Medical Record Technician Program
East Los Angeles College
1301 Brooklyn Avenue
Monterey Park, California 91754

Medical Record Technician Program
San Diego Mesa College
7250 Mesa College Drive
San Diego, California 92111

Medical Record Technician Program
City College of San Francisco
50 Phelan Avenue
San Francisco, California 94112

COLORADO

Medical Record Technician Program
Arapahoe Community College
5900 South Sante Fe Drive
Littleton, Colorado 80120

FLORIDA

Medical Record Technician Program
Daytona Beach Community College
P.O. Box 1111
Daytona Beach, Florida 32015

Medical Record Technician Program
Miami-Dade Community College
Medical Center Campus
950 N.W. 20th Street
Miami, Florida 33127

Medical Record Technician Program
Pensacola Junior College
Warrington Campus
5555 Highway 98 West
Pensacola, Florida 32507

GEORGIA

Medical Record Technician Program
Armstrong State College
11935 Abercorn Street
Savannah, Georgia 31419-1997

IDAHO

Medical Record Technician Program
Boise State University
1910 University Drive
Boise, Idaho 83725

ILLINOIS

Medical Record Technician Program
Belleville Area College
2500 Carlyle Road
Belleville, Illinois 62221

Medical Record Technician Program
Truman College
1145 West Wilson Avenue
Chicago, Illinois 60640

Medical Record Technician Program
Oakton Community College
1600 East Golf Road
Des Plaines, Illinois 60016

Medical Record Technician Program
College of DuPage
22nd and Lambert Roads, IC-1028
Glen Ellyn, Illinois 60137

Medical Record Technician Program
College of Lake County
19351 West Washington Street
Grayslake, Illinois 60030

Medical Record Technician Program
Moraine Valley Community College
6201 West 115th Street
Worth, Illinois 60482

INDIANA

Medical Record Technician Program
Indiana University Northwest
3400 Broadway
Gary, Indiana 46408

Medical Record Technician Program
Vincennes University
1002 North First Street
Vincennes, Indiana 47501-9986

IOWA

Medical Record Technician Program
Kirkwood Community College
6301 Kirwood Blvd., S.W.
P.O. Box 2068
Cedar Rapids, Iowa 52406

Medical Record Technician Program
Indiana Hills Community College
Grandview and Elm
Ottumwa, Iowa 52501

KANSAS

Medical Record Technician Program
Hutchinson Community College
Davis Hall
815 N. Walnut Street
Hutchinson, Kansas 67501

Medical Record Technician Program
Washburn University of Topeka
17th and College Streets
Topeka, Kansas 66621

KENTUCKY

Medical Record Technician Program
Western Kentucky University
Academic Complex 210
Bowling Green, Kentucky 42101

Medical Record Technician Program
Eastern Kentucky University
Richmond, Kentucky 40475

LOUISIANA

Medical Record Technician Program
Louisiana Tech University
P.O. Box 3171
Ruston, Louisiana 71272-0001

MARYLAND

Medical Record Technician Program
Community College of Baltimore
2901 Liberty Heights Avenue
Baltimore, Maryland 21215

Medical Record Technician Program
Prince George's Community College
301 Largo Road
Largo, Maryland 20772

MASSACHUSETTS

Medical Record Technician Program
Catherine Laboure' College
2120 Dorchester Avenue
Boston, Massachusetts 02124

Medical Record Technician Program
Northern Essex Community College
100 Elliot Street
Haverhill, Massachusetts 01830

Medical Record Technician Program
Holyoke Community College
303 Homestead Avenue
Holyoke, Massachusetts 01040

Medical Record Technician Program
Massachusetts Bay Community College
50 Oakland Street
Wellesley, Massachusetts 02181

MICHIGAN

Medical Record Technician Program
Ferris State College
VFS 402
Big Rapids, Michigan 49307

Medical Record Technician Program
Henry Ford Community College
22586 Ann Arbor Trail
Dearborn Heights, Michigan 48127

Medical Record Technician Program
Mercy College of Detroit
8200 West Outer Drive, Box 8
Detroit, Michigan 48219

Medical Record Technician Program
Schoolcraft College
1751 Radcliff Street
Garden City, Michigan 48135-1197

Medical Record Technician Program
Muskegon Business College
141 Hartford
Muskegon, Michigan 49442

MINNESOTA

Medical Record Technician Program
Anoka Area Vocational Technical Institute
1355 West Main Street
Anoka, Minnesota 55303

Medical Record Technician Program
St. Mary's Campus of the College of St. Catherine
2500 South Sixth Street
Minneapolis, Minnesota 55454

Medical Record Technician Program
Moorhead Area Vocational Technical Institute
1900 28th Avenue South
Moorehead, Minnesota 56560

MISSISSIPPI

Medical Record Technician Program
Meridian Junior College
5500 Highway 19 North
Meridian, Mississippi 39305

Medical Record Technician Program
Hinds Junior College
P.O. Box 428 HJC
Raymond, Mississippi 39154-0999

MISSOURI

Medical Record Technician Program
St. Mary's College of O'Fallon, Inc.
200 North Main Street
O'Fallon, Missouri 63366

NEW HAMPSHIRE

Medical Record Technician Program
New Hampshire Vocational-Technical College
Hanover Street Extension
Claremont, New Hampshire 03743

NEW JERSEY

Medical Record Technician Program
Union County College
1033 Springfield Avenue
Cranford, New Jersey 07016

Medical Record Technician Program
Hudson County Community College
2039 Kennedy Blvd.
Jersey City, New Jersey 07305-1597

NEW YORK

Medical Record Technician Program
State University of New York
Agricultural and Technical College
Alfred, New York 14802

Medical Record Technician Program
Broome Community College
P.O. Box 1017
Binghamton, New York 13902

Medical Record Technician Program
Borough of Manhattan Community College
199 Chambers Street
New York, New York 10007

Medical Record Technician Program
Monroe Community College
1000 East Henrietta Road
Rochester, New York 14623

Medical Record Technician Program
National Technical Institute for the Deaf
One Lomb Memorial Dr., Bldg. LBJ-1261
P.O. Box 9887
Rochester, New York 14623-0887

Medical Record Technician Program
Mohawk Valley Community College
1101 Sherman Drive
Utica, New York 13501

NORTH CAROLINA

Medical Record Technician Program
Central Piedmont Community College
P.O. Box 35009
Charlotte, North Carolina 28235-5009

NORTH DAKOTA

Medical Record Technician Program
North Dakota State School of Science
800 North Sixth Street
Wahpeton, North Dakota 58075

OHIO

Medical Record Technician Program
Stark Technical College
6200 Frank Avenue, N.W.
Canton, Ohio 44720

Medical Record Technician Program
Cincinnati Technical College
3520 Central Parkway
Cincinnati, Ohio 45223

Medical Record Technician Program
Cuyahoga Community College
2900 Community College Avenue
Cleveland, Ohio 44115

Medical Record Technician Program
Sinclair Community College
444 W. Third Street
Dayton, Ohio 45402

Medical Record Technician Program
Bowling Green State University-Firelands College
901 Rye Beach Road
Huron, Ohio 44839

Medical Record Technician Program
Hocking Technical College
Route 1
Nelsonville, Ohio 45764

OREGON

Medical Record Technician Program
Central Oregon Community College
2600 N.W. College Way
Bend, Oregon 97701

Medical Record Technician Program
Portland Community College
12000 S.W. 49th Avenue
Portland, Oregon 97219

PENNSYLVANIA

Medical Record Technician Program
Gwynedd-Mercy College
Sumneytown Pike
Gwynedd, Pennsylvania 19437

Medical Record Technician Program
Community College of Philadelphia
1700 Spring Garden Street
Philadelphia, Pennsylvania 19130

Medical Record Technician Program
Community College of the Allegheny
County - Allegheny Campus
808 Ridge Avenue
Pittsburgh, Pennsylvania 15212

SOUTH DAKOTA

Medical Record Technician Program
Dakota State College
6 Heston Hall
Madison, South Dakota 57042-1799

TENNESSEE

Medical Record Technician Program
Chattanooga State Technical Community College
4501 Amnicola Highway
Chattanooga, Tennessee 37406

Medical Record Technician Program
Volunteer State Community College
Nashville Pike
Gallatin, Tennessee 37066

Medical Record Technician Program
Roane State Community College
Patton Lane
Harriman, Tennessee 37748

TEXAS

Medical Record Technician Program
Tarrant County Junior College
Northeast Campus
828 Harwood Road
Hurst, Texas 76054

Medical Record Technician Program
South Plains College
1302 Main Street
Lubbock, Texas 79401

Medical Record Technician Program
St. Philip's College
2111 Nevada Street
San Antonio, Texas 78203

Medical Record Technician Program
Temple Junior College
2600 South First Street
Temple, Texas 76501

Medical Record Technician Program
Wharton County Junior College
911 Boling Highway
Wharton, Texas 77488

VIRGINIA

Medical Record Technician Program
Northern Virginia Community College
8333 Little River Turnpike
Annandale, Virginia 22003

Medical Record Technician Program
Central Virginia Community College
3506 Wards Road
Lynchburg, Virginia 24502

Medical Record Technician Program
Tidewater Community College
1700 College Crescent
Virginia Beach, Virginia 23456

WASHINGTON

Medical Record Technician Program
Shoreline Community College
16101 Greenwood Avenue North
Seattle, Washington 98133

Medical Record Technician Program
Spokane Community College
N. 1810 Green Street MS 2090
Spokane, Washington 99207

Medical Record Technician Program
Tacoma Community College
5900 S. 12th Street-Bldg. 19
Tacoma, Washington 98465

WEST VIRGINIA

Medical Record Technician Program
Fairmont State College
Locust Avenue
Fairmont, West Virginia 26554

WISCONSIN

Medical Record Technician Program
District One Technical Institute
620 West Clairemont Avenue
Eau Claire, Wisconsin 54701

Medical Record Technician Program
Western Wisconsin Technical Institute
6th and Vine Streets
La Crosse, Wisconsin 54601

Medical Record Technician Program
Moraine Park Techical Institute
2151 North Main Street
P.O. Box 617
West Bend, Wisconsin 53095-0617

PUERTO RICO

Medical Record Technician Program
Puerto Rico Junior College
Box 21373
Rio Piedras, Puerto Rico 00928

Medical Record Clerk

Under supervision of a medical record technician, the *medical record clerk* performs routine clerical tasks in the maintenance of medical information systems. The clerk assembles, verifies, and provides to the hospital staff the non-technical data in medical records. Other duties of a medical record clerk may include data entry, typing, filing, and related clerical duties.

Besides working in a hospital, the medical record clerk may also be employed in a smaller health care facility such as a nursing home. The medical record clerk may be solely responsible for the medical records, under the supervision of a medical record consultant; (one who is credentialed as a Registered Record Administrator (RRA), or an Accredited Record Technician (ART)). The medical record clerk should enjoy working in an office setting since there is no direct patient contact.

Persons interested in training as a medical record clerk should be high school educated and possess basic secretarial skills. Training may be done on the job, and is approximately three to six months in duration.

Medical record clerks with several years experience advance to the technician level after successfully completing the American Medical Record Association's Independent Study Program, obtaining 30 credit hours of appropriate college course work and passing the national accreditation examination to become an ART (Accredited Record Technician). Refer back to the chapter under Medical Record Technician for more details on the Independent Study Program.

Salaries for medical record clerks are similar to full-time clerical and data entry positions in other service industries. Annual salaries vary because of geographic location, experience level and size of facility, but generally range from $8,500 for entry level positions to $15,000 for clerks with several years experience.

SOURCES:
American Medical Record Association
Occupational Outlook Handbook

Medical Transcriptionist

The *medical transcriptionist* is the allied health professional who transcribes, edits, and types physicians' dictated notes of patients' medical procedures and treatment. The medical transcriptionist must have sharp listening skills to translate the physicians' oral comments into well-organized and accurate typewritten statements. The physician records patients' cases onto tape-recording devices and submits the cassettes to the medical transcriptionist for transcription. As a medical terminology specialist, the medical transcriptionist transcribes each report accurately, ensuring that the meaning does not change. The medical terminologist correctly translates complex medical terms, being sure to use correct usage, spelling and punctuation. The medical transcriptionist is able to detect discrepancies in dictation and edit them accordingly. The medical transcriptionist is a proficient typist, familiar with a variety of medical documents, including medical histories, physicals, consultations and operative reports.

Medical transcriptionists must be organized, prompt, able to type quickly and accurately, and not easily distracted.

Medical transcriptionists work independently, with little supervision. They work in office settings in hospitals, clinics, laboratories, physicians' offices, insurance companies, and with medical transcribing services. Some medical transcriptionists concentrate in one particular area of the medical profession such as radiology, pathology, or emergency room medicine. The medical transcriptionist may transcribe for one or a few physicians in a small medical practice, or for several hundred in a large healthcare facility.

Formal training programs for medical transcription are offered through universities, colleges, community and junior colleges, vocational-technical institutes, and adult education programs. Programs generally include classroom and clinical experience and last from 9 months for a certificate program up to two years for associate degree education. Graduates of these programs develop an extensive knowledge of medical terminology, and demonstrate an understanding of anatomy and physiology, medical supplies, equipment, drugs, surgical procedures, medicolegal issues, and laboratory procedures and results.

The American Association for Medical Transcription indicates a demand for experienced and highly skilled medical transcriptionists.

At present, the American Association for Medical Transcription is compiling a list of known educational institutions offering training programs in medical transcription. In the interim, the Association recommends that individuals contact educational institutions in their community to determine where such programs exist.Individuals interested in becoming certified in medical transcription may take the American Association of Medical Transcription-sponsored certification examination, and if successfully passed, apply for the credential of Certified Medical Transcriptionist (CMT). Examination applicants must have a minimum of three years comprehensive medical transcription experience in a variety of medical specialties.

For further information on certification or a career as a medical transcriptionist, write to the American Association for Medical Transcription, P.O. Box 6187, Modesto, California 95355.

SOURCES:

American Association for Medical Transcription
Occupational Outlook Handbook

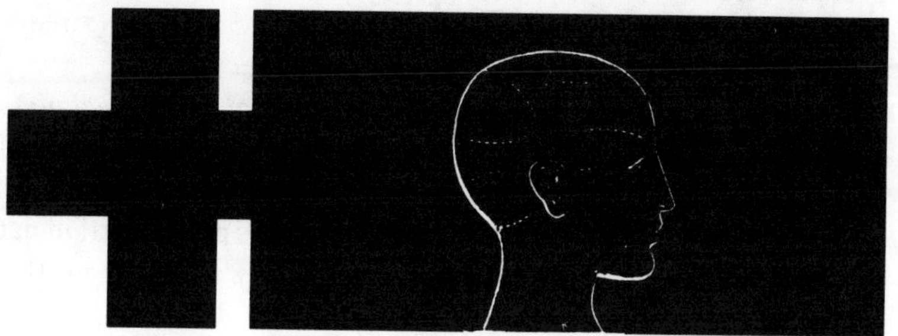

MENTAL HEALTH

Mental health is the medical profession concerned with the diagnosis, prevention, treatment and rehabilitation of human mental disorders.

The *psychiatrist,* a physician trained in the specialized field of psychiatry, diagnoses and treats disorders of the mind. The psychiatrist must graduate from an accredited medical school and complete extensive additional training in psychiatry.

The *psychologist* is a highly trained professional with doctorate degree training who studies and assesses human behavior and works in the prevention and treatment of emotional and mental disorders. The majority of psychologists specialize in clinical psychology, helping those with emotional or mental disorders adjust to everyday life, while others specialize in counseling, research or education.

Counselors help individuals deal with personal or social problems. The *mental health counselor* helps individuals resolve marriage and family conflicts, deal with substance abuse problems and improve interpersonal relationships. The *rehabilitation counselor* helps physically, mentally, emotionally, or socially impaired individuals become self sufficient. A master's degree in rehabilitation counseling, or psychology is generally the minimum educational requirement for a career as a counselor.

Social workers in mental health help individuals and families find ways to deal with their mental health problems. The social worker interviews clients, plans treatment plans, refers clients to other healthcare professionals, and provides information on community resources. A master's degree in social work is generally the minimum requirement for a career in social work.

The psychiatrist, psychologist, counselor, and social worker work as part of a mental health team along with other healthcare professionals including psychiatric nurses, therapeutic recreation specialists and occupational specialists, whose career descriptions are listed elsewhere in this handbook.

In the practice of mental health there are also several allied health careers, and since the occupational titles and training requirements for the allied mental health careers may vary among the different mental health programs of each state, careers in allied mental health will be discussed collectively in the following section.

Described below are the careers of the *mental health technician,* the *human services technician* and the *psychiatric aide.* These positions are available in mental healthcare programs managed by hospitals and/or by federal, state, and local agencies. The reader should remember that the following descriptions are general in nature and that individual job classifications and responsibilities may vary among the different state mental health programs.

For further information on careers in psychiatry write to the American Psychiatric Association, 1400 K Street, N.W., Washington, D.C. 20005; for careers in psychology to the American Psychological Association, 1200 17th Street, N.W., Washington, D.C. 20036; for mental health or rehabilitation counseling careers to the American Association for Counseling and Development, 5999 Stevenson Avenue, Alexandria, Virginia 22304 or the National Rehabilitation Counseling Association, 633 South Washington Street, Alexandria, Virginia 22314; and for careers in social work contact the National Association of Social Workers, 7981 Eastern Avenue, Silver Spring, Maryland 20910.

Mental Health Technician
Human Services Technician
Psychiatric Aide

The *mental health technician* works with mentally retarded, emotionally disturbed, or psychiatric patients under the supervision of a psychiatrist, psychologist, social worker, or nurse. Trained as a generalist in a number of mental health fields and employed in a variety of health institutions, the mental health technician provides physical and mental rehabilitation for patients through recreational, occupational, and readjustment activities. The technician participates in group therapy with patients and their families, refers patients to community agencies, and visits patients after their release from an institution.

Working with the mentally retarded, the mental health technician attends to patients' physical needs and well being. The technician also assists, under supervision, in the rehabilitation of patients through teaching and recreation activities. Mental health technicians are also employed in private and public mental hospitals or on the psychiatric wards of general hospitals, mental health clinics and human services programs. In a hospital setting, the mental health technician may perform routine nursing tasks such as taking pulse, blood pressure and respiration rates. Mental health technicians observe and counsel patients and help in their treatment plan.

The mental health technician also may work as community health worker in a variety of agencies that rehabilitate and resocialize people, and may be referred to as a *human services technician.* The human services technician is trained as a generalist, but with emphasis in community mental health as opposed to institutional mental health, and thus uses the noncustodial approach in an attempt to rehabilitate those who have problems responding to their social environment. Under supervision of a healthcare professional, the human services technician interviews and counsels clients, administers psychological tests, and participates in group activities. He or she may be primarily concerned with drug and alcohol abuse, parental effectiveness, the elderly, and/or interpersonal relationships. Human services technicians work in social welfare departments, child care centers, preschool nurseries, vocational rehabilitation workshops, and schools for the learning disabled, emotionally disturbed, and mentally handicapped.

The *psychiatric aide* works as a type of nursing aide/orderly performing routine nursing tasks and caring for the patients' eating, sleeping, and personal hygiene habits. He or she also takes temperatures, blood pressure, pulse and respiration counts in addition to providing rehabilitation assistance in the patient's development of social relationships and vocational responsibilities. The psychiatric aide also spends time talking with patients and accompanying them to activities and games.

The psychiatric aide works in state, and county mental hospitals, psychiatric departments of general hospitals, private psychiatric facilities, community mental health and substance abuse treatment programs.

Education for a career as a mental health or human services technician usually involves completion of a two-year associate degree program in mental health technology or psychology, offered through community colleges, vocational-technical schools or other post-secondary educational institutions.

Training programs for the psychiatric aide are usually six-to-eight weeks in length and are usually held on-the-job. Formal nursing aide training programs are offered through community colleges, vocational-technical schools and post-secondary educational institutions. For more information on the career of nursing aide refer to the chapter titled Nursing Aide/Orderly.

For further information on the careers of mental health technician, human services technician or psychiatric aide, interested persons should contact the National Mental Health Association, 1021 Prince Street, Alexandria, Virginia 22314, their local Mental Health Association or community mental health program, or state, community, or local mental health facilities.

SOURCES:

American Psychiatric Association
United States Department of Health and Human Services
Occupational Outlook Handbook

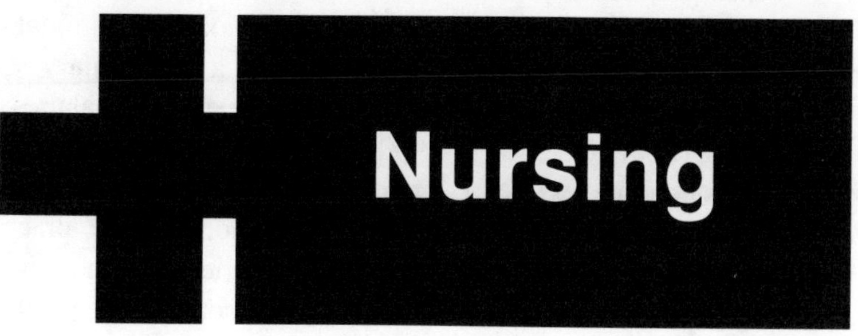

NURSING

Nursing is the healthcare profession concerned with patient care. The professional nurse handles a variety of tasks relating to both health and illness. Providing direct patient care is the most common job responsibility.

Nursing is a growing field and nurses with appropriate education and experience may find expanding opportunities in the clinical, managerial, academic and entrepreneurial fields.

Nurses are employed in a variety of settings, including hospitals, clinics, nursing homes, community agencies, public and private schools, health maintenance organizations, outpatient care facilities, colleges and universities, overseas, and in the Armed Forces.

Training requirements vary depending upon the type of nursing career desired. Training for the nursing aide involves six-to-eight weeks on-the-job training with formal training programs available through community or junior colleges, vocational-technical institutes, hospitals, and other post-secondary institutions. Licensed practical nurses must graduate from a state approved nursing training program which generally lasts one year, and is offered in post-secondary educational institutes around the country. Registered nurse training programs last from two-to-five years beyond high school and award an associates degree for a two year program to a bachelor's degree for four to five year programs. Master's degree programs are available in numerous colleges and universities for nurses who want advanced education. Some nursing specialties, such as the professional nurse practitioner require a master's degree.

All nurses must be licensed and licensure requirements include graduating from an approved school of nursing and passing a national examination administered by each state. Certification in addition to licensure is required for some nursing specialties. Some states require nursing aides to be certified. Each state's Board of

Licensing can provide further details on licensure requirements for nurses.

Salaries for nurses vary by geographic location, amount of education, employer, and years of experience. According to a 1987 salary survey conducted by the University of Texas Medical Branch, starting annual salaries for the licensed practical nurse (LPN) averaged $14,900, while those with experience averaged $20,100. Staff registered nurses (RNs) started at $21,000 for entry level positions and experienced professionals earned $30,000. Professional nurse practitioners earned starting salaries of $25,700 and those with experience earned average annual salaries of $34,000. Nurses who were recently promoted to the position of head nurse earned salaries of $26,300, while those in the position for several years earned $36,400. The highest salary of the nursing professions surveyed was for the nurse anesthetist who earned average annual salaries of $33,400 for starting positions, and $44,400 for those with several years experience.

This chapter provides a summary of the varied opportunities in the nursing field. For information on educational programs, financial aid, career opportunities and licensure requirements, write to either the respective nursing associations listed in this chapter, the National League for Nursing, 10 Columbus Circle, New York, New York 10019, the American Nurses' Association, 2420 Pershing Road, Kansas City, Missouri 64108, or to the Canadian Nurses Association, 50 The Driveway, Ottawa, Ontario, Canada K2P 1E2.

SOURCES:

American Hospital Association
Alperin Stanley, *Careers in Nursing,* Ballinger Publishing Company, Cambridge, Massachusetts
Occupational Outlook Handbook

The Registered Nurse

The *registered nurse* (RN) is a person who has received training in techniques for delivering nursing services to patients found in hospitals, clinics, health agencies, physicians' offices, private homes, and many other places where people need medical attention.

These nurses take temperatures, pulse rates, blood pressure readings, and check other vital signs to evaluate the patient's progress. They record data from these observations on the patient's chart and notify the supervisor or physician of any change indicating the need for special attention.

The nurse prepares the patient for examination and assists the physician during examination and treatment. Registered nurses administer medications and treatments under the direction of the physician.

The nurse's duties vary according to the size and staffing of the place of employment. In a large, well-staff hospital with many nursing aides (assistants), the nurse's duties may be almost exclusively patient treatment, but in a smaller institution with less support staff, the nurse may also sterilize instruments, make beds, feed and bathe patients, and prepare rooms for occupancy. The experienced nurse may have some supervisory duties over the nursing aides (assistants).

Registered nurses may be assigned to work in a special section in the hospital, such as surgery, pediatrics, obstetrics, psychiatry, or the admitting office. The nurse who works in several of the special sections of the hospital gets a good overview of the scope of nursing specialties and is able to make a more informed decision regarding further study and specialization.

For more information on a career as a registered nurse, write to the National League for Nursing, 10 Columbus Circle, New York, New York 10019.

The Air Force Nurse

The *Air Force nurse* works in hospitals, medical centers, and clinics to deliver nursing and health services to Air Force personnel and their families.

Air Force nurses perform the same duties as a civilian registered nurse. Working under the direction of a licensed physician, they administer prescribed medication and treatment; check vital signs such as pulse, respiration, and blood pressure; and perform other nursing duties to aid the patient's comfort and recovery. As in civilian nursing, Air Force nurses may specialize in such areas as surgery, intensive care, and flight nursing aboard an aircraft.

Further information regarding a nursing career in the Air Force is available from the nearest Air Force recruiter, listed in the telephone directory under U.S. Government, Air Force.

The Army Nurse

Army nurses work in Army hospitals, health centers, clinics, and physicians' offices to deliver nursing services to Army personnel and their dependents.

Army nurses perform the same duties as civilian registered nurses. Working under the direction of a licensed physician, they administer prescribed medication and treatment; check such vital signs as pulse, respiration, and blood pressure; and perform other nursing duties to aid the patient's comfort and recovery. Army nurses may specialize in surgical nursing, midwifery, pediatrics, community health, anesthesiology, psychiatric nursing, intensive care, and obstetric and gynecologic nursing.

For details regarding a career in the Army Nurse Corps, contact the nearest Army Recruiting Office, listed in the telephone directory under U.S. Government, Army.

The Community Health Nurse

Community health nurses, sometimes called *public health nurses,* are registered nurses (RNs) who visit homes to provide nursing services and health education to patients and their families. These nurses are stationed in public health departments, visiting nurse associations, voluntary health agencies, school health programs, and occupational health programs.

Community health nurses work with the patient in the home to develop a plan of treatment and rehabilitation and involve the family in assisting in the patient's recovery, as well as providing education in the prevention of disease and the maintenance of good health for the entire family. These nurses work under the instruction of the physician to administer needed medication and treatment. In the case of a patient who is attended by a licensed practical nurse (LPN), the community health nurse instructs and supervises the treatment to be given by the LPN. Part of the duties of the community health nurse include instruction in home nursing and child care.

The community health nurse must be able to assess the needs of the patient who may need referral for professional help with emotional problems, and must maintain a good relationship with other community agencies where ancillary services may be available.

This nurse works with the physician, the family and the patient, and other community health personnel to find accommodations in nursing homes or other rehabilitative facilities when the patient must be cared for outside the home.

The community health nurse is very involved in the entire health services delivery system for the community, working with other agencies in assessing community health needs and planning for meeting those needs. This nurse also participates actively in programs to improve the health of the children of the community, often working with the school system to assist in immunization campaigns and educating school students about good health habits. He or she may also conduct group instruction for parents regarding community health programs. Since community health nurses are involved in a wide area of practice, they also often participate in the conduct of surveys and research projects. By virtue of experience and continuing education, these nurses may specialize in one phase of nursing, for example, pediatrics or geriatrics.

The Emergency Room Nurse

The *emergency room nurse* is a registered nurse (RN) who works in the emergency room in hospitals, clinics, or other healthcare agencies to furnish to persons who, because of accidents or acute illness, are in need of immediate expert medical care.

The emergency room nurse works with persons who are victims of automobile accidents, drowning, drug overdoses, assaults, burns, heart attacks, strokes, diabetic comas, and many other conditions. In these cases, the speed and competence of the emergency room staff may make the difference between life and death.

Emergency room nurses clean wounds or cuts; stop minor bleeding; take temperatures, pulse rates, and blood pressure; and record this information on patient charts. They apply bandages, splints, tape, slings, and cervical collars; insert tubes into tracheotomy openings, perform electrocardiograms, defibrillate cardiac patients; remove stitches; and may suture minor cuts. In some hospitals, under the physician's supervision, more complicated procedures may be performed.

For further details on a career as an emergency room nurse, write to the Emergency Nurses Association, 230 E. Ohio Street, Chicago, Illinois 60611.

The Diabetes Nurse

The *diabetes nurse* is a registered nurse (RN) who has received special training to work with the diabetic patient. This nurse must be able to assist in treatment from the admission to the hospital in which the patient may be in a diabetic coma, to the time of discharge after the patient has been taught how to care for the diabetes at home.

The diabetes nurse must have a thorough knowledge of nutrition and its relation to diabetes and must educate the patient and family to care for the condition at home. This involves teaching the patient how to administer insulin, the importance of exercise and weight control, side effects of medications, care of the feet, and how to recognize and react to complications. The patient must be taught the importance of taking care to avoid acidosis and coma, which are life threatening.

For more information on a career as a diabetes nurse, write to the National League for Nursing, 10 Columbus Circle, New York, New York 10019.

The Family Nurse Clinical Specialist

The *family nurse clinical specialist* works with family groups in hospitals, clinics, nursing homes, schools, health maintenance organizations, health centers, and physicians' offices to provide nursing and healthcare services to family groups.

This nurse provides nursing services to family groups, including young families consisting of parents and young children, and the older family of adults, some of whom may be elderly. Family health nurses assess the health of members of families by physical examination and taking medical histories. They counsel and teach the patients in order to promote health maintenance and disease prevention, making referrals to other medical services when indicated. These nurses are prepared to understand the structure and function of families and the psychological effect on health that may result from the interaction in the group. They also evaluate the service being provided to family groups, and make recommendations and implement changes needed to improve the service.

Family nurse clinical specialists utilize research skills in collection and evaluation of data to work with community health planners to establish or improve health delivery systems. They participate in the management of critical health situations such as epidemics, floods, or severe winter storms. They also spend some time in instruction in nurse education programs in addition to regular duties.

The General Duty Nurse

General duty nurses, also called *staff nurses,* are registered nurses (RNs) employed in the hospital, infirmary, nursing home, community health agency, or other similar institution giving general nursing care to patients. They work under the supervision of nursing supervisors and physicians.

The general duty nurse observes the condition of the patient, takes temperature, pulse rate, blood pressure, and any other vital signs needed to evaluate the progress of the patient. The nurse records data from these observations on patients' charts and notifies the supervisor or physician of any change indicating the need for special attention. These nurses prepare the patient for examination, assist the physician during examination and treatment, and administer medications and treatments under the direction of the physician.

Duties will vary according to the size and type of institution. In a large, fully staffed hospital with many nursing aides (assistants), the nurse's duties may be almost exclusively patient treatment. In a smaller institution with less support staff, duties may include sterilization of instruments, bed making, feeding and bathing patients, and preparation of rooms for occupancy.

The general duty nurse may be assigned to work in a special section of the hospital, such as surgery, pediatrics, obstetrics, psychiatry, or the admitting office. The nurse who works in several of these sections gets a broad scope of nursing specialties and is able to make a more informed decision as to which of the clinical areas to choose for further study and specialization.

Persons who enter the career field of nursing should have a genuine liking for people, and should be emotionally stable, enabling them to cope with ill patients and their distressed families. They should be able to work under pressure, be responsible and resourceful, be able to direct the activities of the nursing aides (assistants), as well as be able to take precise orders from superiors and execute them exactly. The general duty nurse needs a lot of physical stamina as the occupation requires much walking and standing as well as lifting and moving patients. During periods of disaster or epidemics, the nurse may be required to work prolonged shifts until the emergency passes.

The Geriatric Nurse

The *geriatric nurse* is a registered nurse who has been trained in the aging process and how it affects the healthcare needs of the older person. Geriatric nurses deliver nursing care in hospitals, nursing homes, clinics, and physicians' offices, and some are visiting nurses taking nursing services to the homes of the patients.

Geriatric nurses work with physicians and other medical staff to assess the condition of the patient and to devise an individual healthcare plan, then seeing that that plan is implemented. They also keep records showing the patient's condition, amount and times of medication, and other treatments such as physical therapy or radiation treatment.

Nursing care for the elderly has a large counseling component. Nurses must help patients understand the aging process and how it affects their health and life-styles. The nurse helps the patient find ways of adjusting to these changes in a manner that will allow for a life-style as comfortable as the situation will permit. Great care must be taken to recognize and take care of the psychological needs of the patient.

Patience is one of the greatest assets a geriatric nurse can have. Assisting patients with such basic needs as dressing, eating, and bathing calls for infinite amounts of patience and tact. Because of age and ill health, elderly patients may be very slow in performing routine tasks, but the help of understanding nurses enable these patients to do things for themselves and retain some feelings of independence and self esteem. Many elderly patients have been depersonalized by the treatment of society and their families and the task of geriatric nurses is to bring a personal touch to nursing to motivate these patients to utilize what capacities they have to live as normally as possible.

The visiting geriatric nurse works under the supervision of the physician, but, since the physician is not always readily available, some independent action is necessary. These nurses work without the technical equipment in a hospital and must improvise to provide treatment in whatever setting the patient resides. Obviously, the visiting geriatric nurse must be resourceful and able to work with all types of people. Some nurses derive great job satisfaction from working as a visiting nurse because of the close involvement with patients and their families.

The Gynecologic Nurse

The *gynecologic nurse* is a registered nurse (RN) especially trained to work with women with problems relating to their reproductive and sexual lives and the relationship of those systems to the complete health of the women.

This nurse may work in hospitals, physicians' offices, public health departments, clinics, and community agencies.

The gynecologic nurse takes medical histories of patients, performs pregnancy tests and Pap smears, participates in the family planning program by counseling women in the use of contraceptives, and may fit diaphragms. In the hospital, the gynecologic nurse administers medications, dresses surgical wounds, and removes sutures. They assist with patients who have had mastectomies, hysterectomies, sterilizations, or abortions.

This nurse has been very instrumental in programs promoting the early detection of breast cancer and may perform breast examinations and instruct women in the technique of self examination. They also play an important part in the education of the general public in campaigns for the control of venereal disease and may participate in programs for the testing of venereal disease.

The gynecologic nurse needs to have a good command of counseling skills in order to help rape victims, women who are considering abortion or giving their babies up for adoption, and women who are having difficulty adjusting to sexual problems. This nurse must be very aware of the psychological problems that can attend some gynecologic procedures and be able to give counseling to those patients and be aware of referral sources to which the patient can be referred to at the level of counseling or psychiatric care indicated.

Write for more information to the Nurses Association of the American College of Obstetricians and Gynecologists, 600 Maryland Avenue, S.W., Washington, DC 20024.

The Head Nurse

The *head nurse* is an experienced registered nurse in charge of the nursing activities in a hospital unit, instructing the nurses, and coordinating the work of the unit to secure the best care for its patients.

The head nurse observes the work of the staff nurses and assistants to see that care is being given to patients as directed and that the physicians' instructions are being followed. This nurse makes assignments to duties, evaluates the performance of the nursing staff, plans needed changes to upgrade the service, and makes sure that rooms and wards are kept clean and comfortable. The head nurse also directs staff in keeping patient records and makes rounds with physicians to keep abreast of any special instructions for patients. Drugs and supplies are either ordered by or at the direction of the head nurse who also is responsible for keeping records of the supply and distribution of narcotics in the unit. This nurse takes care of such problems as conflicts between staff members and resolves these differences or refers to higher authority in order to maintain smooth personnel relations.

The Intensive Care Nurse

The *intensive care nurse* is a registered nurse who provides nursing services to patients admitted to the hospital in such a critical state that specific, immediate, and expert care will make the difference in whether the patient lives or dies.

In the intensive care unit, staffed by nurse-physician teams, constant monitoring and assessment of the patient is coupled with treatment administered by trained staff experts. In this unit treatment is available constantly and immediately when needed. The nurse in the intensive care unit is trained in the use of the newest, most sophisticated medical life-support equipment.

The nursing service is under the direction of the physician. The nurse clinician has the responsibility of determining the nursing needs of the patient, devising a nursing plan for each individual, making sure that such plans are carried out, and coordinating tests and other diagnostic procedures. The nurse communicates to the family appropriate information on the patient's condition. Preparation of the family is very important; studies have shown that family anxiety transfers to the patient.

The intensive care nurse is trained to recognize danger signals calling for initiation of emergency procedures and the techniques of administering that treatment. The nurse observes the behavior of patients to determine their psychological state and provides the support and reassurance necessary to enable patients to participate in their own recovery.

Nurses receive special preparation for work in the particular unit in which they will be stationed. There are intensive care units for heart failure, stroke, kidney failure, diabetic coma, shock, pediatric problems, respiratory failure, newborns, burns, surgical complications, and others. Each type of unit has its own particular lifesaving equipment and procedures. Nurse preparation includes understanding the function of the machines, being able to operate them, and knowing the techniques of administration of lifesaving procedures.

Perhaps the best known of the intensive care units is the coronary care unit, where patients are placed to recover from heart attacks. These attacks are a major cause of deaths in the United States. As soon as patients arrive in the unit, they are in the hands of professionals, well trained in the use of the life-support systems and the most important methods of communication, emotional support, and reassurance to allay the panic of the patients. As patients improve, the nurse becomes both counselor and teacher, helping patients to understand their conditions and learn what must be done to adjust to a new life-style compatible with their new state of health.

There is probably no specialty in nursing that has as strong an emotional impact on the nurse as intensive care nursing. In any such unit, there is an atmosphere of crisis much of the time. The nurses must be strong and stable emotionally and need constantly to reexamine their own feeling toward events that arise in life and death situations. The patient, often fearing that death is imminent, depends on the nurse for reassurance. The intensive care nurses must be very emotionally involved with their patients, understanding their need to be angry, fearful, and uncooperative because of the threatening situation in which they are involved. The patient is often connected to strange machines on which life depends and the nurse is the means of conveying to the patient that there is a human, caring presence.

Licensed Practical Nurses

Licensed practical nurses (LPNs), known in Texas and California as *licensed vocational nurses,* work under the supervision of physicians and registered nurses in hospitals, convalescent and nursing homes, clinics, schools, public health agencies, and private homes to deliver nursing services to the ill and injured. The LPN performs many of the same nursing tasks as the registered nurse (RN), but does not receive the same level of academic and clinical preparation. The length of the training period for LPNs is twelve to eighteen months, compared to two to four years for the RN. Upward mobility for the LPN is considerably less than that for the RN.

Licensed practical nurses employ the techniques and principles of nursing to perform such duties as dressing wounds, taking temperatures and pulse and respiration rates, giving prescribed medication, and recording the results of these activities on the patients' records. They administer enemas and douches, carry out catheterization, and may perform routine laboratory procedures such as urinalysis. They answer patients' calls, observe patients, and report any changes of condition to supervisory staff on duty. They supply patients with ice bags and hot water bottles and give massages or alcohol rubs as directed. They sometimes make beds and clean rooms. They may be assigned to special duty stations such as the geriatric unit of the hospital. Licensed practical nurses may supervise assist in the supervision of nurse's aides, orderlies, and attendants. For more information on a career as a licensed practical nurse, write to the National League for Nursing, 10 Columbus Circle, New York, New York 10019, or the National Federation of Licensed Practical Nurses, P.O. Box 11038, Durham, North Carolina 27703.

The Navy Nurse

Navy nurses work in naval hospitals, clinics, and dispensaries delivering nursing services to Navy personnel and their families. Navy nurses perform the same duties as civilian registered nurses. Working under the direction of a licensed physician, they administer prescribed medication and treatment; check such vital signs as pulse, respiration, and blood pressure; and perform other nursing duties for the patient's comfort and recovery. In the Navy, the nurse may also specialize in such areas as pediatrics, family practice, and obstetrics.

For details regarding a career in the Navy Nurse Corps, contact the nearest Navy Recruiting Office, listed in the telephone directory under U.S. Government, Navy.

The Neonatal Nurse

The *neonatal nurse* works in the hospital nursery and has the responsibility of constantly monitoring the newborns to make sure that they are making normal progress. This nurse evaluates the condition of the patients; keeps records of vital signs; and if a change should develop warranting it, alerts the physician.

An important duty of the neonatal nurse is the care of premature infants and those born with defects that may endanger their normal developmental progress. Some neonatal nurses may specialize in these problems and be assigned to the high-risk nursery. Neonatal nurses are responsible for initiating lifesaving procedures and administering complicated medical treatment under the supervision of the physician.

Another function of the neonatal nurse is the education and counseling of parents in the care of the infant and the awareness of the developmental progress to be expected in the normal growth of the infant. The neonatal nurse usually works with the obstetric nurse assigned to postpartum care in the counseling and education of the parents and other members of the family.

For more information on a career as a neonatal nurse, write to the Nurses Association of the American College of Obstetricians & Gynecologists, 600 Maryland Avenue, S.W., Washington, D.C. 20024.

The Nephrology Nurse

The *nephrology nurse* is a registered nurse who works in a renal dialysis center, a community health agency, or in the home to provide nursing services to patients with kidney diseases, kidney transplants, or abnormalities producing kidney dysfunction. The nephrology nurse is part of a team that includes the physician, other health services personnel, and the patients and their families.

The nephrology nurse participates in setting up individualized plans of care for each patient. The patient is examined and evaluated so that appropriate treatment and other services can be arranged. Counseling and emotional support are provided to lessen the patient's anxiety over a condition that often poses a real threat to life and requires long-term care.

The nephrology nurse working with kidney transplant patients will be involved in preparing both the donor and the recipient physically and emotionally for the surgery and the postoperative recovery period. The nurse, as well as the other members of the team, will be trained to recognize and handle the psychological problems that arise in kidney transplant cases.

The nephrology nurse checks the dialysis equipment and ensures that it is operating properly, making adjustments or having them made by maintenance personnel. During the dialysis, the patient and the equipment are monitored carefully and the patient is taught to monitor his or her own dialysis equipment. This nurse teaches the patient proper care between dialysis to avoid infections, and instructs the patient on matters of diet. The nephrology nurse also receives training in the management of acute renal failure and other emergency conditions such as massive blood loss, shock, or equipment failure.

The nephrology nurse will need some teaching skills in order to instruct the patient and members of the family in the patient's home care. The patient may need to adopt a new life-style compatible to his or her altered physical state and will need the nurse's instruction and support. This nurse will also keep comprehensive records of the schedule and type of treatment and changes in the condition of the patient.

Persons interested in entering this specialty may get further information by contacting the American Nephrology Nurses Association, 4903 Glenmeadow Drive, Houston, Texas 77096.

The Neurosurgical/Neurological Nurse

The *neurosurgical/neurological nurse* is a registered nurse who has been specially trained to furnish nursing services to persons who, by injury or disease, are suffering physical or mental disorders due to dysfunction of the nervous system.

The progress of the neurological patient is best assessed by close monitoring at periodic intervals of vital signs, responsiveness, and motor ability; as well as subtle changes in the physiological, behavioral, and emotional conditions of the patient. Pain and hyperactivity must be controlled with minimum sedation so as not to suppress the responses necessary in evaluation of the patient's state. The nurse must be able to interpret the significance of these changes in light of treatment and prognosis. Using reports, records, interviews, and physical examinations, the nurse assesses the condition and nursing needs of the patient, then implements, under the physician's direction, emergency or other measures designed to work toward the rehabilitation of the patient.

The aim of the neurosurgical nurse is to return the patient to a condition that is as nearly normal as possible, given the extent of injury or deterioration of the nervous system. This nurse must have knowledge of rehabilitation nursing skills. The problems of the neurosurgical patient range from disturbance of the most basic bodily functions to the most complicated functions of the human mind. This requires a thorough understanding of the physiological and neurological function of the mind and body on the part of the nurse.

Persons interested in further information on this career, should contact the National League for Nursing, 10 Columbus Circle, New York, New York 10019.

The Nurse Anesthetist

The *nurse anesthetist* is the oldest of the nursing specialties and has grown to the extent that today more than 50 percent of the anesthesia used is administered by nurse anesthetists.

The anesthetist is an important part of the surgical team and must offer psychological assurance and support to the patient as well as perform the highly technical and scientific part of the operation. Since all situations in which anesthesia is required have a certain amount of stress, the person who enters this specialty must be able to work under pressure and to maintain control of their mind and emotions at all times.

Most anesthetists are employed by hospitals, but some work in group practice and there are those who independently contract their services where needed. Some anesthetists are employed by dentists who perform dental surgery.

Nurse anesthetists administer intravenous, spinal, and other anesthetics as needed for surgical operations, deliveries, and other medical and dental procedures. They control the flow of the gases or injected fluids to maintain the needed anesthetic state of the patient.

Anesthetists monitor such vital signs as blood pressure, pulse, and color to assess the condition of the patient and administer emergency measures when indicated to prevent the patient from going into shock. They keep the physician apprised of the patient's condition and keep records of the preoperative and postoperative condition of the patient and all anesthesia and medication administered. Nurse anesthesiologists may, under the direction of the physician, give postoperative care. Because of their intensive training in respiratory and cardiopulmonary function, nurse anesthetists are often called upon to assist in the resuscitation of patients in intensive care, coronary care, and other emergency situations.

Write to the American Association of Nurse Anesthetists at 216 Higgins Road, Chicago, Illinois 60068, for more information on this career.

The Nurse Consultant

Nurse consultants are registered nurses who have extensive experience and a high level of academic preparation in the nursing field. They work in a consulting role with schools of nursing, industrial organizations, hospitals, and public health agencies to solve problems in nursing and other health services.

These nurses assist nursing education programs by reviewing curricula and making suggestions for changes to be made to improve the programs. They also assist in preparation of manuals and procedures and the setting up of staff development programs for hospitals, schools, and agencies. Nurse consultants review nursing programs in hospitals, nursing homes, and clinics and make recommendations for changes in nursing techniques, administration, and procedures to increase efficiency in the delivery of nursing services. They also work with industrial and community groups by preparing educational materials, participating in setting up educational programs, and advising these organizations about community resources in the nursing and healthcare field. Some consulting may be with nursing associations and organizations regarding nursing education and professional development programs. Increasingly, as in the entire nursing field, nurse consultants participate in surveys and research studies aimed at planning for establishing policies and programs to improve the quantity and quality of nursing services for the community.

The Nurse Instructor

The *nurse instructor* is a registered nurse who may work in a college, university, or hospital nursing school. The employment may be part time while the nurse is employed in a nursing capacity or it may be full time as a member of a college or university faculty.

The nurse instructor conducts classroom instruction in such nursing-related subjects as physiology, anatomy, and psychology and supervises nursing students in the performance of laboratory work. The instructor prepares and administers examinations to evaluate the progress of the students and monitors students' progress in the clinical work experience part of the training.

Nurse instructors work with the medical and nursing staff to plan curricula and to evaluate and improve training programs. They may assist in setting up seminars and workshops for the continuing education of the hospital staff. These nurses work under the supervision of the medical and nursing staff in a hospital and under the department head in a college or university. They may specialize in a particular subject in the nursing curriculum, such as nutrition, physiology, or anatomy or in a special field of nursing, such as surgical nursing or gynecologic nursing.

The Nurse-Midwife

The *nurse-midwife* works as a part of a medical team in the prenatal, delivery, and postnatal care of women with normal pregnancies.

The nurse-midwife participates in the initial examination of the pregnant woman and works in collaboration with the physician to determine responsibilities during the period of the pregnancy, labor, and delivery. The nurse-midwife's responsibilities include periodic examinations during the term of the pregnancy and instructing the patient in proper care, nutrition, and exercise to insure a delivery as normal and comfortable as possible, producing a healthy baby. This nurse monitors the results of laboratory tests to assure that the patient is making normal progress. If evidence of complication does appear, in collaboration with the obstetrician, the nurse works out corrective procedures to alleviate the complication.

The nurse-midwife stays with the patient during labor and delivery providing emotional support and care of physical needs, including administration of needed medication. Under supervision of the obstetrician, the nurse-midwife delivers babies if the delivery is uncomplicated. In the case of complications, the nurse-midwife administers emergency measures and sees that the obstetrician is notified immediately.

Following the delivery of the baby, the nurse-midwife performs routine examinations of the patient, instructs the new mother in infant care, and may conduct classes for mothers and other family members in the care of the newborn. Postpartum care may include home visits to monitor progress of the mother and the child. Information and advice on contraception and family planning are part of the aftercare.

For further career information, write to the American College of Nurse-Midwives, 1522 "K" Street, N.W., Washington, D.C. 20005.

The Nurse Nuclear Medical Technologist

The nurse who becomes a *nuclear medical technologist* (NMT) has received special training in the use of radioactive materials for diagnosis and treatment.

The nuclear medical technologist, working under the direction of a radiologist, performs analyses of biological specimens such as blood and urine by combining them with radioactive drugs (also called radiopharmaceuticals) to detect such substances as hormones, drugs, or other chemicals.

The NMT also administers radioactive materials that localize in a particular organ, and is then photographed or "imaged" by scanners or cameras so that the physician can study the structure and function of the organ to diagnose disease or structural abnormalities. This procedure subjects the patient to minimal radiation and is not painful.

This nurse administers radioactive materials in the treatment of disease. Other responsibilities include assuring radiation safety; preparation, administration, and disposal of radioactive materials; use of nuclear instruments; and the preparation of specimens for laboratory study. The data from these studies are prepared for the physician's use in diagnosis.

The Nurse Practitioner

The *nurse practitioner* is usually defined as a registered nurse (RN) with education and experience enabling nursing performance in an expanded role. The extent of this expanded role has not been uniformly established, and can vary considerably with the job. This nurse is competent to work without supervision in many of the nursing services. Though the term "nurse practitioner" is relatively new, the concept of the nurse working independently is not. For many years in rural areas, ghettos, and other places where a physician is not readily available, nurses have worked with independence, being the main source of medical care in some isolated regions. The nurse practitioner works in many settings, including clinics, health centers, public health agencies, physicians' offices, emergency departments, nursing homes, prisons, industry, and isolated rural areas.

The nurse practitioner assesses the health status of patients by taking health histories, performing physical examinations, and ordering and interpreting diagnostic tests. This nurse consults with the physician and plans treatment, establishes a healthcare plan including preventive and maintenance measures, and, with approval of the physician, implements such plans. The nurse recommends medication and other types of treatment such as physical therapy or psychotherapy. This nurse may make referrals to specialists for treatment of conditions beyond the scope of the nurse practitioner and maintains records of patient's condition, treatment, and prognosis.

Nurse practitioners have a teaching and counseling role in helping patients in maintaining health and preventing illness, assisting parents to develop better physical and emotional health for their children, and counseling the elderly in maintaining good health during the aging process. These nurses may counsel the terminally ill and their families to help them through the death of the patient. They may manage the care of women with normal pregnancies.

Nurse practitioners work with and under the guidance of a licensed physician. However, there are some states in which the state law permits them to engage in independent practice. Persons interested in this career should contact their state licensure board to determine what a nurse practitioner can do in their state.

For more information, write to the National Association of Pediatric Nurse Associates & Practitioners, 1101 Kings Highway North, Cherry Hill, New Jersey 08034.

The Nurse Supervisor

The *nurse supervisor* works in a hospital or health agency supervising the delivery of nursing services for patient care units, assuring that the staff provides quality care to the patients, and administering medication and treatment according to physicians' instructions and institutional policy. The supervisor coordinates the nursing activities on a unit as well as coordinating activities with other units in the hospital.

The nurse supervisor evaluates the performance of the unit nursing staff, participates in planning in-service training and education programs to insure staff development, and offers guidance for nurses seeking ways of advancing in their profession. The supervisor is also involved in preparation of the budget for the unit or units supervised and may participate in studies or surveys to contribute to nursing research designed to promote better nursing programs.

The nurse supervisor may be in charge of a unit specializing in a particular area of nursing, such as obstetrics, coronary care, or surgery. The nurse who supervises such a specialty unit will need to have experience as well as special academic preparation in the specialty.

The Obstetric Nurse

The *obstetric nurse* is a registered nurse (RN) who works in hospitals, physicians' offices, public health departments, family planning clinics, homes, and community agencies furnishing nursing services to women during pregnancy, delivery, and the postpartum period.

Obstetric nurses may begin to work with patients in early pregnancy, counseling them on diet, exercise, and the physical changes that will take place as the pregnancy progresses. They help prepare mothers for the processes of labor and delivery and may conduct classes in natural childbirth that include the fathers and any other members of the family who may want to be a part of the birth experience. In this phase of obstetric care, nurses may work with high-risk patients and have responsibility for the close monitoring of these patients to ascertain any conditions that may require the care of the physician.

The obstetric nurse may work in the delivery room to assist the mother in having a delivery that is as safe and comfortable as possible. Duties may include administering medications, blood transfusions, and emergency measures necessary in the case of such conditions as hemorrhage or shock. Since childbirth is certainly an emotional and may be a difficult time, the role of the nurse in offering support and comfort for the patient is a vital one.

Following the birth of the baby, these nurses assist the mother during the healing process. They assess the mother's physical and emotional condition and lend whatever assistance the mother needs in adapting to her new baby and its needs. Counseling and education for the mother in this situation may also include the father and siblings.

For further information, write to the American College of Obstetricians & Gynecologists, 600 Maryland Avenue, S.W., Washington, D.C. 20024.

The Occupational Health Nurse

Occupational health nurses, formerly called *industrial nurses,* provide nursing services to workers in department stores, factories, large office complexes, or other places of employment that have large numbers of employees in one place.

The most important objectives of the occupational health nurse are the prevention of illness and the maintenance of the highest possible level of good health for the work force. Since employee ill health and its accompanying absentee rate are very costly to the employer, the role of the occupational health nursing staff in the counseling and education of employees in matters of good health cannot be overestimated.

The occupational health nurse works closely with the personnel department to discover and deal with such problems as alcoholism, chronic health problems, and emotional and mental instability in an effort to prevent them from progressing to insolubility.

It is important for the occupational health nurse to maintain cooperative relationships with local physicians, community health centers, and other health agencies. These may be needed for referral of clients for care beyond the scope of the nurse.

Occupational health nurses render competent nursing care to persons who may become ill or injured at the place of employment. After administering first aid in the case of an accident, they see that patients are transported to a physician or hospital for needed additional care. After treatment by a physician, these nurses may, under direction of the physician, apply subsequent dressings to wounds.

The nurse may visit homes of employees to determine cause of prolonged absence and need for referral services, and to give guidance to employees and their families in health care. It is necessary to keep complete records of treatment given employees and to prepare accident reports and other reports for worker's compensation, insurance coverage, and so forth.

The occupational health nurse organizes or participates in programs of accident prevention, health examination, or group immunization. The nurse who enters this field of work must be prepared to view the prevention of accidents and illness and the maintenance of good health as important as treatment of the patient after the onset of ill health. The occupational health nurse may be called upon to participate in seminars for supervisors and managers aimed at education on the early detection of physical or mental conditions and behavior patterns that may point to impending greater health problems and their resulting absenteeism. The nurse in this profession must exercise exceptionally good human relations skills.

For further details, write to the American Association of Occupational Health Nurses, 3500 Piedmont Road, N.E., Atlanta, Georgia 30305

The Office Nurse

The *office nurse* who is employed in a busy physician's office fills many roles, functioning at times like a physician's assistant, at others like a laboratory technician, and even, at times, like a secretary, bookkeeper, or receptionist.

The office nurse prepares patients for examination, assists the physician during examination, and instructs the patient regarding medication or home care following office treatment. The office nurse may, under instructions from the physician, administer injections or other medication, dress wounds, and remove stitches.

Office nurses assist the doctor with minor surgical procedures performed in the office and maintain office records of patient diagnosis, treatment, and prognosis. They check and requisition supplies, clean and sterilize equipment, and may develop x-rays and perform routine laboratory tests such as urinalyses and blood counts.

The duties of the office nurse vary with the employment situation. In a small office with limited staff the office nurse may perform receptionist and secretarial duties and send out the monthly bills; in an office with more help, these duties will be performed by clerical staff.

The office nurse works under the supervision of the physician and may, in turn, supervise nursing assistants or clerical help. This nurse may be allowed to work with varying degrees of independence, depending on the nurse's experience and the inclination of the employing physician. Some persons prefer this one-boss arrangement to the layers of supervision and management in a hospital setting.

Persons entering this field of nursing need to be emotionally stable, able to handle emergencies in the absence of the doctor, have the ability to work well with people, and have a genuine liking for people. This nurse will often deal with many members of the same family over a period of years and may be called upon to give counseling and reassurance to the patient and family.

Some nurses derive a high degree of job satisfaction from this work. They become a valued assistant to the physician, relied upon by the patients to take care of their minor problems when the doctor is not available.

The Oncology Nurse

The oncology section of the hospital is where patients with tumors are treated. Since most of these patients are cancer patients, this chapter will discuss the nurse involved in the care of cancer patients.

Oncology nurses perform many traditional nursing duties besides those special duties peculiar to the disease. They take temperatures, blood pressure readings, and pulse rates; bathe patients; feed those who are unable to eat; persuade others to eat, and give medications as directed by the physician. They work to keep the patient clean and odor-free and give special care to the skin before and after radiation treatment.

The oncology nurse prepares the cancer patient, both physiologically and psychologically for surgery. Following surgery, the nurse assists the patient through the postoperative period by giving medication, comfort, and reassurance. The nurse cares for the tracheostomy, laryngectomy, mastectomy, and colostomy and teaches the patient home care of these conditions.

There is probably no nursing specialty that requires as much warmth and understanding on the part of the nurse. The disease is so threatening that family relationships may become very strained. The nurse is often the intermediary for communication between patient and family as well as between patient and doctor. This nurse must be able to communicate with the family so that they understand the situation and how important their support is to the patient at this time.

The cancer patient sometimes must undergo mutilating surgery resulting in cosmetic damage and severe emotional trauma. The oncology nurse will need to help the patient work through this adjustment and begin rehabilitation therapy. Sometimes the patient has suffered trauma requiring change of vocation and will need to be referred to a vocational counselor.

When the patient is ready for discharge, this nurse instructs the patient and family in home care. The nurse also counsels the family on its attitude toward the patient and the necessity of maintaining a positive outlook, along with tolerance for the behavior of the patient trying to adjust to a very traumatic situation. The family must be made to understand the importance of the patient's return to activity that is as nearly normal as possible.

Some hospitals are now organizing their oncology care units using the primary care system, where the staff nurse has responsibility for a small group of patients from their time of entry into the hospital until discharge. The primary nursing system in the cancer ward seems to cut down on the high turnover rate usual in this nursing specialty. The close nurse-patient relationship seems to lead to greater job satisfaction.

For more information, write to the Oncology Nursing Society, 1016 Greentree Road, Pittsburgh, Pennsylvania 15220.

The Orthopedic Nurse

The *orthopedic nurse* is a registered nurse who has received special training in the care and treatment of musculoskeletal difficulties, deformities, and chronic diseases of the joints and spine.

Orthopedic nurses work with patients who have arthritis, bursitis, poliomyelitis, fractures, dislocations, and congenital deformities. Before the introduction of the Salk vaccine in 1955, a large part of orthopedic nursing was devoted to work with patients crippled by poliomyelitis. Following the virtual disappearance of polio, the emphasis shifted to working with birth defects and with orthopedic conditions in the elderly.

The orthopedic nurse assesses the patient data available and identifies the nursing needs of the patient, then devises and implements a nursing care plan. Working under the direction of the physician, the plan is implemented, evaluated, and changed as needed.

This nurse teaches the patient to use crutches, walkers, braces, and other equipment in the orthopedic unit. For patients who have had orthopedic surgery, the nurse helps care for the patient while in the hospital and instructs the patient in home care upon discharge.

Orthopedic patients frequently have conditions that require a change in life-style and it is the orthopedic nurse's responsibility to prepare them for this change, working with the family so that they are ready for the patient's return and are prepared to share in the adjustments they may have to make to accommodate the patient's new life-style. The orthopedic nurse must be prepared to give psychological support to patients while they make these changes.

In the case of patients who may have a prolonged stay in the hospital, the orthopedic nurse may be involved in providing craft classes or other diversions and arranging for school or tutoring for those patients who are school age.

The Pediatric Nurse

Pediatric nurses are registered nurses specially trained to furnish nursing services to infants, children, and adolescents. They may work in hospitals, public health agencies, well-child clinics, family clinics, and physicians' offices.

Pediatric nurses perform traditional nursing functions such as taking temperatures, blood pressures, and respiratory rates and recording this data. They bathe patients, weight them, feed them or persuade them to eat, and give medication as prescribed by the physician. Pediatric nurses must thoroughly understand the growth and development patterns of the child in order to assess the significance of behavior in relation to the child's illness.

The pediatric nurse must be able to communicate with the child and be able to understand his or her nonverbal communication since the patient may be too young to talk or just too intimidated by the situation to complain. This increases the importance of close observation of appearance and behavior. A large part of pediatric nursing is allaying the anxiety of the children by explaining the procedures being used and reassuring and supporting them. The pediatric nurse's training in child psychology enables him or her to assess the behavior of the patient under treatment.

Hospitalized children who are physically able to do so, may participate in play program. Play experience is a part of the training for this specialty. These nurses have the responsibility of making the children's stay as pleasant as possible, and keeping them occupied and diverted from dwelling on being absent from home and the fear of painful treatment.

The pediatric nurse must also be able to reassure and support the parents as well as explain to them the procedures being used to treat their child. This avoids having fearful parents transfer anxiety to their children.

Pediatric nurses may work in the nursery in the care of the new-born, with older children, or with adolescents from twelve to fourteen years of age. Adolescents often resent being placed in the children's ward and some hospitals now separate this age group in a separate ward. Nurses working this area must have a thorough understanding of the physical and emotional development of the adolescent.

The Private Duty Nurse

The *private duty nurse* is a registered nurse (RN) who makes a private contract to furnish nursing services at home or in a hospital. Usually this will be for nursing one patient only.

The private duty nurse works under the supervision of a physician to administer prescribed medication and other treatment to the patient. The nurse monitors the patient, noting changes in condition, evaluates and records these changes, initiates emergency measures if needed, and notifies the physician immediately of the patient's condition.

The private duty nurse instructs the patient and family in the procedures needed to restore and maintain the patient in a state of good health. If the nurse is working in a private home, they may supervise the diet of the patient. This nurse cooperates with any community agencies furnishing services to the family.

The Psychiatric Nurse

The *psychiatric nurse* is a registered nurse who delivers nursing service to patients having mental health problems. The psychiatric nurse may work in mental hospitals, the psychiatric wards of general hospitals, health clinics, community mental health centers, nursing homes, and private homes.

The psychiatric nurse performs many of the same nursing functions as the general duty nurse, such as administering medication prescribed by the physician, and taking and recording temperatures, pulse rates, blood pressures, and other vital signs affecting the physical health of the patient. In addition, the psychiatric nurse works with individual patients and with groups to assist them in understanding their problems, developing better self concepts, and learning the coping skills necessary to move back toward mental health.

The psychiatric nurse observes and assesses the behavior of the patient and, on the basis of this observation and assessment, forms a nursing diagnosis. Then, working with the physician and other members of the nursing team, the nurse devises a nursing plan for each individual patient.

The psychiatric nurse must be both teacher and counselor in addition to being a nurse in the traditional sense. Working with the patients in a warm accepting manner helps them make a more socially acceptable adjustment to their environment and the people with whom they come in contact. This nurse is trained in listening and communication skills, to assist the client in socializing with others and developing better interpersonal relations skills.

The psychiatric nurse works under a skilled psychotherapist to learn and practice the principles of psychotherapy to enable the patient to return to a more normally functioning state. this nurse evaluates the nursing care the patient is receiving and monitors the progress of the patient to determine if the results are satisfactory or if the nursing plan needs revision.

The Rehabilitation Nurse

The *rehabilitation nurse* is a registered nurse who provides services to persons needing restoration of physical or mental functioning to a state as nearly normal as possible. These patients have suffered trauma as a result of disease, birth defects, or accidental injury.

Rehabilitation nurses work in hospitals, rehabilitation centers, nursing homes, community health agencies, insurance companies, schools, clinics, and hospices. They perform many tasks performed by regular staff nurses, such as administering medication prescribed by the physician; taking temperatures, blood pressures, pulse rates, and other vital signs; and keeping records of patient care. In addition, they are especially trained in rehabilitation nursing techniques, including assisting the patient in use of prostheses, physical therapy, and special exercises to restore function in impaired body parts.

Some of the conditions the rehabilitation nurse will work with include arthritis, drug addiction, birth defects, cerebral palsy, cancer, epilepsy, spinal cord injuries, alcoholism, blindness, deafness, and handicaps resulting from deteriorating disease processes and accidental injuries.

The rehabilitation nurse is trained in the use of a wide variety of machines and equipment designed to help the patient's recovery. The nurse instructs the patient in the use of such aids as braces, walkers, respirators, and artificial limbs and other prostheses.

Being a rehabilitation nurse calls for good counseling skills, since, if the patient has psychological problems related to his or her handicap, they must be worked through so they will not stand in the way of rehabilitation and resumption of a nearly normal life. Teaching skills are necessary to teach the patient the use of new equipment, new methods of doing things, and sometimes, a whole new life-style compatible with the patient's capabilities.

This nurse must be infinitely patient, able to derive encouragement from the patient's minimal improvement and able to persuade the patient to share this encouragement. Patients who have been handicapped from birth or early childhood may have built up such highly defensive behavior that it interferes with socialization or employment. The nurse assists the patient in developing a better self-concept by setting achievable goals and assisting the patient in reaching these goals.

The Respiratory Therapy Nurse

The *respiratory therapy nurse* is a registered nurse who has been trained to administer diagnostic and treatment procedures to persons with cardiopulmonary problems that affect their ability to breathe normally. Most respiratory therapy nurses are employed in hospitals, but some will be found in medical clinics, nursing homes, industry, military service, and physicians' office.

The respiratory therapy nurse is a member of the critical care staff, working with patients who require life-support measures to maintain clear airways. They provide artificial ventilation for patients who cannot breathe normally. This requires highly specialized knowledge in the use of very sophisticated ventilation equipment as well as a thorough understanding of the underlying physiology involved in cardiopulmonary dysfunctions.

In addition to management of critical cases in which life is threatened, the respiratory nurses work in the routine care of patients with respiratory disorders. They administer oxygen, supervise exercises, and perform cardiopulmonary resuscitation.

Respiratory nurses treat such conditions as cardiac failure, emphysema, stroke, asthma, drowning, and shock. They conduct such diagnostic procedures as screening of lungs, measurement of lung capacity, and securing of secretion samples for cancer diagnosis.

The School Nurse

The *school nurse* is a registered nurse (RN) who is employed in an elementary school, junior high school, high school, or college. The school nurse works more with healthy than with sick patients, a large part of this job being preventive medicine-such as assisting in immunization and safety programs, counseling, and educating the student body regarding the maintenance of good health.

School nurses perform physical examination, give vision and hearing tests, render first aid following accidents on the school property, and refer students to a physician if treatment beyond first aid is indicated.

Students who are having problems in classes, such as inattention, disruptive behavior, drug abuse, or apparent emotional instability may be referred to the school or college nurse so that the underlying physical or emotional condition that may be responsible for the student's inappropriate behavior may be discovered. Duties of the college nurse will also include sex education and contraceptive information.

The school nurse works with school administrative officials to establish standards and policies for a school health program, then monitors and evaluates that program. Part of the work of these nurses is health education and they may instruct classes in home health-care, child care, and the general maintenance of good health.

School nurses are usually involved in the community and work with its agencies to plan activities for children outside the school. They may also be involved in devising special programs designed to aid handicapped children.

These nurses need to have counseling skills, a liking for youth of the age with which they work, and good interpersonal relations skills. Persons considering entering this field would do well to examine their attitudes toward the elementary school child, the adolescent, and the college student. While nursing skills for all groups may be the same, relating to the attitudes and emotions of the various age groups requires different approaches incorporating a good understanding of developmental psychology.

The Surgical Nurse

The *surgical nurse* is a registered nurse (RN) who has special training and experience working with patients hospitalized for surgery. The work of the surgical nurse falls into three phases-preoperative nursing, operating room duties, and postoperative care.

The goal of the preoperative phase is to prepare the patient physically and psychologically for surgery. The nurse interviews the patient in depth to uncover any indications of problems that might surface during surgery or in the postoperative period. All available previous medical records are reviewed by the nurse to alert the physician to any past medical history that might impinge on the planned procedures. The importance of this interview cannot be overemphasized. Such things as allergies to medication, unreasonable fears of anesthesia, and emotional pressures will surface in the good interview, offering the nurse the opportunity to explain to patients each procedure they can expect to experience. The manner in which this interview is handled by the nurse will determine to a great extent the degree of anxiety patients will take with them to the operating room. Communicating with the families of patients is important to allay their anxiety, since their fears may be transferred to the patient. This nurse needs counseling skills so that the fears and anxieties of the patient can be acknowledged as normal for the situation, and the patient can be allowed to talk through these fears to the extent possible. The nurse should be sensitive to the spiritual needs of the patient and should react to the patient's suggestions, however veiled, that the services of a clergyman would be welcome.

The second phase of surgical nursing is the operating room phase. The scrub nurse, who must be experienced and know what equipment the surgeon will need for each specific procedure, sees that such equipment is in place before the surgery. During the surgery this nurse hands the instruments, sutures, sponges, and other needed supplies to the physician. The efficient scrub nurse observes the surgeon closely to know what is needed before it is requested. The maneuvers must be accomplished with careful speed so that no time is wasted but no accidents occur due to undue haste or carelessness. It is also the responsibility of the scrub nurse to see that sterile conditions are maintained in the operating room.

In addition to the scrub nurse, there is the circulating nurse who supervises the preparation of the operating room, insuring that the room and all its equipment are scrupulously clean and properly prepared for the surgery. Following the operation, the circulating nurse supervises clean-up and preparation for the next scheduled patient. This nurse is usually a senior nurse with several years of experience.

The third phase of surgical nursing is the postoperative phase. It starts with the recovery room (or the intensive care unit if the patient has complications) and includes care of the surgical wound, measurements to guard against infection, support and reassurance for the patient, and the teaching of home care after hospital discharge.

Additional information can be obtained through the Association of Operating Room Nurses, 10170 E. Mississippi Avenue, Denver, Colorado 80231.

Foreign Nurses

Due to the severe shortage of nurses in this country, persons who are licensed nurses in foreign countries are given preference status by the immigration system to come to the United States to practice nursing. Admitted into the states on this basis, nurses get work permits and may work as registered nurses (RNs) as soon as they pass the state board nursing examination. Foreign nurses receive no special status regarding citizenship, however. To become a citizen of the United States, they must wait as long as immigrants who enter the country in the normal manner. Nurses who enter in this way must have a contract with an employing institution in this country before admission.

These nurses must pass the state board examination and become licensed in the state in which they intend to practice. A high percentage have been failing the state examinations and, not able to work as registered nurses, have taken jobs as nurse's aides or nursing assistants at a pay rate much lower than the RN salary. To lessen the likelihood of such exploitation, the Commission on Graduates of Foreign Nursing Schools (CGFNS) has set up a procedure by which foreign nursing school graduates can take a screening examination to determine their chances of passing a state examination in the United States. Upon passing the CGFNS preliminary examination, the nurse is given a certificate to be presented to the U.S. Immigration and Naturalization Service for a preference visa and to the U.S. Labor Department for a work permit.

To qualify to take the screening examination, nurses must have graduated from a government-approved nursing course lasting at least two years and must be licensed to practice nursing in their own country. The examination lasts approximately seven hours, is given twice a year, and covers nursing proficiency and English comprehension. Foreign nursing graduates who hold CGFNS certificates have a 76.9 percent rate in passing state board examinations, while the passing rate for those who do not hold certificates is around 20 percent. The nursing section of the CGFNS examination covers medical, obstetric, psychiatric, pediatric, and surgical nursing just as U.S. state board examinations do.

Application to take the examination may be made by contacting a U.S. embassy or consulate, national nurses' associations, or writing to CGFNS for application forms. A fee is required for taking the examination the first time. Each applicant is notified of passing or failing within ninety days of testing. Those who pass will receive certificates that they can present to a U.S. embassy to get information on securing visas and meeting other requirements for entry into the United States.

The CGFNS examination is also given in the United States for foreign nurses already in the country who may need the certificate for an extension of their visa or a change in the status of it. Detailed information on the CGFNS examination, examination sites and dates, and entry into the United States for the purpose of practicing nursing may be obtained by writing to the Commission on Graduates of Foreign Nursing Schools (CGFNS), 3642 Market Street, Philadelphia, Pennsylvania 19104, U.S.A.

Nursing Aide/Orderly

The *nursing aide/orderly* works as an auxiliary employee in an entry-level position in a department of nursing, helping the professional nursing staff in the care of sick, disabled or infirm patients. The title nursing aide generally refers to female workers, while orderly refers to male workers. Nursing aides/orderlies may also be referred to as *nursing assistants, hospital attendants,* or in the case of mental health facilities, nursing homes or home-healthcare agencies, as *psychiatric aides, geriatric aides* or *home-health aides,* respectively. Refer to the chapters titled Mental Health and Homemaker Home-Health Aide Services for more information on the positions of psychiatric aide and home-health aide.

Depending on the type of health facility and the type of patient being cared for, the duties of the nursing aide/orderly vary from cleaning patients' rooms and other household tasks to assisting in patient care.

Under direct supervision of the nursing staff, the nursing aide performs routine duties such as answering patient bell calls, delivering messages, serving and collecting food trays, feeding patients who are unable to feed themselves, assisting patients with their personal hygiene, giving massages and alcohol rubs, and reporting all unusual conditions and reactions of patients to the nurses in charge. In assisting in basic patient care, the nursing aide may administer catheterization treatments; take and record temperature, blood pressure, pulse, and respiration rates; and accompany patients during exercise periods.

The orderly performs the same functions as the nursing aide, but with emphasis on the personal care of male patients. The orderly also does the lifting and heavy work such as transporting patients in wheelchairs and stretchers, lifting and turning patients in bed, and carrying mattresses to the sterilization room. With special training the orderly may also transport and set up catheterization, sterilization, respiratory, traction, and mobile X-ray equipment.

Most nursing aides/orderlies work in hospitals, while others are employed in nursing homes and other long-term care facilities.

After being hired by a hospital or nursing home, the nursing aide/orderly is trained on-the-job for six-to-eight weeks. Some employers prefer their aides/orderlies to be recent high school graduates, and others, such as nursing homes and psychiatric hospitals, prefer to hire as their aides/orderlies more mature individuals.

Many vocational schools, community colleges, and other post-secondary institutions throughout the United States have training programs for the nursing aide/orderly. Interested students should check with schools in their area for further information.

Some states require that nursing aides/orderlies be certified. Certification generally requires graduating from a state approved nursing aide (nursing assistant) training program and successfully passing a state examination.

A list of state approved training programs can be obtained through the state's Department of Education, Division of Vocational Training.

Salaries for the nursing aide/orderly are higher in hospitals than in nursing homes. Recent annual salaries for nursing aides/orderlies working in Veterans Administration hospitals ranged from $10,700 with no experience to approximately $13,000 with several years experience. The average salary for all aides/orderlies working for the federal government was approximately $15,500 a year.

The nursing aide/orderly has limited opportunities for promotion and better salaries without additional education and training. The nursing aide/orderly may, for example, take specialized courses or on-the-job training and become an cardiographic technician or radiographer (X-ray technician).

For additional information on job opportunities, persons interested in a career as a nursing aide/orderly should contact the Personnel Director of their local healthcare facility or talk with faculty or career counselors at post-secondary educational institutions in their area offering nursing aide/orderly training programs.

SOURCES

American Health Care Association
Occupational Outlook Handbook

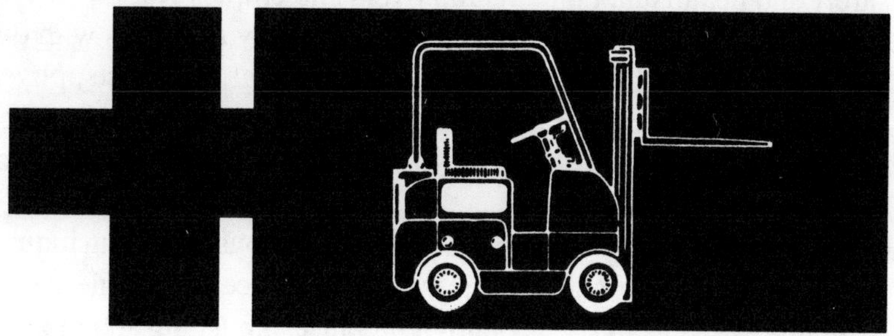

OCCUPATIONAL SAFETY AND HEALTH

Occupational safety and health is concerned with the maintenance of optimal health standards in all of today's working environments. To protect workers from undue hazards and dangerous working conditions in industry, manufacturing, mining, construction, transportation, and scientific research, safety and health regulations are established to prevent or reduce work-related accidents, injuries, and illnesses. In this field of allied health there are several closely related careers, including those of the *safety professional,* the *industrial hygienist,* the *occupational safety* and *health technician,* and the *industrial hygiene technician;* all of these are discussed below.

Safety Professional

Known as a *safety engineer,* a *safety specialist,* or a *safety manager,* the safety professional plans and administers accident-prevention and injury-control programs in industrial and other settings. He or she investigates health and safety conditions and the potential for accidents and for the loss of time, materials, or equipment in working environments. Such hazards as faulty equipment, poor facility design, dangerous materials, unsafe work practices, and the nonobservance of safety and health regulations are all the concern of the safety professional. The safety professional develops and implements programs that will eliminate or reduce the chances of an accident by informing management of problems, by enforcing safety standards, by recommending the use of safer equipment or more stringent control procedures, and/or by conducting intensive educational programs to increase and stimulate awareness and interest in occupational safety and health among both employers and employees.

The safety professional also coordinates safety activities with others who participate in safety and health, including managers, industrial hygienists, physicians, nurses, and fire and security personnel. Finally, as a *safety consultant* he or she offers advice on the design and construction or installation of working facilities or equipment and the safety of manufactured products.

Safety professionals work in a variety of locations including industrial and manufacturing plants, construction and mining sites, insurance companies, research and educational institutions, and in all levels of government, establishing and maintaining safety and health regulations.

Recommended high school courses for students interested in a career as a safety professional include mathematics, biology, chemistry, physics, and English.

The minimum educational requirement for a safety professional is a bachelor's degree in either safety management, safety engineering, or in one of the traditional engineering disciplines with a specialization in safety. Graduate programs are available for those who wish to obtain high level jobs in the various fields of occupational safety and health.

According to a recent salary survey in *Professional Safety* magazine, safety professionals employed as manufacturing managers or supervisors earned average annual salaries of $25,000 and those employed as safety engineers and safety and training supervisors averaged $32,500. Safety professionals with advanced education and experience may earn considerably more. Highest average annual salaries for safety professionals were in the mining, communications, and utilities industries.

For further information on a career as a safety professional, write to the American Society of Safety Engineers, 1800 E. Oakton Street, Des Plaines, Illinois 60018-2187, or the National Institute for Occupational Safety and Health, Robert A. Taft Laboratories, 4676 Columbia Parkway, Cincinnati, Ohio 46226.

Below is a list of bachelor's degree programs in occupational safety and health, compiled from data from the National Institute for Occupation Safety and Health.

SOURCES:

American Society of Safety Engineers
National Institute for Occupational Safety and Health

Safety Professional Programs

ARIZONA

Occupational Safety and Health Program
University of Arizona
Health Sciences Center
Tucson, Arizona 85724

CALIFORNIA

Occupational Safety and Health Program
California State University, Fresno
Department of Health Science
School of Health and Social Work
Shaw and Cedar Avenue
Fresno, California 93740

Health and Safety Studies Program
California State University, Los Angeles
Department of Health and Safety Studies
5151 State University Drive
Los Angeles, California 90032

Occupational Safety and Health Program
University of Southern California
Institute of Safety and Systems Management
University Park
Los Angeles, California 90089-0021

Occupational Health and Safety Program
National University
4141 Camino del Rio South
San Diego, California 92108

COLORADO

Occupational Health and Safety Program
Metropolitan State College
Department of Chemistry
Box 52, 1006 11th Street
Denver, Colorado 80204

CONNECTICUT

Occupational Safety and Health Program
University of New Haven
School of Professional Studies
and Continuing Education
300 Orange Avenue
West Haven, Connecticut 06516

FLORIDA

Occupational Safety and Health Program
University of Miami
Department of Industrial Engineering
School of Engineering and Architecture
Coral Gables, Florida 33124

IDAHO

Industrial Technology Program
University of Idaho
Idaho Falls Center of Higher Education
Box 778
Idaho Falls, Idaho 83402

ILLINOIS

Occupational Health and Safety Program
University of Illinois at Urbana-Champaign
Department of Health and Safety Studies
College of Applied Life Sciences
120 Huff Gymnasium
Champaign, Illinois 61820

Industrial Safety Program
Northern Illinois University
Department of Industry and Technology
College of Professional Studies
Still Gym
DeKalb, Illinois 60115

Occupational Safety Studies Program
Illinois State University
Department of Industrial Technology
Normal, Illinois 61761

INDIANA

Occupational Safety Program
Indiana University
Hazard Control Technology
The Poplars
400 E. Seventh Street
Bloomington, Indiana 47405

Industrial Health and Safety Management Program
Indiana State University
Department of Health and Safety
School of Health, Physical Education, and
Recreation
Terre Haute, Indiana 47809

Environmental and Occupational Safety
and Health Program
Purdue University
School of Health Sciences and School of
Pharmacy and Pharmaceutical Sciences
West Lafayette, Indiana 47907

IOWA

Occupational Safety Program
Iowa State University
Safety Education Laboratory
Ames, Iowa 50011

Occupational Safety and Health Program
University of Dubuque
Department of Safety
College of Liberal Arts
Dubuque, Iowa 52001

KENTUCKY

Occupational Safety and Health Program
Murray State University
Department of Safety Engineering and Health
Murray, Kentucky 42071

LOUISIANA

Occupational Safety and Health Program
Louisiana State University
Department of Industrial and Technical Education
Baton Rouge, Louisiana 70803

Environment Science Program
Moneese State University
Department of Biological and
Environmental Sciences
Lake Charles, Louisiana 70609

Occupational Safety and Health Program
Our Lady of Holy Cross College
Division of Business and Economics
4123 Woodland Drive
New Orleans, Louisiana 70114

MICHIGAN

Occupational Safety and Health Program
Ferris State College
School of Allied Health
Big Rapids, Michigan 49307

Occupational Safety and Health
Management Program
Grand Valley State College
148 Lake Michigan Hall
Allendale, Michigan 49401

Occupational Safety and Health/Fire
Science Program
Madonna College
Division of Natural Sciences and Mathematics
36600 Schoolcraft Road
Livonia, Michigan 48150

Industrial Health and Safety Program
Oakland University
Center for Health Sciences
Rochester, Michigan 48063

MISSOURI

Occupational Safety Program
Central Missouri State University
Department of Industrial Safety and Hygiene
College of Applied Science and Technology
Warrensburg, Missouri 64093

MONTANA

Occupational Safety and Health Program
Montana College of Mineral Science
and Technology
Environmental Engineering Department
Butte, Montana 59701

NEW HAMPSHIRE

Safety Studies Program
Keene State College
Safety Center
229 Main Street
Keene, New Hampshire 03431

NEW YORK

Occupational Safety and Health Program
Mercy College
555 Broadway
Dobbs Ferry, New York 10522

Occupational Safety and Health Program
New York University
Department of Occupational Health and Safety,
School of Education, Health, Nursing, and Arts
Professions
715 Broadway
New York, New York 10003

NORTH CAROLINA

Occupational Safety and Health Program
North Carolina Agricultural and
Technical State University
Department of Occupational Safety and Health,
and Safety and Driver Education
Greensboro, North Carolina 27411

Environmental Health Program
East Carolina University
Department of Environmental Health
School of Allied Health and Social Work
Greenville, North Carolina 27834

Occupational Health and Safety Program
Saint Augustine's College
Department of Chemistry
1315 Oakwood Avenue
Raleigh, North Carolina 27611

OHIO

Occupational Safety and Health Program
Wright State University
Department of Biological Sciences
College of Science and Engineering
Dayton, Ohio 45235

OKLAHOMA

Fire Protection, Safety and Loss
Prevention Program
Oklahoma State University
Division of Engineering Technology
Stillwater, Oklahoma 74078

OREGON

Safety Studies Environmental Health Program
Oregon State University
Department of Health
Corvallis, Oregon 97331

PENNSYLVANIA

Safety Science Program
Indiana University of Pennsylvania
Safety Sciences Department
Indiana, Pennsylvania 15705

Occupational Safety and Health Program
Millersville University of Pennsylvania
School of Education
Myers Hall
Millersville, Pennsylvania 17551

SOUTH CAROLINA

Occupational Safety and Health Program
Clemson University
College of Industrial Management
and Textile Science
Clemson, South Carolina 29631

TEXAS

Environmental Science Program
Lamar University
Environmental Science Department
P.O. Box 10208
Beaumont, Texas 77710

Radiation Protection Engineering Program
Texas A&M University
Department of Nuclear Engineering
College Station, Texas 77843

Safety Engineering Program
Texas A&M University
Department of Industrial Engineering
College Station, Texas 77843

UTAH

Occupational Safety and Health Program
Utah State University
Department of Biology and Industrial Technology
Colleges of Science and Engineering, UMC 53,
Logan, Utah 84322

VIRGINIA

Safety Engineering Program
Virginia Polytechnic Institute and State University
Department of Industrial Engineering and
Operations Research
Blacksburg, Virginia 24061

WASHINGTON

Occupational Safety and Health Program
Central Washington University
Central Safety Center
Edison Building
Ellensburg, Washington 98926

Occupational Safety and Health Program
Eastern Washington University
Washington Safety Center
Cheney Hall
Cheney, Washington 99004

WEST VIRGINIA

Engineering Technology Program
Salem College
Industrial Technology Department
Salem, West Virginia 26426

WISCONSIN

Occupational Safety and Health
Education Program
University of Wisconsin-Madison
Department of Education
225 North Mills Street
Madison, Wisconsin 53706

Industrial Safety Program
Milwaukee School of Engineering
College of Engineering, Engineering Technology,
and Management
Evening College
1025 N. Milwaukee Street
Milwaukee, Wisconsin 53201

Occupational Safety Program
University of Wisconsin-Platteville
Department of Industrial Studies
College of Business, Industry, and Communication
Platteville, Wisconsin 53818

Safety Education and Occupational Safety Program
University of Wisconsin-Whitewater
Department of Safety Studies
School of Education
800 West Main Street
Whitewater, Wisconsin 53190

Industrial Hygienist

As a member of the occupational safety team, the *industrial hygienist* recognizes, evaluates, and controls environmental factors that affect the safety and health of workers. The industrial hygienist performs many duties similar to the safety professional, such as conducting safety and health inspections, recommending changes to equipment or to processes, implementing control procedures, and advising on the design and construction of new facilities. Where their respective duties differ however is in the industrial hygienist's particular concern with the controlling of chemical, physical, and biological agents that cause illness, injuries, discomfort, and fatigue to workers. Agents the industrial hygienist strives to minimize include radiation, fungi, air and noise pollution, vibration, poor lighting and other unsanitary, unhealthy, and hazardous working conditions. In a large industrial location the industrial hygienist may be part of an occupational health program that includes physicians, nurses, bacteriologists, chemists, physicians, and engineers; whereas in a smaller setting he or she may have sole responsibility for ensuring the health, safety, and comfort of workers.

A bachelor's degree in industrial hygiene is the minimum educational requirement for the industrial hygienist, and continued professional development is available through a number of graduate degree programs. It should be noted that individual courses in industrial hygiene are usually offered as part of degree-granting programs in occupational safety and health.

For further information on a career as an industrial hygienist, write to the American Industrial Hygiene Association, 475 Wolf Ledges Parkway, Akron, Ohio 44311-1087

Below is a list of bachelor's degree programs in industrial hygiene, compiled from information from the American Industrial Hygiene Association and the National Institute for Occupational Safety and Health.

SOURCES:

American Industrial Hygiene Association
National Institute for Occupational Safety and Health

Industrial Hygienist Programs

ALABAMA

Industrial Hygiene Program
University of North Alabama
Department of Chemistry
Box 5159
Florence, Alabama 35632

CALIFORNIA

Industrial Hygiene Program
University of Southern California
Institute of Safety and Systems Management
University Park
Los Angeles, California 90089-0021

Environmental and Occupational Health Program
California State University, Northridge
Department of Health Science
School of Communication and Professional Studies
18111 Nordhoff Street
Northridge, California 91330

COLORADO

Environmental Health Program
Colorado State University
Occupational Health and Safety Section
Fort Collins, Colorado 80523

CONNECTICUT

Industrial Hygiene Program
Quinnipiac College
Department of Biological Sciences
School of Allied Health and Natural Sciences
Mt. Carmel Avenue
Hamden, Connecticut 06518

ILLINOIS

Industrial Hygiene Program
Illinois State University
Department of Health Sciences
College of Applied Science and Technology
Normal, Illinois 61761

KANSAS

Radiation Biophysics Department
University of Kansas
Department of Radiation Biophysics
140 Nuclear Reactor Center
West Fifteenth Street
Lawrence, Kansas 66044

KENTUCKY

Industrial Hygiene Program
Western Kentucky University
Department of Engineering Technology
Bowling Green, Kentucky 42101

MASSACHUSETTS

Environmental Health Program
University of Massachusetts at Amherst
Division of Public Health
School of Health Sciences
Amherst, Massachusetts 01003

MISSISSIPPI

Environmental Health Program
Mississippi Valley State University
Environmental Health Program
Biological Sciences Department
Itta Bena, Mississippi 38941

MICHIGAN

Environmental Health Program
Oakland University
Environmental Health Program
College of Arts and Sciences
Rochester, Michigan 48063

MISSOURI

Industrial Hygiene Program
Central Missouri State University
Department of Industrial Safety and Hygiene
College of Applied Science and Technology
Warrensburg, Missouri 64093

NEW YORK

Environmental Health Science Program
City University of New York, York College
Department of Natural Sciences
Jamaica, New York 11451

OHIO

Industrial Hygiene Program
Ohio University
College of Arts and Sciences
Department of Chemistry
Athens, Ohio 45701

Environmental Health Program
Bowling Green State University
College of Health and Community Services
Bowling Green, Ohio 43403

OREGON

Industrial Hygiene Program
Oregon State University
Department of Health
Waldo Hall 321
Corvallis, Oregon 97331

OKLAHOMA

Environmental Science Program
East Central Oklahoma State University
Department of Environmental Science
School of Mathematics and Sciences
Ada, Oklahoma 74820

TENNESSEE

Environmental Health Program
East Tennessee State University
Department of Environmental Health
School of Public and Allied Health
Johnson City, Tennessee 37601

UTAH

Industrial Hygiene Program
Utah State University
Department of Biology
College of Science, UMC 53
Logan, Utah 84322

WISCONSIN

Industrial and Environmental Hygiene Program
University of Wisconsin-Parkside
Science Division, Allied Health Discipline
Kenosha, Wisconsin 53141

Occupational Safety and Health Technician
Industrial Hygiene Technician

The *occupational safety and health technician* and the *industrial hygiene technician* support and work in the same locations as the safety professional and the industrial hygienist, respectively. Both technicians are concerned with maintenance of safety and health standards and with accident prevention and perform such duties as inspecting working conditions; collecting samples of physical, chemical, and biological agents for testing; operating instruments that detect and measure levels of noise, radiation, air flow, light, and gas; keeping records of the amounts of hazardous agents to which workers could be exposed; and investigating work-related accidents. Both technicians also teach workers the principles and techniques of disease and accident prevention.

An associate degree in arts, science, or applied science is generally the minimum educational requirement for both the occupational safety and health technician and also the industrial hygiene technician. Some one-year certificate programs are available for high school graduates.

Below is a list of associate degree and certificate programs in occupational health and safety and in industrial hygiene, compiled from information from the American Industrial Hygiene Association and the National Institute for Occupational Safety and Health. The two fields are closely related, and most programs, whatever their title, offer courses in both. Persons interested in a specific program should contact it directly and inquire about its particular specialties and degree offered.

SOURCES:

American Industrial Hygiene Association
American Society of Safety Engineers
National Institute for Occupational Safety and Health

Occupational and Industrial Safety and Health Technician Programs

CALIFORNIA

Occupational Safety and Health
Technology Program
Orange Coast College
Department of Occupational Safety and Health
2701 Fairview Road
Costa Mesa, California 92626

Safety Operations Technology Program
California State University, Long Beach
Department of Industrial Technology
School of Applied Arts and Science
1250 Bellflower Blvd.
Long Beach, California 90840

Occupational Safety and Health
Technology Program
San Diego City College
1313 Twelfth Avenue
San Diego, California 92101

COLORADO

Risk and Safety Management Program
Pikes Peak Community College
5675 South Academy Blvd.
Colorado Springs, Colorado 80906

CONNECTICUT

Occupational Safety and Health Program
University of New Haven
School of Professional Studies and Continuing
Education
300 Orange Avenue
West Haven, Connecticut 06516

FLORIDA

Environmental Control Engineering
Technology Division
Brevard Community College
1519 Clearlake Road
Cocoa, Florida 32922

HAWAII

Occupational Safety and Health
Technology Program
Honolulu Community College of the
University of Hawaii
Department of Occupational Safety and Health
874 Dillingham Blvd.
Honolulu, Hawaii 96817

IDAHO

Industrial Safety Technology Program
University of Idaho
Idaho Falls Center for Higher Education
Box 778
Idaho Falls, Idaho 83402

ILLINOIS

Occupational Safety and Health Technology Program
Rock Valley College
Division of Technology
3301 North Mulford Road
Rockford, Illinois 61101

INDIANA

Hazard Control Technology Program
Indiana University
Hazard Control Technology
The Poplars
400 E. Seventh Street
Bloomington, Indiana 47405

KENTUCKY

Health and Safety Program
Western Kentucky University
Department of Health and Safety
Bowling Green Kentucky 42101

Occupational Safety and Health Technology and Industrial Hygiene Technology Program
Murray State University
Department of Safety Engineering and Health
Murray, Kentucky 42071

LOUISIANA

Occupational Safety and Health Technology Program
Delgado Community College
Occupational Safety and Health Department
Building Technology and Safety Division
615 City Park Avenue
New Orleans, Louisiana 70119

MARYLAND

Occupational Safety and Health Technology Program
Catonsville Community College
Natural Science Department
800 South Rolling Road
Catonsville, Maryland 21228

MICHIGAN

Safety Management Technology Program
Detroit College of Business
Department of Management-Marketing
4801 Oakman Blvd.,
Dearborn, Michigan 48216

Occupational Safety and Health/Fire Science Program
Madonna College
Division of Natural Sciences and Mathematics
36600 Schoolcraft Road
Livonia, Michigan 48150

MINNESOTA

Occupational Safety and Health Technology Program
Inver Hills Community College
8445 College Trail
Inver Grove Heights, Minnesota 55075

NEW HAMPSHIRE

Safety Studies Technology Program
Keene State College
Safety Center
229 Main Street
Keene, New Hampshire 03431

NEW YORK

Industrial Hygiene Technology Program
Broome County Community College
P.O. Box 1017
Binghamton, New York 13902

Safety Technology Program
City University of New York, College of Staten Island
Mechanical Technology Department
Occupational Safety and Health
715 Ocean Terrace
Staten Island, New York 10301

NORTH CAROLINA

Industrial Safety and Health Technology Program
Cleveland County Technical Institute
Management, Mathematics and Sciences Department
137 South Post Road
Shelby, North Carolina 28150

OHIO

Occupational Safety and Health
Technology Program
University of Cincinnati
University College
Clifton Campus, Department of
Mathematics and Applied Science
562 French Hall
Cincinnati, Ohio 45221

Environmental Control and Protection
Technology Program
Technical Science and Mathematics Department
University of Toledo
University Community and Technical College
2801 W. Bancroft
Toledo, Ohio 43606

OKLAHOMA

Safety Technology Program
Tulsa Junior College
909 South Boston Avenue
Tulsa, Oklahoma 74119

OREGON

Occupational Safety and Health
Technology Program
Mount Hood Community College
Trades and Service Occupations Division
36000 S.E. Stark Street
Gresham, Oregon 97030

TEXAS

Occupational Safety and Health
Technology Program
Texas State Technical Institute, Waco Campus
Waco, Texas 76705

VIRGINIA

Occupational Safety and Health
Technology Program
Northern Virginia Community College
Alexandria Campus
Division of Health and Public Service
3001 N. Beauregard Street
Alexandria, Virginia 22311

Occupational Safety and Health
Technology Program
Thomas Nelson Community College
Division of Public Services Technologies
and Social Sciences
Department of Occupational Safety and Health
P.O. Box 9407
Hampton, Virginia 23670

WEST VIRGINIA

Occupational Safety and Health Technology
Marshall University
Community College
Huntington, West Virginia 25701

Occupational Safety and Health
Technology Program
Salem College
Industrial Technology Department
Salem, West Virginia 26426

WISCONSIN

Industrial Hygiene Technology Program
Western Wisconsin Technical Institute
Trade and Industrial Division
Sixth and Vine Streets
La Crosse, Wisconsin 54601

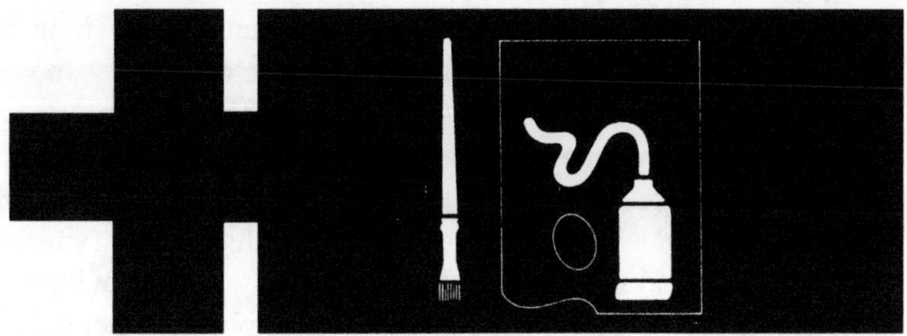

OCCUPATIONAL THERAPY

Occupational therapy is a health profession concerned with the physical and psychological rehabilitation of individuals who suffer from injury or illness, or from emotional, mental, or developmental problems. In occupational therapy, rehabilitation employs the use of educational, vocational, and recreational activities or "occupations". There are three career classifications in occupational therapy: *occupational therapist, occupational therapy assistant,* and *occupational therapy aide*.

Occupational Therapist

The *occupational therapist* attempts to restore a medical patient's health, independence, and self-reliance by first evaluating the patient's needs, and then teaching the patient to understand and compensate for their disability through planned activities and therapy. By teaching specially designed occupations such as manual and creative activities, the occupational therapist can, for example, help a patient restore the mobility and coordination of an injured limb. For the mentally ill or emotionally disturbed, the occupational therapist can create a social environment through group activities that will help the patient experience and adjust to social relationships and interaction. By concentrating on the patient's strengths and downplaying his or her weaknesses, the occupational therapist can give the patient the opportunity to accomplish tasks and acquire skills that will help restore self-confidence and emotional stability. The occupational therapist may also work in keeping the elderly occupied with interesting activities and hobbies. The occupational therapist also assists with the physical, psychological, and social development of physically and mentally handicapped children and children with learning disabilities. A common therapy involves helping the disabled child develop sensory, motor, and perceptual skills, all essential for further growth and development. No matter what the impairment or disability, whether mental or physical, occupational therapy attempts to rehabilitate and to provide restorative services so that the patient may achieve full or partial functional independence and learn to lead, or return to leading, a satisfying productive life.

The occupational therapist has the opportunity to work with a variety of members of a professional health team, including physicians, physical therapists, psychologists, nurses, speech pathologist, teachers, and others. Although most work in hospitals, the occupational therapist can also work in community mental health centers, public school systems, schools for handicapped children and the mentally retarded, home healthcare services, and nursing homes.

Occupational therapists may advance to supervisory positions with accountability for physical therapy assistants and physical therapy aides. A master's degree is usually the minimum requirement for teaching, research, and administrative positions.

An individual can become an occupational therapist by one of the following ways: (1) obtain a bachelor's degree with four years in a college or university occupational therapy program; (2) attend a liberal arts college or university for two years and then attend a college or university occupational therapy program for two years; (3) obtain a master's degree; or (4) obtain a certificate of proficiency in occupational therapy after completing a bachelor's degree in a related field of science or liberal arts. In all four cases, as part of the educational program, a six to nine month supervised clinical internship is included in the curriculum. Specific questions regarding admission or transfer requirements should be directed to those individual colleges or universities listed at the end of this chapter.

Upon completion of an accredited educational program graduates are eligible to take a national certification examination, conducted by the American Occupational Therapy Association, to become a registered occupational therapist (OTR) and to practice occupational therapy.

Many states also require occupational therapists to be licensed. Licensure applicants must generally complete an accredited occupational therapy program and successfully pass the American Occupational Therapy Association's national certification examination. Contact the state's occupational therapy licensing division for more specifics on licensure.

High school students who are interested in a career in occupational therapy should take courses in biology, chemistry, mathematics, health, social sciences, and crafts. They also should try to maintain above-average grades, especially in the science fields.

According to a 1986 salary survey compiled by the American Occupational Therapy Association of its members, OTRs (Registered Occupational Therapists) certified one year or less earned average annual salaries of $21,000, those certified 3-4 years averaged $24,000 and those certified 10 or more years, averaged $30,000.

The job outlook for occupational therapists is expected to be excellent through the mid-1990's with nearly a 60% increase in job openings, as predicted by the U. S. Bureau of Labor Statistics. Employment opportunities in private practice and home healthcare will continue to increase.

For further information on occupational therapy careers as well as financial aid and scholarship information for occupational therapy students, write to the American Occupational Therapy Association, Inc., at 1383 Piccard Drive, Rockville, Maryland 20850.

Below is a list of educational programs in occupational therapy accredited by the Committee on Allied Health Education and Accreditation of the American Medical Association, in collaboration with the American Occupational Therapy Association.

Key:

(1) Bachelor's degree program.

(2) Post-baccalaurate certificate program for students with a degree other than occupational therapy.

(3) Master's degree for students with a degree other than in occupational therapy.

(4) Master's degree program for occupational therapists.

(5) Programs accepting students and seeking accreditation.

SOURCES:

American Occupational Therapy Association
Occupational Outlook Handbook

Occupational Therapist Programs

ALABAMA

Occupational Therapy Program (1,4)
University of Alabama in Birmingham
Regional Technical Institute
University Station
Birmingham, Alabama 35294

Occupational Therapy Program (1)
Tuskegee Institute
Division of Allied Health School of Nursing and Allied Health
Tuskegee Institute, Alabama 36088

ARKANSAS

Occupational Therapy Program (1)
University of Central Arkansas
P.O. Box U1761
Conway, Arkansas 72032

CALIFORNIA

Occupational Therapy Program (1,2,3,4)
University of Southern California
12933 Erickson Avenue
Downey, California 90242

Occupational Therapy Program (1)
Loma Linda University
School of Allied Health Professions
Loma Linda, California 92350

Occupational Therapy Program (1,2,4)
San Jose State University
School of Applied Arts and Sciences
One Washington Square
San Jose, California 95192-0001

COLORADO

Occupational Therapy Program (1,3,4)
Colorado State University
100 Humanities Building
Fort Collins, Colorado 80523

CONNECTICUT

Occupational Therapy Program (1)
Quinnipiac College
School of Allied Health and Natural Sciences
Hamden, Connecticut 06518

DISTRICT OF COLUMBIA

Occupational Therapy Program (1)
Howard University
College of Allied Health Sciences
6th & Bryant Sts, NW
Washington, DC 20059

FLORIDA

Occupational Therapy Program (1,4)
University of Florida
Box J164, JHMHC
Gainesville, Florida 32610

Occupational Therapy Program (1)
Florida International University
Miami, Florida 33199

GEORGIA

Occupational Therapy Program (1,4)
Medical College of Georgia
School of Allied Health Sciences
Augusta, Georgia 30912

ILLINOIS

Occupational Therapy Program (1)
Chicago State University
College of Allied Health
95th Street at King Drive
Chicago, Illinois 60628

Occupational Therapy Program (3,4)
Rush University
Rush-Presbyterian-St. Luke's Medical Center
1753 West Congress Parkway
Chicago, Illinois 60612

Occupational Therapy Program (1,4)
University of Illinois at Chicago
College of Associated Health Professions
Health Sciences Center
1919 West Taylor Street
Chicago, Illinois 60612

INDIANA

Occupational Therapy Program (3,5)
Indiana Central University
1400 East Hanna Avenue
Indianapolis, Indiana 46227

Occupational Therapy Program (1)
Indiana University School of Medicine
Division of Allied Health Sciences
1140 West Michigan Street
Indianapolis, Indiana 46223

KANSAS

Occupational Therapy Program (1)
University of Kansas
318 Blake Hall
Lawrence, Kansas 66045

KENTUCKY

Occupational Therapy Program (1)
Eastern Kentucky University
Wallace Building
Richmond, Kentucky 40475

LOUISIANA

Occupational Therapy Program (1)
Northeast Louisiana University
School of Allied Health Sciences
Monroe, Louisiana 71209

Occupational Therapy Program (1)
Louisiana State University Medical Center
School of Allied Health Professions
1732 Canal Street, Suite 265
New Orleans, Louisiana 70112

MAINE

Occupational Therapy Program (1)
University of New England
College of Health Sciences
Biddeford, Maine 04005

MARYLAND

Occupational Therapy Program (1,4)
Towson State University
Lida Lee Tall Building
Towson, Maryland 21204

MASSACHUSETTS

Occupational Therapy Program (1,3,4)
Boston University
Sargent College of Allied Health Professions
University Road
Boston, Massachusetts 02215

Occupational Therapy Program (1,3,4)
Tufts University-Boston
School of Occupational Therapy
Medford, Massachusetts 02155

Occupational Therapy Program (1,5)
Worcester State College
486 Chandler Street
Worcester, Massachusetts 01602

MICHIGAN

Occupational Therapy Program (1,2,4)
Wayne State University
College of Pharmacy and Allied Health Professions
Detroit, Michigan 48202

Occupation Therapy Program (1,3,4)
Western Michigan University
Kalamazoo, Michigan 49008

Occupational Therapy Program (1)
Eastern Michigan University
Department of Associated Health Professions
328 King Hall
Ypsilanti, Michigan 48197

MINNESOTA

Occupational Therapy Program (1)
University of Minnesota
Health Sciences Center
Box 388, Mayo Building
Minneapolis, Minnesota 55455

Occupational Therapy Program (1,2)
College of Saint Catherine
2004 Randolph Avenue
St. Paul, Minnesota 55105

MISSOURI

Occupational Therapy Program (1)
University of Missouri
Health Related Professions
124 Lewis Hall
Columbia, Missouri 65212

Occupational Therapy Program (1)
Washington University
School of Medicine
4567 Scott Avenue
St. Louis, Missouri 63110

NEBRASKA

Occupational Therapy Program (1,5)
Creighton University
School of Pharmacy and Allied Health Professions
California at 24th Street
Omaha, Nebraska 68178

NEW HAMPSHIRE

Occupational Therapy Program (1)
University of New Hampshire
School of Health Studies
Hewitt Hall
Durham, New Hampshire 03824

NEW JERSEY

Occupational Therapy Program (1,2)
Kean College of New Jersey
Willis 311
Morris Avenue
Union, New Jersey 07083

NEW YORK

Occupational Therapy Program (1)
State University of New York
Downstate Medical Center
450 Clarkson Avenue
Brooklyn, New York 11203

Occupational Therapy Program (1,4)
University at Buffalo
State University of New York
515 Stockton Kimball Tower
3435 Main Street
Buffalo, New York 14214

Occupational Therapy Program (1)
York College of the City
University of New York
Jamaica, New York 11451

Occupational Therapy Program (3,4)
Columbia University
College of Physicians & Surgeons
630 West 168th Street
New York, New York 10032

Occupational Therapy Program (1,3,4)
New York University
Division of Health
34 Stuyvesant Street
New York, New York 10003

Occupational Therapy Program (1)
Dominican College of Blauvelt
10 Western Highway
Orangeburg, New York 10962

Occupational Therapy Program (1)
Utica College of Syracuse University
Division of Allied Health
Burrstone Road
Utica, New York 13502

NORTH CAROLINA

Occupational Therapy Program (3)
University of North Carolina
Medical School, Wing E 222H
Chapel Hill, North Carolina 27514

Occupational Therapy Program (1)
East Carolina University
School of Allied Health and Social Work
Greenville, North Carolina 27834

NORTH DAKOTA

Occupational Therapy Program (1)
University of North Dakota
Box 8036, University Station
Grand Forks, North Dakota 58202

OHIO

Occupational Therapy Program (1,2)
Cleveland State University
Fenn Tower, 704
1983 East 24th Street
Cleveland, Ohio 44115

Occupational Therapy Program (1,2,4)
Ohio State University
School of Allied Medical Professions
1583 Perry Street
Columbus, Ohio 43120

OKLAHOMA

Occupational Therapy Program (1)
University of Oklahoma Health Sciences Center
College of Allied Health
P.O. Box 26901
Oklahoma City, Oklahoma 73190

OREGON

Occupational Therapy Program (1,5)
Pacific University
2043 College Way
Forest Grove, Oregon 97116

PENNSYLVANIA

Occupational Therapy Program (1)
College of Misericordia
Division of Allied Health Professions
Dallas, Pennsylvania 18612

Occupational Therapy Program (1)
Elizabethtown College
Elizabethtown, Pennsylvania 17022

Occupational Therapy Program (1,2,3,4)
Temple University
College of Allied Health Professionals
Health Sciences Campus
3307 North Broad Street
Philadelphia, Pennsylvania 19140

Occupational Therapy Program (1,2)
Thomas Jefferson University
College of Allied Health Sciences
Edison Building
130 South 9th Street
Philadelphia, Pennsylvania 19107

Occupational Therapy Program (1)
University of Pittsburgh
School of Health Related Professions
270 Thackeray Hall
Pittsburgh, Pennsylvania 15260

PUERTO RICO

Occupational Therapy Program (1)
University of Puerto Rico
Medical Sciences Campus
College of Health Related Professions
GPO Box 5067
San Juan, Puerto Rico 00936

SOUTH CAROLINA

Occupational Therapy Program (1,4)
Medical University of South Carolina
College of Allied Health Sciences
171 Ashley Avenue
Charleston, South Carolina 29425

TEXAS

Occupational Therapy Program (1,2,3,4)
Texas Woman's University
Box 23718, TWU Station
Denton, Texas 76204

Occupational Therapy Program (1)
University of Texas Medical Branch at Galveston
School of Allied Health Sciences
Galveston, Texas 77550

Occupational Therapy Program (1)
Texas Tech University Health Sciences Center
School of Allied Health
Lubbock, Texas 79430

Occupational Therapy Program (1)
University of Texas Health Science Center at San Antonio
7703 Floyd Curl Drive
San Antonio, Texas 78284

VIRGINIA

Occupational Therapy Program (1,3,4)
Virginia Commonwealth University
Box 8, MCV Station
Richmond, Virginia 23298

WASHINGTON

Occupational Therapy Program (1,4)
University of Washington
School of Medicine
Dept. of Rehabilitation Medicine, RJ-30
Seattle, Washington 98195

Occupational Therapy Program (1,2,3)
University of Puget Sound
1500 North Warner
Tacoma, Washington 98416

WISCONSIN

Occupational Therapy Program (1,4)
University of Wisconsin-Madison
1300 University Avenue
Madison, Wisconsin 53706

Occupational Therapy Program (1)
Mount Mary College
2900 N. Menomonee
River Parkway
Milwaukee, Wisconsin 53222

Occupational Therapy Program (1)
University of Wisconsin-Milwaukee
School of Allied Health Professions
P.O. Box 413
Milwaukee, Wisconsin 53201

Occupational Therapy Assistant

The *occupational therapy assistant* works under the supervision of the professional occupational therapist and helps in the planning and implementing of rehabilitation programs. The occupational therapy assistant teaches self-care and creative and work-related skills. They may be involved in the making of such items as simple splints and adaptive equipment and contribute observations to clinical records. Although requiring supervision in carrying out remedial programs, the occupational therapy assistant can work independently when conducting a maintenance therapy program.

Most occupational therapy assistants work in hospitals while others may work in schools for handicapped children and the mentally retarded, rehabilitation centers, nursing homes, and community mental health centers.

To become an occupational therapy assistant, one can complete either a two-year associate degree program or certificate program in a community or junior college or vocational-technical school. A certificate program is generally for returning students with several years of related healthcare experience or education. At least two months supervised practical experience is also required in both these educational programs. Physical sciences, health, social sciences, and crafts are subjects recommended for high school students if they are interested in a career as an occupational therapy assistant.

Graduates of an accredited educational program are eligible to take the American Occupational Therapy Association's examination to become a certified occupational therapy assistant (COTA).

According to a 1986 salary survey compiled by the American Occupational Therapy Association of its members, COTAs (Certified Occupational Therapy Assistants) certified one year or less earned average annual salaries of $14,000, those certified 3-4 years averaged $15,000 and those certified 10 or more years averaged $18,000.

For more information about becoming an occupational therapy assistant, write to the Occupational Therapy Association, Inc., 1383 Piccard Drive, Rockville, Maryland 20850.

Below is a list provided by the American Occupational Therapy Association, of approved educational facilities that offer occupational therapy assistant programs.

KEY:

(1) Occupational therapy assistant associate degree program

(2) Occupational therapy assistant certificate program

(3) Programs accepting students and seeking approval

SOURCES:

American Occupational Therapy Association
Occupational Outlook Handbook

Occupational Therapy Assistant Programs

ALABAMA

Occupational Therapy Assistant Program (1)
University of Alabama in Birmingham
Regional Technical Institute
University Station
Birmingham, Alabama 35294

CALIFORNIA

Occupational Therapy Assistant Program (1,2)
Los Angeles City College
855 North Vermont Avenue
Los Angeles, California 90029

COLORADO

Occupational Therapy Assistant Program (1)
Pueblo Community College
900 West Orman Avenue
Pueblo, Colorado 81004

CONNECTICUT

Occupational Therapy Assistant Program (1)
Manchester Community College
P.O. Box 1046, M.S., 19
Manchester, Connecticut 06040

FLORIDA

Occupational Therapy Assistant Program (1)
Palm Beach Junior College
4200 South Congress Avenue
Lake Worth, Florida 33461

GEORGIA

Occupational Therapy Assistant Program (1,3)
School of Allied Health Sciences
Augusta, Georgia 30912

HAWAII

Occupational Therapy Assistant Program (1)
Kapiolani Community College
Allied Health Department
4303 Diamond Head Road
Honolulu, Hawaii 96816

ILLINOIS

Occupational Therapy Assistant Program (1,3)
Parkland College
2400 West Bradley Avenue
Champaign, Illinois 61821

Occupational Therapy Assistant Program (1)
Chicago City-Wide College
Cook County Hospital
Health Services Institute at Cook County
1900 W. Polk Street
Chicago, Illinois 60612

Occupational Therapy Assistant Program (1)
Illinois Central College
East Peoria, Illinois 61635

Occupational Therapy Assistant Program (1)
Thornton Community College
15800 South State Street
South Holland, Illinois 60473

INDIANA

Occupational Therapy Assistant Program (1)
Indiana University School of Medicine
Division of Allied Health Sciences
Coleman Hall-311
1140 West Michigan Street
Indianapolis, Indiana 46223

IOWA

Occupational Therapy Assistant Program (1)
Kirkwood Community College
P.O. Box 2068
6301 Kirkwood Boulevard
Cedar Rapids, Iowa 52406

KANSAS

Occupational Therapy Assistant Program (1,2)
Barton County Community College
Great Bend, Kansas 67530

Occupational Therapy Assistant Program (2)
University of Kansas
318 Blake Hall
Lawrence, Kansas 66045

LOUISIANA

Occupational Therapy Assistant Program (1)
Northeast Louisiana University
School of Allied Health Sciences
College of Pharmacy and Health Sciences
Monroe, Louisiana 71209

MARYLAND

Occupational Therapy Assistant Program (1,3)
Catonsville Community College
800 S. Rolling Road
Baltimore, Maryland 21228

MASSACHUSETTS

Occupational Therapy Assistant Program (1)
North Shore Community College
3 Essex Street
Beverly, Massachusetts 01915

Occupational Therapy Assistant Program (1,3)
Mount Ida College
Junior College Division
777 Dedham Street
Newton Centre, Massachusetts 02159

Occupational Therapy Assistant Program (1)
Becker Junior College
61 Sever Street
Worcester, Massachusetts 01609

Occupational Therapy Assistant Program (1,2)
Quinsigamond Community College
670 West Boylston Street
Worcester, Massachusetts 01606

MICHIGAN

Occupational Therapy Assistant Program (1)
Wayne County Community College
1001 W. Fort Street
Detroit, Michigan 48226

Occupational Therapy Assistant Program (1)
Grand Rapids Junior College
143 Bostwick, N.E.
Grand Rapids, Michigan 49503

Occupational Therapy Assistant Program (1)
Schoolcraft College
18600 Haggerty Road
Livonia, Michigan 48152

MINNESOTA

Occupational Therapy Assistant Program (1)
Anoka Area Vocational Technical Institute
1355 West Main Street
Anoka, Minnesota 55303

Occupational Therapy Assistant Program (1,3)
Austin Community College
1600 Eighth Ave., NW
Austin, Minnesota 55912

Occupational Therapy Assistant Program (1)
Duluth Area Vocational Technical Institute
2101 Trinity Road
Duluth, Minnesota 55811

Occupational Therapy Assistant Program (1)
St. Mary's Junior College
2500 South Sixth Street
Minneapolis, Minnesota 55454

MISSOURI

Occupational Therapy Assistant Program (1)
Penn Valley Community College
32301 Southwest Trafficway
Kansas City, Missouri 64111

Occupational Therapy Assistant Program (1)
St. Louis Community College at Meramec
11333 Big Bend Boulevard
St. Louis, Missouri 63122

NEW HAMPSHIRE

Occupational Therapy Assistant Program (1)
New Hampshire Vocational Technical College
Hanover Street Extension
Claremont, New Hampshire 03743

NEW JERSEY

Occupational Therapy Assistant Program (1)
Union County College
1033 Springfield Avenue
Cranford, New Jersey 07016

Occupational Therapy Assistant Program (1)
Atlantic Community College
Allied Health Division
Mays Landings, New Jersey 08330

NEW YORK

Occupational Therapy Assistant Program (1)
Maria College
700 New Scotland Avenue
Albany, New York 12208

Occupational Therapy Assistant Program (1)
Erie Community College
Main Street and Youngs Road
Buffalo, New York 14221

Occupational Therapy Assistant Program (1)
Herkimer County Community College
Herkimer, New York 13350

Occupational Therapy Assistant Program (1)
LaGuardia Community College
31-10 Thomson Avenue
Long Island City, New York 11101

Occupational Therapy Assistant Program (1)
Orange County Community College
115 South Street
Middletown, New York 10940

Occupational Therapy Assistant Program (1)
Rockland Community College
145 College Road
Suffern, New York 10901

Occupational Therapy Assistant Program (1)
Maria Regina College
1024 Court Street
Syracuse, New York 13208

NORTH CAROLINA

Occupational Therapy Assistant Program (1)
Stanly Technical College
Route 4, Box 55
Albermarle, North Carolina 28001

Occupational Therapy Assistant Program (1)
Caldwell Community College and Technical Institute
1000 Hickory Boulevard
Hudson, North Carolina 28638

NORTH DAKOTA

Occupational Therapy Assistant Program (1)
North Dakota State School of Science
Wahpeton, North Dakota 58075

OHIO

Occupational Therapy Assistant Program (1)
Stark Technical College
6200 Frank Avenue, NW
Canton, Ohio 44720

Occupational Therapy Assistant Program (2)
Columbia Public Schools
North Adult Education Center
100 Arcadia Avenue
Columbus, Ohio 43202

Occupational Therapy Assistant Program (1)
Cuyahoga Community College
2900 Community College Ave.
Cleveland, Ohio 44115

Occupational Therapy Assistant Program (1)
Shawnee State Community College
940 Second Street
Portsmouth, Ohio 46552

Occupational Therapy Assistant Program (1)
Lourdes College
6832 Convent Boulevard
Sylvania, Ohio 43560

OKLAHOMA

Occupational Therapy Assistant Program (1)
Oklahoma City Community College
7777 South May Avenue
Oklahoma City, Oklahoma 73159

OREGON

Occupational Therapy Assistant Program (1)
Mount Hood Community College
26000 SE Stark Street
Gresham, Oregon 97030

PENNSYLVANIA

Occupational Therapy Assistant Program (1)
Harcum Junior College
Bryn Mawr, Pennsylvania 19010

Occupational Therapy Assistant Program (1)
Mount Aloysius Junior College
Cresson, Pennsylvania 16630

Occupational Therapy Assistant Program (1)
Community College of Alleghney County
Boyce Campus
595 Beatty Road
Monroeville, Pennsylvania 15146

Occupational Therapy Assistant Program (1)
Lehigh County Community College
2370 Main Street
Schnecksville, Pennsylvania 18078

PUERTO RICO

Occupational Therapy Assistant Program (1)
Humacao University College
CUH Postal Station
Humacao, Puerto Rico 00661

Occupational Therapy Assistant Program (1)
Ponce Technological University College
University of Puerto Rico
P.O. Box 7186
Ponce, Puerto Rico 00732

TENNESSEE

Occupational Therapy Assistant Program (1)
Nashville State Technical Institute
120 White Bridge Road
Nashville, Tennessee 37209

TEXAS

Occupational Therapy Assistant Program (1)
Austin Community College
Health Sciences Center
Brackenridge Campus
707 E. 14th Street
Austin, Texas 78701

Occupational Therapy Assistant Program (2)
Academy of Health Sciences, U.S. Army
Medicine & Surgery Division
Fort Sam Houston, Texas 78234

Occupational Therapy Assistant Program (2)
Houston Community College
3100 Shenandoah
Houston, Texas 77021

Occupational Therapy Assistant Program (1)
St. Phillip's College
2111 Nevada Street
San Antonio, Texas 78203

WASHINGTON

Occupational Therapy Assistant Program (1)
Green River Community College
12401 S.E. 320th Street
Auburn, Washington 98002

Occupational Therapy Assistant Program (1,3)
Yakima Valley Community College
16th Avenue and Nob Hill Blvd.
P.O. Box 1647
Yakima, Washington 98907

WISCONSIN

Occupational Therapy Assistant Program (1)
Fox Valley Technical Institute
1825 North Bluemound Drive
P.O. Box 2277
Appleton, Wisconsin 54913

Occupational Therapy Assistant Program (1)
Madison Area Technical College
211 North Carroll Street
Madison, Wisconsin 53703

Occupational Therapy Assistant Program (1)
Milwaukee Area Technical College
1015 North 6th Street
Milwaukee, Wisconsin 53203

Occupational Therapy Aide

The *occupational therapy aide* performs mostly routine work, ordering supplies, maintaining the work area, preparing work materials, transporting patients, and maintaining the tools and equipment used the therapy. The occupational therapy aide generally has no direct patient care responsibilities.

Occupational therapy aides are employed mainly in hospitals, but they may also work in other healthcare facilities where occupational therapy is conducted.

Training to become an occupational therapy aide is done on-the-job in hospitals and other healthcare facilities. The length and content of training programs depends upon the duties for which the aide will be responsible. Persons interested in becoming occupational therapy aides should contact the Chief Occupational Therapist or the Personnel Director of their local hospital.

SOURCE:

Dictionary of Occupational Titles

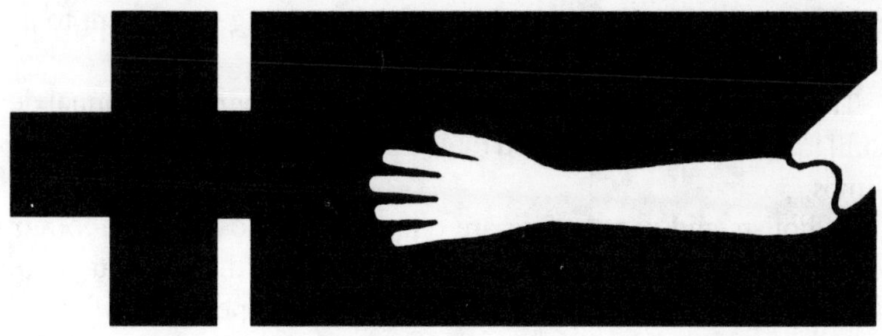

ORTHOTIC AND PROSTHETIC TECHNOLOGY

Orthotics and prosthetics are allied health professions concerned with the making and fitting of orthopedic braces and other supportive appliances (orthoses) and of artificial limbs (prostheses). The orthotist and prosthetist are members of a healthcare rehabilitation team, which may incorporate skills of a physician, surgeon, physical and occupational therapist and social worker. An individual can be trained as either an orthotist, prosthetist or both. Summarized below are two career classifications in each profession: *orthotist* and *prosthetist* and *orthotic technician* and *prosthetic technician.*

Orthotist And Prosthetist

The *orthotist/prosthetist* designs, fabricates, fits, and repairs orthoses and prostheses. These appliances are designed to support or replace a patient's limbs or other bodily features that have been disable or lost through injury, abnormality, or disease.

Following the physician's prescription the orthotist/prosthetist selects an appliance, taking into consideration function, efficiency, and comfort as well as cosmetic appearance. In deciding upon the correct prescription for a specific patient, the physician will often consult with the orthotist/prosthetist on the design and material of the orthoses/prostheses. After the appliance has been made and approved by the physician, the orthotist/prosthetist is responsible for evaluating its performance and also for initially assisting the physical therapist and/or occupational therapist in training the patient to use and care for the new orthoses/prostheses.

The orthotist/prosthetist must possess a high degree of manual dexterity and mechanical skill to operate the specialized tools that are used in the manufacture of braces and artificial limbs.

Orthotists and prosthetists are employed in hospitals, laboratories, and rehabilitation centers. Responsibilities of the orthotist/prosthetist may vary depending upon the size of the healthcare facility. In a small office or department, the orthotist/prosthetist may design, fabricate, and fit the appliance. In a larger facility, the orthotist/prosthetist may only be responsible for designing, measuring and fitting the appliance and hire technicians to fabricate the orthoses or prostheses.

A practitioner of orthotics/prosthetics can become certified by the American Board for Certification in Orthotics and Prosthetics as either a certified orthotist (CO), a certified prosthetist (CP), or a certified prosthetist-orthotist (CPO).

There are several options available concerning the amount of training and work experience required to take the American Board for Certification in Orthotics and Prosthetics certification exam. At present, applicants for certification must have either (1) a bachelor's degree in orthotics/prosthetics from an accredited program, plus one year's work experience, or (2) a bachelor's degree in any field plus a certificate obtained by successfully completing an accredited long term certificate program and one year's work experience in the selected discipline (orthotics or prosthetics), or (3) an associate degree in any field, a certificate obtained by successfully completing an accredited long term certificate program, plus four years of orthotic and/or prosthetic experience. At least one year of the experience must be obtained after completing the certificate program.

Annual salaries for certified orthotists/prosthetists depend upon responsibility and size of the healthcare facility but range from between $15,000 to $19,000 for starting positions. Some orthotists/prosthetists can earn salaries in the high 20's with several years experience.

Below is a list of orthotic and prosthetic educational programs accredited or pending accreditation by the American Board for Certification in Orthotics and Prosthetics. For more information on training programs contact either the individual schools or the American Board for Certification in Orthotics and Prosthetics at 717 Pendleton Street, Alexandria, Virginia 22314.

KEY:

(1) Bachelor of science degree

(2) Long term certificate program

SOURCES:

American Board for Certification in Orthotics and Prosthetics
Occupational Outlook Handbook
Occupation Outlook Quarterly

Orthotist And Prosthetist Programs

CALIFORNIA

Orthotic/Prosthetic Program (1)
California State University
Dominquez Hills
Carson, California 90747

Orthotic Department (2)
Rancho Los Amigos Hospital
7450 Leeds Street
Downey, California 90242

Department of Prosthetics (2)
University of California at Los Angeles
1000 Veteran Avenue
Los Angeles, California 90024

FLORIDA

Orthotic/Prosthetic Program (2)
Prosthetic Program (2)
Florida International University
Tamiami Campus
Miami, Florida 33199
(provisional accreditation)

ILLINOIS

Prosthetic Orthotic Center (2)
Northwestern University Medical School
345 East Superior Street
Chicago, Illinois 60611

NEW YORK

Department of Prosthetics and Orthotics (1,2)
New York University Medical School
317 East 34th Street
New York, New York 10016

MINNESOTA

Orthotic/Prosthetic Program (2)
Prosthetic Program (2)
Northeast Metro Technical Institute
3300 Century Avenue North
White Bear Lake, Minnesota 55110

TENNESSEE

Orthotic/Prosthetic Program (2)
Shelby State Community College
P.O. Box 4568
Memphis, Tennessee 38104

TEXAS

Prosthetics and Orthotics Department (1)
University of Texas
School of Allied Health Sciences
5323 Harry Hines Boulevard
Dallas, Texas 75235

WASHINGTON

Division of Prosthetics and Orthotics (1)
University of Washington School of Medicine
Seattle, Washington 98195

WISCONSIN

Orthotic/Prosthetic Program (2)
Northeast Wisconsin Technical Institute
Service Trade Division
2740 West Mason Street
Green Bay, Wisconsin 54303

Orthotic and Prosthetic Technician

Supervised by the orthotist/prosthetist, the *orthotic/prosthetic technician* aids in the fabricating, maintenance and repair of orthoses and prostheses. The orthotic/prosthetic technician is employed in the same locations as the orthotist/prosthetist, and must similarly possess the mechanical skills needed to use specialized device-making tools.

Registration as an *orthotic technician,* a *prosthetic technician,* or an *orthotic/prosthetic technician* requires that the candidate possess at least a high school degree or equivalent; have completed an accredited training program, or applicable experience; and have successfully passed the technician examination.

Salaries for orthotic/prosthetic technicians are just below the salary levels of orthotic/prosthetic practitioners.

For further information on the technician examination, training facilities and career opportunities contact the American Board for Certification in Orthotics and Prosthetics, Inc., 717 Pendleton Street, Alexandria, Virginia 22314.

SOURCES:

American Board for Certification in Orthotics and Prosthetics, Inc.

Orthotic and Prosthetic Technician Programs

PENNSYLVANIA

Orthotic/Prosthetic Technician Program
Harmerville Rehabilitation Center, Inc.
P.O. Box 11460
Guys Run Road
Pittsburg, Pennsylvania 15238

WASHINGTON

Orthotic/Prosthetic Technician Program
Spokane Falls Community College
W3140 Fort George Wright Drive
Spokane, Washington 99204-5288

WISCONSIN

Orthotic/Prosthetic Technician Program
Northeast Wisconsin Technical Institute
2740 West Mason Street
Green Bay, Wisconsin 54303

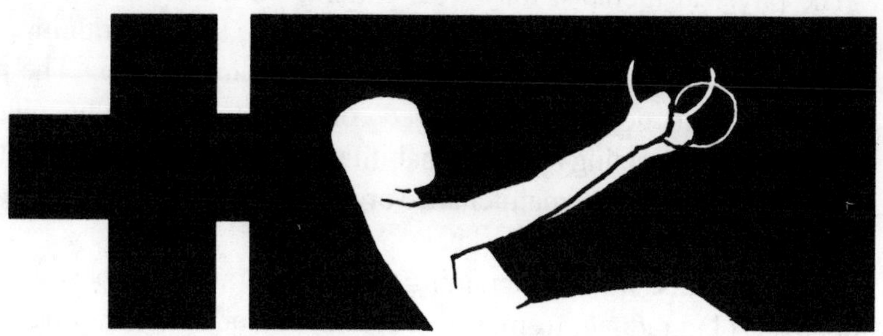

PHYSICAL THERAPY

Physical therapy is the allied health profession concerned with the rehabilitation of individuals who have been physically disabled by disease or accident, or who are born with a physical handicap. By attempting to restore function and prevent further disability, physical therapy assists patients in reaching their maximum performance in learning to live a normal life within the limits of their capabilities. There are two levels of physical therapy practitioners: the professionally qualified *physical therapist* and the *physical therapist assistant.* Both require graduation from an accredited training program, with on-the-job-training offered by some hospitals for the non-professional position of *physical therapy aide* (listed at the end of this chapter).

Physical Therapist

Upon referral by a physician, the *physical therapist* evaluates the extent of the patient's disability in such areas as neuromuscular, musculoskeletal, sensorimotor, cardiovascular, and respiratory functions. The physical therapist then plans, implements and evaluates an appropriate treatment program that may include one or more of the following: exercises for increasing muscle strength, endurance and coordination; electrical stimulation to activate paralyzed muscles; instruction in the use of assistive devices; and the application of massage, heat, cold, sound, water, ultrasound, or electricity; all of which are designed to relieve pain or to change the patient's physiological condition. The physical therapist must also be supportive and sensitive to a patient's emotional as well as physical well-being.

The physical therapist may treat patients with a wide variety of disabilities, or may specialize in geriatrics, pediatrics, orthopedics, athletic training, (refer to chapter titled Athletic Training), neurology or cardiopulmonary disease. The physical therapist most often works in general, specialized, or long-term care hospitals, but may also find employment in nursing homes, rehabilitation or research centers, schools for handicapped children, clinics, health maintenance organizations, home-health agencies, school systems, and private practice.

There are three ways of obtaining the proper training to become a professional physical therapist: (1) graduate from a four year bachelor's degree program; (2) graduate from a twelve to twenty-four month certificate program after completion of a bachelor's degree in a field related to physical therapy, or (3) obtain a master's degree in physical therapy after completion of a bachelor's degree in a related field. All three professional programs provide clinical experience and education in the direct care of patients in a healthcare facility.

Recommended high school subjects include mathematics, health, biology, chemistry, physics and social sciences. Admission into physical therapy programs is competitive, and applicants should have good grades in the above courses.

Licensure or registration is required in all fifty states, the District of Columbia, and Puerto Rico, and can be attained by graduating from an accredited physical therapy program and passing an examination in the state in which the physical therapist wishes to practice. Contact the state licensing board (located in the state capitol) for more information on licensing requirements.

The following list of sources of financial aid is supplied by the American Physical Therapy Association and is restricted to students enrolled in physical therapy education programs. Contact the source directly on other application restrictions.

Sources of Financial Aid Physical Therapy Education

COLORADO

Dorothy Hoag Student Aid Fund
P.O. Box 6380
Cherry Creek Station
Denver, Colorado 80206

GEORGIA

Georgia Chapter Arthritis Foundation
1038 W. Peachtree St. N.W.
Atlanta, Georgia 30309

KENTUCKY

Scholarship Governing Committee
Kentucky Chapter-APTA
Physical Therapy Dept. Children's Hospital
226 Chestnut Street
Louisville, Kentucky 40404

MARYLAND

Student Loan Fund.
Maryland Chapter-APTA
University of Maryland School of Physical Therapy
32 South Green Street
Baltimore, Maryland 21201

MINNESOTA

Minnesota Chapter-APTA.
Scholarship Committee
860 Mayo
University of Minnesota
Minneapolis, Minnesota 55455

NEW HAMPSHIRE

New Hampshire Chapter-APTA.
Catholic Medical Center
100 McGregor Street
Manchester, New Hampshire 03102

NORTH CAROLINA

North Carolina Physical Therapy Association, Inc.
P.O. Box 10387
Raleigh, North Carolina 27605

OREGON

Oregon Physical Therapy Association.
P.O. Box 12945
Salem, Oregon 97309

WISCONSIN

Wisconsin Chapter-APTA
Revolving Loan Fund
Director Student Financial Aid
University of Wisconsin
Madison, Wisconsin 53706

Phi Theta Loan Fund at Briggs Memorial
Loan Fund
Director, Student Financial Aids
University of Wisconsin
Madison, Wisconsin 53706

According to the American Physical Therapy Association, annual salaries of recent graduates of accredited bachelor or certificate programs range between $20,000. and $25,000. Salaries may vary because of geographic location, level of experience and type of facility.

Outlook for physical therapy employment is good. The U. S. Department of Labor has projected more than a 50% increase in jobs to be filled by the 1990's. For more information on physical therapy careers or certification requirements, write to the American Physical Therapy Association, 1111 North Fairfax Street, Alexandria, Virginia 22314.

Below is a list of college and university physical therapy programs accredited by the American Physical Therapy Association.

KEY:

(1) Bachelor's degree program.

(2) Certificate program.

(3) Bachelor's degree available from affiliating college or university.

(4) Master's degree program (bachelor's degree with science course emphasis required - does not require prerequisite in physical therapy).

(5) Accepts women students only

SOURCES:

American Physical Therapy Association
Occupational Outlook Handbook

Physical Therapist Programs

ALABAMA

Division of Physical Therapy (4)
University of Alabama at Birmingham
Birmingham, Alabama 35294

Department of Physical Therapy (1)
University of South Alabama
Mobile, Alabama 36688

ARIZONA

Dept. of Physical Therapy (1)
Northern Arizona University
C.U. Box 15105
Flagstaff, Arizona 86011

ARKANSAS

Dept. of Physical Therapy (1)
University of Central Arkansas
1211 Wolfe Street, Suite 235
Little Rock, Arkansas 72202

CALIFORNIA

Department of Physical Therapy (4)
University of Southern California
Rancho Los Amigos Center
12933 Erickson Ave.
Downey, California 90242

Physical Therapy Program (1)
California State University at Fresno
Fresno, California 93740

Department of Physical Therapy (1)
Loma Linda University
School of Allied Health Professions
Loma Linda, California 92350

Physical Therapy Dept. (1)
California State University at Long Beach
School of Allied Arts and Sciences
1250 Bellflower Boulevard
Long Beach, California 90840

School of Physical Therapy (4)
Children's Hospital of Los Angeles
Box 54700
Los Angeles, California 90027

Department of Physical Therapy (1,5)
Mount Saint Mary's College
12001 Chalon Road
Los Angeles, California 90049

Physical Therapy Program (1)
California State University at Northridge
Health Science Department, ENG 220
18111 Nordhoff Street
Northridge, California 91330

Curriculum in Physical Therapy (1,2)
University of California
School of Medicine, Room U-512
San Francisco, California 94143

COLORADO

Curriculum in Physical Therapy (1)
University of Colorado
Health Science Center
4200 E. Ninth Avenue, Box C244
Denver, Colorado 80262

CONNECTICUT

Dept. of Physical Therapy (1)
Quinnipiac College
School of Allied Health & Natural Sciences
Hamden, Connecticut 06518

Program in Physical Therapy (1)
University of Connecticut
School of Allied Health Professions
U 101
Storrs, Connecticut 06268

DELAWARE

Physical Therapy Program (1)
University of Delaware
School of Life and Health Sciences
049 McKinly Laboratory
Newark, Delaware 19716

DISTRICT OF COLUMBIA

Department of Physical Therapy (1)
Howard University
College of Allied Health Sciences
6th & Bryant Streets, N.W.
Washington, DC 20059

FLORIDA

Programs in Physical Therapy (1,4)
University of Miami
5801 Red Road
Coral Gables, Florida 33143

Department of Physical Therapy (1)
University of Florida
College of Health Related Professions
POB J-154, JHMHC
Gainesville, Florida 32610

Department of Physical Therapy (1)
Florida International University
School of Health Sciences
Miami, Florida 33199

Division of Physical Therapy (1)
Florida A&M University
Tallahassee, Florida 32307

GEORGIA

Division of Physical Therapy (4)
Emory University
1441 Clifton Road, S.E.
Atlanta, Georgia 30322

Department of Physical Therapy (1)
Georgia State University
University Plaza
Atlanta, Georgia 30303

Department of Physical Therapy (1)
Medical College of Georgia
Augusta, Georgia 30912

ILLINOIS

Programs in Physical Therapy (1)
Northwestern University
Medical School
345 East Superior Street
Chicago, Illinois 60611

Department of Physical Therapy (1)
University of Illinois at Chicago
College of Associated Health Professions
1919 W. Taylor
Chicago, Illinois 60612

Physical Therapy Program (1)
Northern Illinois University
School of Allied Health Professions
DeKalb, Illinois 60115

Physical Therapy Program (1)
School of Related Health Sciences
University of Health Sciences Chicago Medical School
3333 Green Bay Road North
North Chicago, Illinois 60064

INDIANA

Physical Therapy Program (1)
University of Evansville
1800 Lincoln Avenue
Evansville, Indiana 47722

Physical Therapy Program (1)
Indiana University
Division of Allied Health Sciences
School of Medicine
1140 West Michigan Street, CF326
Indianapolis, Indiana 46223

Physical Therapy Program (4)
University of Indianapolis
1400 East Hanna Avenue
Indianapolis, Indiana 46227

IOWA

Physical Therapy Education (4)
University of Iowa
2600 Steindler Building
Iowa City, Iowa 52242

KANSAS

Dept. of Physical Therapy Education (1)
University of Kansas Medical Center
School of Allied Health
College of Health Sciences and Hospital
503-HINCH
Kansas City, Kansas 66103

Department of Physical Therapy (1)
Wichita State University
College of Health Related Professions
Box 43
Wichita, Kansas 67208

KENTUCKY

Physical Therapy Department (1)
University of Kentucky Medical Center
HP 500
Lexington, Kentucky 40536-0084

Physical Therapy Program (1)
University of Louisville
Division of Allied Health Science
Carmichael Bldg.
525 E. Madison St.
Louisville, Kentucky 40292

LOUISIANA

Department of Physical Therapy (1)
Louisiana State University Medical Center
School of Allied Health Professions
P.O. Box 33932
Shreveport, Louisiana 71130-3932

MAINE

Department of Physical Therapy (1)
University of New England
11 Hills Beach Road
Biddeford, Maine 04005

MARYLAND

Department of Physical Therapy (1)
University of Maryland
School of Medicine
32 South Greene Street
Baltimore, Maryland 21201

Department of Physical Therapy (1)
University of Maryland Eastern Shore
P.O. Box 1061
Princess Anne, Maryland 21853

MASSACHUSETTS

Department of Physical Therapy (1,4)
Boston University
Sargent College of Allied Health Professions
One University Road
Boston, Massachusetts 02215

Department of Physical Therapy (1)
Northeastern University
308 Robinson Hall
360 Huntington Avenue,
Boston, Massachusetts 02115

Department of Physical Therapy (1,5)
Simmons College
300 The Fenway
Boston, Massachusetts 02115

Program in Physical Therapy (1)
University of Lowell
Weed Hall-South Campus
Lowell, Massachusetts 01854

MICHIGAN

Physical Therapy Program (1)
Grand Valley State College
School of Health Sciences
Allendale, Michigan 49401

Department of Physical Therapy (1)
Wayne State University
College of Pharmacy and Allied Health Professions
Detroit, Michigan 48202

University of Lowell
University of Michigan-Flint
School of Health Sciences
Flint, Michigan 48503-2186

Program in Physical Therapy (1)
Oakland University
School of Health Sciences
Rochester, Michigan 48063

MINNESOTA

Department of Physical Therapy(1)
College of St. Scholastica
1200 Kenwood Avenue
Duluth, Minnesota 55811

Department of Physical Therapy (1)
University of Minnesota
Box 388 UMHC
Minneapolis, Minnesota 55455

Department of Physical Therapy (2,3)
Mayo Foundation
108 Guggenheim Building
Rochester, Minnesota 55905

MISSISSIPPI

Department of Physical Therapy (1)
University of Mississippi Medical Center
School of Health Related Professions
2500 N State Street
Jackson, Mississippi 39216

MISSOURI

Department of Physical Therapy (1)
University of Missouri-Columbia
School of Health Related Professions
120 Lewis Hall
Columbia, Missouri 65211

Department of Physical Therapy (1)
Rockhurst College
5225 Troost Avenue
Kansas City, Missouri 64110

Department of Physical Therapy (1)
Maryville College
13550 Conway Road
St. Louis, Missouri 63141

Department of Physical Therapy (1)
St Louis University Medical Center
1504 South Grand Boulevard
St Louis, Missouri 63104

Department of Physical Therapy (1)
Washington University
School of Medicine
660 South Euclid Avenue
Box 8083
St. Louis, Missouri 63110

MONTANA

Department of Physical Therapy (1)
University of Montana
Missoula, Montana 59812

NEBRASKA

Department of Physical Therapy (1)
University of Nebraska Medical Center
College of Medicine
42nd and Dewey Avenue
Omaha, Nebraska 68105

NEW JERSEY

Department of Physical Therapy (1,2)
Kean College of New Jersey
University of Medicine and Dentistry
of New Jersey
School of Allied Health Related Professions
Martlind Building
100 Bergen Street
Newark, New Jersey 07103

NEW MEXICO

Department of Physical Therapy (1)
University of New Mexico
School of Medicine
Albuquerque, New Mexico 87131

NEW YORK

Department of Physical Therapy (1)
Daemen College
4380 Main Street
Amherst, New York 14226

Department of Physical Therapy (4)
Long Island University
University Plaza
Brooklyn, New York 11201

Department of Physical Therapy
State University of New York
Health Science Center at Brooklyn
Box 16,
450 Clarkson Avenue
Brooklyn, New York 11203

Department of Physical Therapy
State University of New York at Buffalo
416 Kimball Tower-Main Street Campus
Buffalo, New York 14214

Department of Physical Therapy (1)
Ithaca College
Ithaca, New York 14850

Department of Physical Therapy (4)
Columbia University
College of Physicians and Surgeons
630 W 168th Street
New York, New York 10032

Department of Physical Therapy (1,2)
Hunter College
School of Health Sciences
425 East 25th Street
New York, New York 10010

Department of Physical Therapy (1)
New York University
433 First Avenue
New York, New York 10010

Department of Physical Therapy
State University of New York at Stony Brook
School of Allied Health Professions
Health Sciences Center
Stony Brook, New York 11794

Department of Physical Therapy
State University of New York
Health Science Center at Syracuse
College of Health Related Professions
708 Irving Avenue
Syracuse, New York 13210

Department of Physical Therapy (1,5)
Russell Sage College
Troy, New York 12180

NORTH CAROLINA

Department of Physical Therapy (1)
University of North Carolina at Chapel Hill
Medical School Wing E
Chapel Hill, North Carolina 27514

Department of Physical Therapy (4)
Duke University Medical Center
Medical Center
POB #3965
Durham, North Carolina 27710

Department of Physical Therapy (1)
East Carolina University
School of Allied Health and Social Professions
Greenville, North Carolina 27834

NORTH DAKOTA

Department of Physical Therapy (1)
University of North Dakota
School of Medicine
Grand Forks, North Dakota 58201

OHIO

Department of Physical Therapy (1)
Ohio University
Convocation Center
Athens, Ohio 45701

Department of Physical Therapy (1)
Cleveland State University
Department of Health Sciences
1983 East 24th Street
Fenn Tower 607
Cleveland, Ohio 44115

Department of Physical Therapy (1)
Ohio State University
306 Allied Medical Professions
1583 Perry Street
Columbus, Ohio 43210

Department of Physical Therapy (1)
Medical College of Ohio In Consortium with
Bowling Green State University and
University of Toledo (1)
Hospital Support Building
C.S. #10008
Toledo, Ohio 43699

OKLAHOMA

Department of Physical Therapy (1)
University of Oklahoma
College of Allied Health
Health Sciences Center
P.O. Box 26901
Oklahoma City, Oklahoma 73190

OREGON

Department of Physical Therapy (1)
Pacific University
2043 College Way
Forest Grove, Oregon 97116

PENNSYLVANIA

Department of Physical Therapy (1,4)
Beaver College
Glenside, Pennsylvania 19038

Department of Physical Therapy (1,4)
Hahnemann University
School of Allied Health Professions
201 N 15th Street
Philadelphia, Pennsylvania 19104

Department of Physical Therapy (4)
Philadelphia College of Pharmacy and Science
43rd Street and Kingsessing Mall
Philadelphia, Pennsylvania 19104

Department of Physical Therapy (1)
Temple University
College of ALlied Health Professions
3307 North Broad Street
Philadelphia, Pennsylvania 19140

Department of Physical Therapy (1)
Thomas Jefferson University
103 S 9th Street
Philadelphia, Pennsylvania 19107

Department of Physical Therapy (1)
University of Pittsburgh
101 Pennsylvania Hall
Pittsburgh, Pennsylvania 15261

Department of Physical Therapy (1)
University of Scranton
5 Jefferson Hall
Scranton, Pennsylvania 18510

PUERTO RICO

Department of Physical Therapy (1)
University of Puerto RIco
College of Health Related Professions
Medical Science Campus
GPO Box 5067
San Juan, Puerto Rico 00936

SOUTH CAROLINA

Department of Physical Therapy (1)
Medical University of South Carolina
171 Ashley Avenue
Charleston, South Carolina 29425

TENNESSEE

Department of Physical Therapy (1)
University of Tennessee
Department of Rehabilitation Sciences
800 Madison Avenue
Memphis, Tennessee 38163

TEXAS

Department of Physical Therapy (1)
University of Texas
Health Science Center at Dallas
School of Allied Health Sciences
5323 Harry Hines Blvd
Dallas, Texas 75235

Department of Physical Therapy (1,4)
Texas Women's University
School of Physical Therapy
Box 22487, TWU Station
Denton, Texas 76204

Department of Physical Therapy (4)
U.S. Army Medical Dept-Baylor University
Academy of Health Sciences
Fort Sam Houston, Texas 78234

Department of Physical Therapy (1)
University of Texas Medical Branch at Galveston
School of Allied Health Sciences
Galveston, Texas 77550

Department of Physical Therapy (1)
Texas Tech University Health Sciences Center
School of Allied Health
Lubbock, Texas 79430

Department of Physical Therapy (1)
Southwest Texas State University
Health Science Center
San Marcos, Texas 78666

UTAH

Department of Physical Therapy (1)
University of Utah
Annex Wing B
Salt Lake City, Utah 84112

VERMONT

Department of Physical Therapy (1)
University of Vermont
School of Allied Health Sciences
Rowell 305
Burlington, Vermont 05401

VIRGINIA

Department of Physical Therapy (1)
Old Dominion University
Department of Community Health Professions
Education Building
Norfolk, Virginia 23508-8544

Department of Physical Therapy (1)
Virginia Commonwealth University
Medical College of Virginia
Box 224
Richmond, Virginia 23298

WASHINGTON

Department of Physical Therapy (1)
University of Washington
Seattle, Washington 98195

Department of Physical Therapy (1)
University of Puget Sound
1500 N Warner
Tacoma, Washington 98416

WEST VIRGINIA

Department of Physical Therapy (1)
West Virginia University Medical Center
School of Medicine Medical Center
PO Box 6302
Morgantown, West Virginia 26505-6302

WISCONSIN

Department of Physical Therapy (1)
University of Wisconsin at LaCrosse
243 Cowley Hall
LaCrosse, Wisconsin 54601

Department of Physical Therapy (1)
University of Wisconsin-Madison
Medical Science Center
1300 University Avenue
Madison, Wisconsin 53706

Department of Physical Therapy (1)
Marquette University
Walter Schroeder Complex
Milwaukee, Wisconsin 53233

CANADA

Department of Physical Therapy (1)
McGill University
3654 Drummond Street
Montreal, Quebec H3G1Y5

Physical Therapist Assistant

The *physical therapist assistant* works under the supervision of a professional physical therapist in the rehabilitation of disabled persons. The assistant helps with complicated therapeutic procedures but may perform routine procedures independently. She or her helps test and evaluate patients' disabilities, applies stimulants, assists patients in performing exercises, trains patients to adapt to splints, braces, and artificial limbs, and observes and reports to the supervising physical therapist, the patient's response.

Most physical therapist assistants work in general and specialized hospitals, while others work in the same range of healthcare facilities as the professional physical therapist, including clinics, health maintenance organizations, nursing homes, rehabilitation centers, schools for handicapped children, and private practices.

The educational requirement to become a physical therapist assistant is the completion of a two year associate degree program at an accredited community or junior college, university, vocational-technical school, or Armed Forces sponsored college program. Some states require physical therapist assistants to be licensed; that is, they must have graduated from an accredited associate degree program and passed a certification examination. Contact the state's licensing board (located in the state capitol) for more information on licensing requirements.

Recommended high school subjects include health, mathematics, and the biological, physical and social sciences.

Recent starting salaries for physical therapist assistants range from $16,000 to $18,000, depending upon location and experience.

Below is a list of educational programs that have received accreditation from the American Physical Therapy Association.

For more information on a career as a physical therapist assistant, write to the American Physical Therapy Association, 1111 North Fairfax Street, Alexandria, Virginia 22314.

SOURCES:

American Physical Therapy Association
Occupational Outlook Handbook

Physical Therapist Assistant Programs

ALABAMA

Physical Therapist Assistant Program
University of Alabama at Birmingham
RTI Building
University Station, Alabama 35294

ARKANSAS

Physical Therapist Assistant Program
University of Central Arkansas
Education Building
12th & Marshall Streets
Little Rock, Arkansas 72201

CALIFORNIA

Physical Therapist Assistant Program
DeAnza Community College
21250 Stevens Creek Blvd.
Cupertino, California 95014

Physical Therapist Assistant Program
Mount St. Mary's College
12001 Chalon Road
Los Angeles, California 90049

Physical Therapist Assistant Program
Cerritos College
Health Occupations Division
11110E Allondra Boulevard
Norwalk, California 90650

Physical Therapist Assistant Program
Los Angeles Pierce College
6201 Winnetka Avenue
Woodland Hills, California 91371

Physical Therapist Assistant Program
San Diego Mesa College
7250 Mesa College Drive
San Diego, California 92111

FLORIDA

Physical Therapist Assistant Program
Broward Community College
Allied Health Center Campus
3501 S.W. Davie Road
Ft. Lauderdale, Florida 33314

Physical Therapist Assistant Program
Miami-Dade Community College
Medical Center Campus
950 N.W. 20th Street
Miami, Florida 33127

Physical Therapist Assistant Program
St. Petersburg Junior College
P.O. Box 13489
St. Petersburg, Florida 33733

GEORGIA

Physical Therapist Assistant Program
Medical College of Georgia
School of Allied Health Sciences
Dept. of Physical Therapy
Augusta, Georgia 30912

ILLINOIS

Physical Therapist Assistant Program
Belleville Area College
2500 Carlyle Road
Belleville, Illinois 62221

Physical Therapist Assistant Program
Southern Illinois University
Clinical Center
Wham 141
Carbondale, Illinois 62901

Physical Therapist Assistant Program
Morton College
3801 South Central Avenue
Cicero, Illinois 60650

Physical Therapist Assistant Program
Oakton Community College
1600 E. Golf Road
Attn: Division of Science Allied Health
Des Plaines, Illinois 60016

Physical Therapist Assistant Program
Illinois Central College
East Peoria, Illinois 61635

INDIANA

Physical Therapist Assistant Program
University of Evansville
P.O. Box 329
Evansville, Indiana 47722

Physical Therapist Assistant Program
Vincennes University
Health Occupations Dept.
Vincennes, Indiana 47591

KANSAS

Physical Therapist Assistant Program
Colby Community College
1255 South Range
Colby, Kansas 67701

Physical Therapist Assistant Program
Washburn University
School of Applied & Continuing Education
Topeka, Kansas 66621

KENTUCKY

Physical Therapist Assistant Program
Jefferson Community College
P.O. Box 1036
Louisville, Kentucky 40201

MARYLAND

Physical Therapist Assistant Program
Community College of Baltimore
2901 Liberty Heights Avenue
Baltimore, Maryland 21215

MASSACHUSETTS

Physical Therapist Assistant Program
North Shore Community College
3 Essex Street
Beverly, Massachusetts 01915

Department of Physical Therapy
Newbury College
129 Fisher Avenue
Brookline, Massachusetts 02146

Physical Therapist Assistant Program
Lasell Junior College
Newton, Massachusetts 02166

Physical Therapist Assistant Program
Springfield Technical Community College
Building 20, One Armory Square
Springfield, Massachusetts 01105

Physical Therapist Assistant Program
Becker Junior College
61 Sever Street
Worchester, Massachusetts 01609

MICHIGAN

Physical Therapist Assistant Program
Kellogg Community College
450 North Avenue
Battle Creek, Michigan 49016

Physical Therapist Assistant Program
Macomb Community College
44575 Garfield Road
Mount Clemens, Michigan 48044-3179

Physical Therapist Assistant Program
Delta College
F-56 Allied Health Building
University Center, Michigan 48710

MINNESOTA

Physical Therapist Assistant Program
St. Mary's Campus of the College of St. Catherine
2500 South Sixth Street
Minneapolis, Minnesota 55454

MISSOURI

Physical Therapist Assistant Program
Penn Valley Community College
3201 Southwest Trafficway
Kansas City, Missouri 64111

Physical Therapist Assistant Program
St. Louis Community College at Meramec
11333 Big Bend Blvd.
St. Louis, Missouri 63122

NEW HAMPSHIRE

Physical Therapist Assistant Program
New Hampshire Vocational-Technical College
Hanover Street Ext.
Claremont, New Hampshire 03743

NEW JERSEY

Physical Therapist Assistant Program
Union County College
1033 Springfield Avenue
Cranford, New Jersey 07016

Physical Therapist Assistant Program
Fairleigh-Dickinson University
285 Madison Avenue
Madison, New Jersey 07940

Physical Therapist Assistant Program
Atlantic Community College
Mays Landing, New Jersey 08330

Physical Therapist Assistant Program
Essex County College
303 University Avenue
Newark, New Jersey 07102

NEW YORK

Physical Therapist Assistant Program
Maria College
700 New Scotland
Albany, New York 12208-1798

Physical Therapist Assistant Program
Nassau Community College
Garden City, New York 11530

Physical Therapist Assistant Program
Orange County Community College
115 South Street
Middletown, New York 10940

Physical Therapist Assistant Program
Institute of Rehabilitation Medicine
New York University Medical Center
400 E. 34th Street
New York, New York 10016

Physical Therapist Assistant Program
Suffolk County Community College
Department of Health Careers
533 College Road
Selden, New York 11784

NORTH CAROLINA

Physical Therapist Assistant Program
Central Piedmont Community College
P.O. Box 35009
Charlotte, North Carolina 28235

Physical Therapist Assistant Program
Fayetteville Technical Institute
P.O. Box 35236
Fayetteville, North Carolina 28303

OHIO

Physical Therapist Assistant Program
Stark Technical College
Allied Health Technologies
6200 Frank Avenue, N.W.
Canton, Ohio 44720

Physical Therapist Assistant Program
University of Cincinnati
L101 University College
ML 168
Cincinnati, Ohio 45221-0168

Physical Therapist Assistant Program
Cuyahoga Community College
2900 Community College Avenue
Cleveland, Ohio 44115

Physical Therapist Assistant Program
Sinclair Community College
444 West Third Street
Dayton, Ohio 45402

OKLAHOMA

Physical Therapist Assistant Program
Oklahoma City Community College
7777 S. May Avenue
Oklahoma City, Oklahoma 73159

Physical Therapist Assistant Program
Tulsa Junior College
909 S. Boston Avenue
Tulsa, Oklahoma 74119

OREGON

Physical Therapist Assistant Program
Mount Hood Community College
26000 S.E. Stark
Gresham, Oregon 97030

PENNSYLVANIA

Physical Therapist Assistant Program
Harcum Junior College
Bryn Mawr, Pennsylvania 19010

Physical Therapist Assistant Program
Pennsylvania State University, Hazelton
Box 704 A
Hazelton, Pennsylvania 18201

Physical Therapist Assistant Program
Lehigh County Community College
2370 Main Street
Schnecksville, Pennsylvania 18078

PUERTO RICO

Physical Therapy Program
Humacao University College
CUH Station
Humacao, Puerto Rico 00661

Physical Therapist Assistant Program
Ponce Technical University College
The University of Puerto Rico
P.O. Box 7186
Ponce, Puerto Rico 00732

SOUTH CAROLINA

Physical Therapist Assistant Program
Greenville Technical College
Box 5616, Station B
Greenville, South Carolina 29606-5616

TENNESSEE

Physical Therapist Assistant Program
Chattanooga State Technical Community College
Division of Life & Health Sciences
4501 Amnicola Highway
Chattanooga, Tennessee 37406

Physical Therapist Assistant Program
Volunteer State Community College
P-205, Nashville Pike
Gallatin, Tennessee 37066

Physical Therapist Assistant Program
Shelby State Community College
Division of Allied Health
P.O. Box 40568
Memphis, Tennessee 40568

TEXAS

Physical Therapist Assistant Program
Amarillo College
P.O. Box 447
Amarillo, Texas 79178

Physical Therapist Assistant Program
Austin Community College
Riverside Campus
5712 East Riverside
Austin, Texas 78741

Physical Therapist Assistant Program
Houston Community College
3100 Shenandoah
Houston, Texas 77021

Physical Therapist Assistant Program
St. Philip's College
2111 Nevada Street
San Antonio, Texas 78203

Physical Therapist Assistant Program
Community College of the Air Force
Group Intermediate Supervisor 913XO Course
School of Health Care Sciences, MSDB
Sheppard Air Force Base, Texas 76311

Physical Therapist Assistant Program
Tarrant County Junior College
Northeast Campus
828 Harwood Road
Hurst, Texas 76054

VIRGINIA

Physical Therapist Assistant Program
Northern Virginia Community College
8333 Little River Turnpike
Annandale, Virginia 22003

Physical Therapist Assistant Program
Tidewater Community College
1700 College Crescent
Virginia Beach, Virginia 23456

WASHINGTON

Physical Therapist Assistant Program
Green River Community College
12401 S.E. 320th Street
Auburn, Washington 98002

WISCONSIN

Physical Therapist Assistant Program
Milwaukee Area Technical College
Health Occupations Division
1015 North 6th Street
Milwaukee, Wisconsin 53203

Physical Therapy Aide

The *physical therapy aide* is a non-licensed employee who works under the supervision of a professional physical therapist. The aide carries out designated routine tasks such as helping patients prepare for treatment, transporting patients to and from treatment area, maintaining, cleaning, and assembling devices and equipment used in treatment, and performing clerical duties. The physical therapy aide generally has no direct patient treatment responsibilities.

Usually a high school graduate or equivalent, the physical therapy aide must be at least eighteen years of age and have completed on-the-job training in a hospital or clinic facility. Length and content of training programs depend upon the duties the aide will be expected to perform. Employers usually prefer that potential aides have some previous hospital experience.

Individuals interested in become physical therapy aides should contact the Chief Physical Therapist or the Personnel Director of their local hospital or healthcare facility.

SOURCES:

American Physical Therapy Association
Occupational Outlook Handbook
Dictionary of Occupational Titles

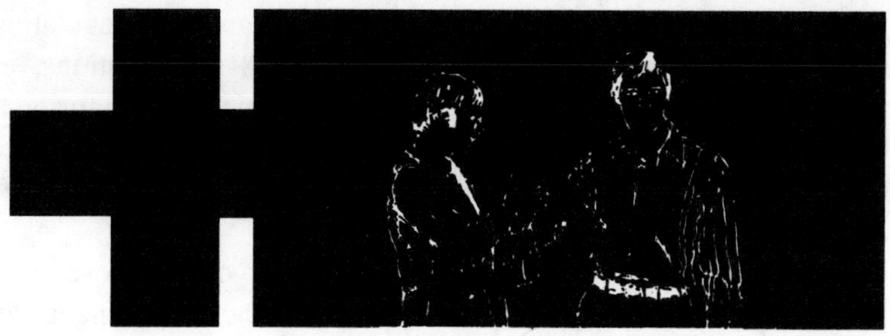

PHYSICIAN EXTENDER SERVICES

Physician extender services provide clinical support to physicians in a wide variety of healthcare settings. Physician extender personnel are trained to function as physician assistants, as surgeon's assistants, or with additional training and education as assistants for various medical specialties including orthopedics, urology, pediatrics and emergency medicine. Two of these careers, *physician assistant* and *surgeon's assistant* are discussed in this chapter. For further information on careers and training of specialized physician assistants, interested persons should contact the American Academy of Physician Assistants, 950 North Washington Street, Alexandria, Virginia 22314. The career of *Surgical Technologist* is listed at the end of this chapter.

Physician Assistant

The physician assistant, sometimes referred to as a *physician associate,* is a skilled health practitioner under the physician's supervision who is qualified by academic and clinical training to provide routine patient services traditionally performed by a licensed physician. By utilizing the skills of the physician assistant, the physician has more time to deal with patients with more complex problems.

The majority of physician assistants work with physicians in primary care specialties, such as family medicine, obstetrics, pediatrics, and general internal medicine. The primary care physician diagnoses and treats slowly progressive and chronic illnesses, provides preventive and emergency services, and offers personal and family counseling.

The wide range of routine medical procedures that the assistant performs depends upon the particular medical practice of the physician and state regulations but usually includes taking medical histories, performing physical examinations, assisting in laboratory procedures, administering injections and immunizations, suturing and caring for wounds, referring patients to other healthcare facilities, counseling patients, and performing emergency medical care. In some states, physician assistants are permitted to prescribe certain medications.

Physician assistants work mainly in physicians' offices, hospitals and clinics. A growing number of physician assistants are employed by health maintenance organizations, student health services, community health centers, and with the Armed Forces. Opportunities are also available in rural communities, nursing homes and correctional facilities.

Medical schools, universities, community colleges, hospitals, and vocational-technical schools offer training programs for the physician assistant. These programs award certificates, associate degrees, and/or bachelor's degrees and have a variety of entrance requirements. The typical program lasts 24 months, although some programs range from 12-24 months, depending upon the type of award offered.

The minimum educational requirement for physician assistant training programs is generally two years of college with course emphasis in the physical and biological sciences and at least one year of experience working in a health profession. This experience requirement usually includes "direct patient contact" experience such as employment as an orderly, nursing aide, emergency medical technician, clinical technician, registered nurse or military medical corpsman. Positions in these programs is competitive and a strong education and experience background is helpful. Training program requirements vary and it is recommended that interested persons contact the program directly and inquire about its particular entrance regulations and awards.

Certification as a "Physician Assistant - Certified" or "PA-C" is awarded by the National Committee on Certification of Physician's Assistants after graduating from an accredited physician assistant training program and successfully passing a national certifying examination. Many states require registration (certification) or licensure for employment and interested persons should inquire with their state's licensing division or board of medical examiners. For additional certification information, write to the National Committee on Certification of Physician's Assistants, 2845 Henderson Mill Road, N.E., Atlanta, Georgia 30341.

Salaries for physician assistants vary because of geographic location, years of experience, education and type of facility, however recent studies indicate that overall average starting annual salaries equalled approximately $24,000. Physician assistants with several years hospital experience may earn from $24,000 to $39,000.

Below is a list provided by the Association of Physician Assistant Programs of physician assistant programs accredited by the American Medical Association's Committee on Allied Health Education and Accreditation.

For further information on physician assistant careers, contact the American Academy of Physician Assistants, 950 North Washington Street, Alexandria, Virginia 22314. The Association of Physician Assistant Programs is located at the same address.

SOURCES:

American Academy of Physician Assistants
Association of Physician Assistant Programs
Occupational Outlook Handbook

Physician Assistant Programs

CALIFORNIA

MEDEX Physician Assistant Program
Charles R. Drew Postgraduate Medical School
1621 East 120th Street
Los Angeles, California 90059

Primary Care Physician Assistant Program
USC School of Medicine
1975 Zonal Avenue
Los Angeles, California 90033

Primary Care Physician Assistant Program
Stanford University Medical Center
703 Welch Road
Palo Alto, California 94304

Physician Assistant Program
Department of Family Practice
Sacramento Medical Center
2221 Stockton Blvd., Trailer 1532
Sacramento, California 95817

COLORADO

Child Health Associate Program
University of Colorado
Health Sciences Center
4200 East 9th Avenue
Denver, Colorado 80262

CONNECTICUT

Physician Associate Program
Yale University School of Medicine
382 Congress Avenue
P.O. Box 3333
New Haven, Connecticut 06510

DISTRICT OF COLUMBIA

Physician Assistant Program
George Washington University
School of Medicine and Health Sciences
2300 Eye Street, N.W.
Washington, DC 20037

Physician Assistant Program
Howard University
Sixth and Bryant Streets, N.W.
Washington, DC 20059

FLORIDA

Physician Assistant Program
College of Health Related Professions
Box J-176
University of Florida
Gainesville, Florida 32610

GEORGIA

Physician Associate Program
Emory University School of Medicine
Post Office Drawer XX
Atlanta, Georgia 30322

Physician Assistant Program
Medical College of Georgia
August, Georgia 30912

IOWA

Physician Assistant Program
College of Medicine
University of Iowa
Iowa City, Iowa 52242

Physician Assistant Program
University of Osteopathic Medicine and Health Sciences
3200 Grand Avenue
Des Moines, Iowa 50312

KANSAS

Physician Assistant Program
The Wichita State University
Wichita, Kansas 67208

KENTUCKY

Physician Assistant Program
Department of Physician Assistant Studies
Albert B. Chandler Medical Center
University of Kentucky
Lexington, Kentucky 40536-0080

MARYLAND

Physician Assistant Program
Essex Community College
Baltimore County, Maryland 21237

MASSACHUSETTS

Physician Assistant Program
Northeastern University
360 Huntington Avenue
Boston, Massachusetts 02115

MICHIGAN

Physician Assistant Program
Mercy College of Detroit
8200 West Outer Drive
Detroit, Michigan 48219

Physician Assistant Program
Western Michigan University
Kalamazoo, Michigan 49008

MISSOURI

Physician Assistant Program
Saint Louis University
School of Allied Health Professions
1504 South Grand Boulevard
St. Louis, Missouri 63104

NEBRASKA

Physician Assistant Program
University of Nebraska Medical Center
42nd Street and Dewey Avenue
Omaha, Nebraska 68105

NEW JERSEY

Physician Assistant Program
Rutgers Medical School
Box 101
Piscataway, New Jersey 08854

NEW YORK

Physician Assistant Program
Albany Medical College
47 New Scotland Avenue
Albany, New York 12208

Physician Assistant Program
The Brooklyn Hospital
121 DeKalb Avenue
Brooklyn, New York 11201

Physician Assistant Program
Touro College
30 West 44th Street
New York, New York 10036

Physician Assistant Program
CUNY Medical Center
Harlem Hospital Center
506 Lenox Avenue
New York, New York 10037

Physician Assistant Program
Bayley Seton Hospital
Staten Island, New York 10304

Physician Assistant Program
Department of Physician Assistant Education
School of Allied Health Professions
SUNY at Stony Brook
Stony Brook, New York 11794

NORTH CAROLINA

Physician Assistant Program
Duke University Medical Center
Durham, North Carolina 27710

Physician Assistant Program
The Bowman Gray School of Medicine
Wake Forest University
1990 Beach Street
Winston-Salem, North Carolina 27103

NORTH DAKOTA

Family Nurse Practitioner Program
University of North Dakota School of Medicine
Primary Care Training Center
221 South Fourth Street
Grand Forks, North Dakota 58201

OHIO

Physician Assistant Program
Kettering College of Medical Arts
3737 Southern Boulevard
Kettering, Ohio 45429

Physician Assistant Program
Cuyahoga Community College
Western Campus
11000 Pleasant Valley Road
Parma, Ohio 44130

OKLAHOMA

Physician Assistant Program
University of Oklahoma Health Sciences Center
P.O. Box 26901
Oklahoma City, Oklahoma 73190

PENNSYLVANIA

Physician Assistant Program
Gannon University
Erie, Pennsylvania 16541

Physician Assistant Program
Saint Francis College
Loretto, Pennsylvania 15940

Physician Assistant Program
School of Allied Health
Hahnemann University
Broad and Vine Streets
Philadelphia, Pennsylvania 19102

Physician Assistant Program
Department of Allied Health
King's College
133 North River Street
Wilkes-Barre, Pennsylvania 18711

TENNESSEE

Physician Assistant Program
Trevecca Nazarene College
333 Murfreesboro Road
Nashville, Tennessee 37203

TEXAS

Physician Assistant Program
University of Texas
Health Science Center
5323 Harry Hines Boulevard
Dallas, Texas 75235

Physician Assistant Program
Department of Physician Assistant Studies
School of Allied Health Sciences
The University of Texas Medical Branch
Galveston, Texas 77550

Physician Assistant Program
Texas Medical Center
Baylor College of Medicine
Houston, Texas 77030

Physician Assistant Program
Academy of Health Sciences
Fort Sam Houston, Texas 78234

UTAH

Physician Assistant Program
Utah MEDEX Project
University of Utah Medical Center
50 N. Medical Drive, Building 428
Salt Lake City, Utah 84132

WASHINGTON

Physician Assistant Program
MEDEX Northwest
301 Clifford Apts.
3731 University Way, N.E.
Seattle, Washington 98105

WEST VIRGINIA

Physician Assistant Program
Alderson-Broaddus College
Philippi, West Virginia 26416

WISCONSIN

Physician Assistant Program
University of Wisconsin-Madison
1300 University Avenue
Madison, Wisconsin 53706

Surgeon's Assistant

The *surgeon's assistant* is a specialized physician assistant who is qualified by academic and clinical training to provide patient services under the supervision and responsibility of a surgeon. Working in any medical setting for which the surgeon is responsible, the surgeon's assistant gathers diagnostic data for the surgeon and assists the surgeon in appropriate treatment. As such the assistant obtains medical histories, carries out physical examinations, and helps evaluate the effectiveness of the surgery during the postoperative period. The surgeon assistant may also accompany the surgeon during visits to the patients' rooms, record notes on their progress and compile data for case summaries.

Through preparation in surgeon's assistant training programs, the student gains experience in both general and specialty surgical services as well as in emergency room procedures. At present, there are three surgeon's assistant training programs, accredited by the Committee on Allied Health Education and Accreditation of the American Medical Association. These programs are generally two years in length and most often require either (1) two years of college with an emphasis in the sciences and/or (2) prior direct patient care experience in an allied health care position such as an orderly, nursing aide, emergency medical technician, registered nurse, clinical technician or military medical corpsman.

Most states require that surgeon's assistants be licensed, registered, or certified as a Physician Assistant - Certified (PA-C). Certification requirements included graduation from an approved surgeon's assistant program and successful completion of the national certification examination. Contact the state's licensing division or board of medical examiners for more specifics. The examination is administered by the National Committee on Certification of Physician's Assistants at 2845 Henderson Mill Road, N.E., Atlanta, Georgia 30341.

Salaries of surgeon's assistants are similar to those of physician assistants. Refer to the previous section titled Physician Assistant for salary information.

For more information on a career as a surgeon's assistant, contact the Surgical Council, American Association of Physician Assistants, 950 North Washington Street, Alexandira, Virginia 22314.

SOURCES:

American Academy of Physician Assistants
Association of Physician Assistant Programs

Surgeon's Assistant Programs

ALABAMA

Surgeon's Assistant Program
Department of Surgery, School of Medicine
University of Alabama at Birmingham
University Station
Birmingham, Alabama 35294

NEW YORK

Surgeon's Assistant Program
Cornell University Medical College
525 East 68th Street
New York, New York 10021

OHIO

Surgeon's Assistant Program
Cuyahoga Community College
Western Campus
11000 Pleasant Valley Road
Parma, Ohio 44130

Surgical Technologist

The surgical technologist, a member of the surgical healthcare team, provides technical support to surgeons, registered nurses, and anesthesiologists, in an operating room setting.

The *surgical technologist*, also referred to as a *surgical technician* or *operating room technician*, is supervised by a registered nurse and performs tasks that are essential to the continuity of the surgical procedure.

In the operating room the technologist arranges supplies and instruments, keeping an accurate count of the latter at all times; helps the surgical team members scrub and dress for surgery; passes instruments and other sterile supplies to the surgeon during the operation; helps apply dressings; and helps prepare and preserve specimens taken for testing. The technologist if qualified, may also operate sterilizers, lights, suction machines, and diagnostic equipment and may become specialized in certain areas of operating room surgery. After the operation the technologist may transfer the patient and help restock the operating room and maintain its aseptic conditions. Under close supervision the technologist may also assist in patient care in the operating room and in the delivery room.

Surgical technologists work in hospitals and other institutions that have operating rooms, delivery rooms, and emergency room facilities.

Training programs are offered by community and junior colleges, vocational-technical schools, the Armed Forces, as well as some hospital based programs. The programs, include both classroom instruction and clinical training, generally last nine to twelve months, and award certificates. Some community college programs last two years and award associate degrees.

Certification by examination is voluntary and available from the Liaison Council on Certification, the certifying body of the Association of Surgical Technologists, Inc. The credentials of CST (Certified Surgical Technologist) is granted after graduating from an approved academic program and successfully passing a written examination. For further information on certification, contact the Liaison Council on Certification, Association of Surgical Technologists, Inc., 8307 Shaffer Parkway, Littleton, Colorado 80127.

For high school students interested in this career, recommended courses include health and biology. Since operating room procedures require precise work and may last several hours, the surgical technologist should have physical stamina, be able to work quickly and accurately under pressure and be detailed oriented.

Starting salaries for new surgical technologists are $12,700 a year, according to recent figures. Surgical technologists with several years experience earn average annual salaries of approximately $17,000. With experience, technologists may advance to supervisory or administrative positions.

Below is a list, provided by the Joint Review Committee on Education for the Surgical Technologist, of academic programs accredited by the Committee on Allied Health Education and Accreditation of the American Medical Association. All programs are nine-to-twelve months in length, require a high school education or the equivalent, and award a certificate, except ones marked with an asterisk (*), which offer a longer program and award an associate degree.

For further information on training and career opportunities contact the Association of Surgical Technologists, Inc., 8307 Shaffer Parkway, Littleton, Colorado 80127.

SOURCES:

Association of Surgical Technologists, Inc.
Occupational Outlook Handbook

Surgical Technologist Programs

ARKANSAS

Surgical Technologist Program
Westlark Community College
P.O. Box 3649
Fort Smith, Arkansas 72193

Surgical Technologist Program (*)
University of Arkansas
Veterans Administration Hospital
300 E. Roosevelt Road
Little Rock, Arkansas 72206

CALIFORNIA

Surgical Technologist Program
California Paramedical and Technical College
3745 Long Beach Boulevard
Long Beach, California 90807

Surgical Technologist Program
Los Angeles Trade and Technical College
400 W. Washington Boulevard
Los Angeles, California 90015

Surgical Technologist Program
Simi Valley Adult School
3150 School Street
Simi Valley, California 93065

COLORADO

Surgical Technologist Program
Denver Community College
1111 West Colfax
Denver, Colorado 80204

CONNECTICUT

Surgical Technologist Program
Danbury Hospital
24 Hospital Avenue
Danbury, Connecticut 06810

Surgical Technologist Program
Manchester Community College
60 Bidwell Street
Manchester, Connecticut 06040

FLORIDA

Surgical Technologist Program (*)
Daytona Beach Community College
P.O. Box 1111
Daytona Beach, Florida 32015

Surgical Technologist Program
Lindsey Hopkins Technical Education Center
Dade County Public Schools
750 Northwest 20th Street
Miami, Florida 33127

Surgical Technologist Program
Erwin Area Vo-Tech School
2010 E. Hillsborough Avenue
Tampa, Florida 33619

GEORGIA

Surgical Technologist Program
DeKalb Community College
495 N. Indian Creek Drive
Clarkston, Georgia 30021

Surgical Technologist Program
Savannah Area Vo-Tech School
5717 White Bluff Road
Savannah, Georgia 31499

ILLINOIS

Surgical Technologist Program
Central DuPage Hospital
25 N. Winfield Road
Winfield, Illinois 60187

Surgical Technologist Program
Swedish American Hospital
1400 Charles Street
Rockford, Illinois 61108

Surgical Technologist Program
Parkland College
2400 West Bradley
Champaign, Illinois 61820

Surgical Technologist Program
Illinois Central College
P.O. Box 2400
East Peoria, Illinois 61635

Surgical Technologist Program
Moline Public Hospital
635 Tenth Avenue
Moline, Illinois 61265

Surgical Technologist Program
Blessing Hospital
1005 Broadway
Quincy, Illinois 62301

Surgical Technologist Program
Triton College
2000 N. Fifth Avenue
River Grove, Illinois 60171

INDIANA

Surgical Technologist Program
Lutheran Hospital
3024 Fairfield Avenue
Ft. Wayne, Indiana 46807

Surgical Technologist Program
Indiana Vo-Tech College
1315 E. Washington Street
Indianapolis, Indiana 46202

Surgical Technologist Program
Indiana Vo-Tech College
3208 Ross Road
P.O. Box 6299
Lafayette, Indiana 47903

Surgical Technologist Program
Ball Memorial Hospital
2401 University Avenue
Muncie, Indiana 47303

Surgical Technologist Program
Indiana Vo-Tech College
Highway 421
Westville, Indiana 46391

IOWA

Surgical Technologist Program
Des Moines Area Community College
2006 Ankeny Boulevard
Ankeny, Iowa 50021

Surgical Technologist Program
Marshalltown Community College
3700 South Center Street
Marshalltown, Iowa 50158

Surgical Technologist Program
Western Iowa Technical Community College
4647 Stone Avenue
Sioux City, Iowa 51106

KANSAS

Surgical Technologist Program
St. Francis Regional Medical Center
Kansas Newman College
3100 McCormick Avenue
Wichita, Kansas 67213

KENTUCKY

Surgical Technologist Program
Bowling Green State Vo-Tech School
1845 Loop Drive
P.O. Box 6000
Bowling Green, Kentucky 42101

Surgical Technologist Program
Central Kentucky Vo-Tech School
104 Vo-Tech Road
Lexington, Kentucky 40511

Surgical Technologist Program
Madisonville State Vo-Tech
701 North Laffoon Street
Madisonville, Kentucky 42431

Surgical Technologist Program
W. Kentucky Vo-Tech School
P.O. Box 7408
Paducah, Kentucky 42001

LOUISIANA

Surgical Technologist Program
Alton Ochsner Medical Foundation
1516 Jefferson Highway
New Orleans, Louisiana 70121

Surgical Technologist Program
Charity Hospital of Louisiana at New Orleans
1532 Tulane Avenue
New Orleans, Louisiana 70140

Surgical Technologist Program
Our Lady of Lourdes
611 St. Landry
Lafayette, Louisiana 70502

MAINE

Surgical Technologist Program
Maine Medical Center
22 Bramhall Street
Portland, Maine 04102

MASSACHUSETTS

Surgical Technologist Program
Quincy Vo-Tech School
34 Woodward Avenue
Quincy, Massachusetts 02169

Surgical Technologist Program
Springfield Technical Community College
Armory Square
Springfield, Massachusetts 01105

MINNESOTA

Surgical Technologist Program
Anoka Technical Institute
1355 West Highway 10
Anoka, Minnesota 55303

Surgical Technologist Program
East Grand Forks Area Voc-Tech Institute
Highway 220 North
East Grand Forks, Minnesota 56721

Surgical Technologist Program
Rochester Area Vo-Tech Institute
332 16th Street, S.E.
Rochester, Minnesota 55901

Surgical Technologist Program
St. Cloud Area Vo-Tech Institute
1540 Norway Drive
St. Cloud, Minnesota 56301

MISSISSIPPI

Surgical Technologist Program
Hinds Junior College
Vo-Tech Jackson Branch
3925 Sunset Drive
Jackson, Mississippi 39213

MISSOURI

Surgical Technologist Program
Independence Missouri School District
1509 W. Truman Road
Independence, Missouri 64050

Surgical Technologist Program
St. Louis Community College at Forest Park
5600 Oakland
St. Louis, Missouri 63110

MONTANA

Surgical Technologist Program
Missoula Vo-Tech Center
909 South Avenue West
Missoula, Montana 59801

NEBRASKA

Surgical Technologist Program
Southeastern Community College
8800 "O" Street
Lincoln, Nebraska 68520

Surgical Technologist Program
Metropolitan Technical Community College
P.O. Box 3777
Omaha, Nebraska 68103

NEW JERSEY

Surgical Technologist Program
Bergen Community College
400 Paramus Road
Paramus, New Jersey 07652

Surgical Technologist Program
University of Medicine and Dentistry of New Jersey
100 Bergen Street
Newark, New Jersey 07103

NEW YORK

Surgical Technologist Program (*)
Nassau Community College
Stewart Avenue
Garden City, New York 11530

Surgical Technologist Program
Niagara County Community College
P.O. Box 5236
3111 Saunders Settlement Road
Sanborn, New York 14132

Surgical Technologist Program (*)
Onondaga Community College
Syracuse, New York 13215

NORTH CAROLINA

Surgical Technologist Program
Fayetteville Tech Institute
P.O. Box 5236
Fayetteville, North Carolina 28303

Surgical Technologist Program
Coastal Carolina Community College
444 Western Boulevard
Jacksonville, North Carolina 28540

Surgical Technologist Program
Lenoir Community College
P.O. Box 188
Kinston, North Carolina 28501

OHIO

Surgical Technologist Program (*)
Cincinnati Technical College
3520 Central Parkway
Cincinnati, Ohio 45223

Surgical Technologist Program (*)
Sinclair Community College
444 West Third Street
Dayton, Ohio 45402

Surgical Technologist Program (*)
Michael J. Owens Technical College
Caller No. 10,000 - Oregon Road
Toledo, Ohio 43699

OKLAHOMA

Surgical Technologist Program
Tulsa County Area Vo-Tech School
3420 South Memorial Drive
Tulsa, Oklahoma 74145

OREGON

Surgical Technologist Program (*)
Mt. Hood Community College
26000 S.E. Stark Street
Gresham, Oregon 97030

PENNSYLVANIA

Surgical Technologist Program
Sacred Heart Hospital
421 Chew Street
Allentown, Pennsylvania 18102

Surgical Technologist Program
Conemaugh Valley Memorial Hospital
1086 Franklin Street
Johnston, Pennsylvania 15905

Surgical Technologist Program
Delaware County Community College
Media, Pennsylvania 19063

Surgical Technologist Program (*)
Community College of Alleghany
Boyce Campus
595 Beatty Road
Monroeville, Pennsylvania 15146

SOUTH CAROLINA

Surgical Technologist Program
McDuffie Vo High School
Anderson Memorial Hospital
1225 South McDuffie Street
Anderson, South Carolina 29621

Surgical Technologist Program
Midlands Technical College
P.O. Box 2408
Columbia, South Carolina 29202

Surgical Technologist Program
Florence-Darlington Technical College
P.O. Box Drawer F-8000
Florence, South Carolina 29501

Surgical Technologist Program
Greenville Technical College
P.O. Box 5616, Station B
Greenville, South Carolina 29606

Surgical Technologist Program
Spartanburg Technical College
Drawer 4386
Spartanburg, South Carolina 29303

TENNESSEE

Surgical Technologist Program
East Tennessee State University
1000 West E Street
Elizabethton, Tennessee 37643

Surgical Technologist Program
Sea Isle Adult Ed. Center
5250 Sea Isle Road
Memphis, Tennessee 38117

TEXAS

Surgical Technologist Program
Amarillo College
P.O. Box 447
Amarillo, Texas 79178

Surgical Technologist Program
Austin Community College
5712 East Riverside Drive
Austin, Texas 78741

Surgical Technologist Program
Del Mar College
Baldwin and Ayers
Corpus Christi, Texas 78404

Surgical Technologist Program
El Centro College
Main and Lamar Streets
Dallas, Texas 75202

Surgical Technologist Program
El Paso Community College
P.O. Box 20500
El Paso, Texas 79998

Surgical Technologist Program
Galveston College-University of Texas Medical Branch
4015 Avenue Q
Galveston, Texas 77550

Surgical Technologist Program
Houston Community College
3100 Shenandoah
Houston, Texas 77021

Surgical Technologist Program
Tarrant County Jr. College
828 Harwood Road
Hurst, Texas 76053

Surgical Technologist Program
Odessa College
201 West University
Odessa, Texas 79762

Surgical Technologist Program
San Jacinto College
8060 Spencer Highway
Pasadena, Texas 77505

Surgical Technologist Program
St. Philip's College
2111 Nevada Street
San Antonio, Texas 78203

Surgical Technologist Program
South Plains College
1302 Main Street
Lubbock, Texas 79401-3298

Surgical Technologist Program
The Victoria College
2200 East Red River
Victoria, Texas 77901

Surgical Technologist Program
Trinity Valley Community College
Cardinal Drive
Athens, Texas 75751

Surgical Technologist Program
USAF High School Military-Sheppard AFB
Dept. of Health Care Science
Sheppard AFB
Wichita Falls, Texas 76311

VIRGINIA

Surgical Technologist Program
Riverside Hospital and Newport News Public Schools
J. Clyde Morris Boulevard
Newport News, Virginia 23601

Surgical Technologist Program
Winchester Medical Center, Inc.
South Stewart Street
Winchester, Virginia 22601

WASHINGTON

Surgical Technologist Program
Seattle Community College
1701 Broadway
Seattle, Washington 98122

Surgical Technologist Program
Spokane Community College
N. 1810 Greene Street
Spokane, Washington 99207

WEST VIRGINIA

Surgical Technologist Program
West Virginia Northern Community College
College Square
Wheeling, West Virginia 26003

WISCONSIN

Surgical Technologist Program
Moraine Park Technical Institute
235 North National
Fond du Lac, Wisconsin 54935

Surgical Technologist Program
West Wisconsin Technical Institute
Sixth and Vine Streets
LaCrosse, Wisconsin 54601

Surgical Technologist Program
Milwaukee Area Technical College
1015 North Sixth Street
Milwaukee, Wisconsin 53202

Surgical Technologist Program
Waukesha County Area Vo-Tech & Adult Education District
800 Main Street
Pewaukee, Wisconsin 53072

Surgical Technologist Program
Mid-State Vo-Tech & Adult Education District
110 West Third Street
P.O. Box 50
Marshfield, Wisconsin 54449

Surgical Technologist Program
Northeast Wisconsin Technical Institute
2740 W. Mason Street
Green Bay, Wisconsin 54303

PUBLIC HEALTH

Made up of federal, state and local health and environmental agencies, the field of public health is concerned with the maintenance and promotion of high quality health standards in the community. Public health encompasses many varied facets of healthcare and research including biomedical and laboratory sciences, biostatistics, dental public health, environmental health, epidemiology (the study of epidemic disease cause and control), health services administration, health policy and planning, mental health, nutrition, occupational safety and health, population studies, and public health education. Because of its diverse nature the public health work force includes physicians, nurses, planners, administrators, educators, social workers, therapists, technicians, and many more kinds of specialists and paraprofessionals, all of whom work towards conserving and improving the health of the public. Most available careers in public health are discussed in this handbook under their respective occupational title.

Public health professionals are employed in the public sector in health departments, and with voluntary and government health agencies.

Schools of public health are primarily graduate institutions that provide education for the administrative professional positions in public health. Applicants to these schools generally have a health background and several years experience.

There are currently 24 graduate schools of Public Health accredited by the Council on Education for Public Health. These programs are listed as follows. Persons interested in a master's degree program in public health at a specific school should contact the school directly to determine the specific area of public health it specializes in teaching.

For further information on a career in Public Health, write to the Association of Schools of Public Health, 1015 15th Street, N.W., Suite 404, Washington, DC 20005.

SOURCES:

Association of Schools of Public Health

Public Health Programs

ALABAMA

Public Health Program
School of Public Health
University of Alabama-Birmingham
The Medical Center
Birmingham, Alabama 35294

CALIFORNIA

Public Health Program
School of Public Health
University of California-Berkeley
Berkeley, California 94720

Public Health Program
School of Health
Loma Linda University
Loma Linda, California 92350

Public Health Program
School of Public Health
University of California-Los Angeles
Center for Health Sciences
Los Angeles, California 90024

Public Health Program
Graduate School of Public Health
San Diego State University
San Diego, California 92182

CONNECTICUT

Public Health Program
Department of Epidemiology and Public Health
Yale University School of Medicine
P.O. Box 3333
60 College Street
New Haven, Connecticut 06510

FLORIDA

Public Health Program
College of Public Health
University of South Florida
13301 North 30th Street
Tampa, Florida 33612

HAWAII

Public Health Program
School of Public Health
University of Hawaii
1960 East-West Road
Honolulu, Hawaii 96822

ILLINOIS

Public Health Program
School of Public Health
University of Illinois at Chicago
P.O. Box 6998
Chicago, Illinois 60680

LOUISIANA

Public Health Program
School of Public Health and Tropical Medicine
Tulane University
1430 Tulane Avenue
New Orleans, Louisiana 70112

MARYLAND

Public Health Program
School of Hygiene and Public Health
The Johns Hopkins University
615 N. Wolfe Street
Baltimore, Maryland 21205

MASSACHUSETTS

Public Health Program
Division of Public Health
School of Health Sciences
University of Massachusetts
Amherst, Massachusetts 01003-0037

Public Health Program
School of Public Health
Boston University
80 East Concord Street
Boston, Massachusetts 02118

Public Health Program
School of Public Health
Harvard University
677 Huntington Avenue
Boston, Massachusetts 02115

MICHIGAN

Public Health Program
School of Public Health
University of Michigan
109 S. Observatory Street
Ann Arbor, Michigan 48109

MINNESOTA

Public Health Program
School of Public Health
University of Minnesota
420 Delaware Street, S.E.
Minneapolis, Minnesota 55455-0318

NEW YORK

Public Health Program
School of Public Health
Columbia University
600 West 168th Street
New York, New York 10032

NORTH CAROLINA

Public Health Program
School of Public Health
University of North Carolina
Chapel Hill, North Carolina 27514

OKLAHOMA

Public Health Program
College of Public Health
University of Oklahoma
P.O. Box 26901
Oklahoma City, Oklahoma 73190

PENNSYLVANIA

Public Health Program
Graduate School of Public Health
University of Pittsburgh
111 Parran Hall
Pittsburgh, Pennsylvania 15261

PUERTO RICO

Public Health Program
School of Public Health
University of Puerto Rico
G.P.O. Box 5067
San Juan, Puerto Rico 00936

SOUTH CAROLINA

Public Health Program
School of Public Health
University of South Carolina
Columbia, South Carolina 29208

TEXAS

Public Health Program
School of Public Health
University of Texas
P.O. Box 20186
Houston, Texas 77025

WASHINGTON

Public Health Program
School of Public Health and Community Medicine
University of Washington
SC-30
Seattle, Washington 98195

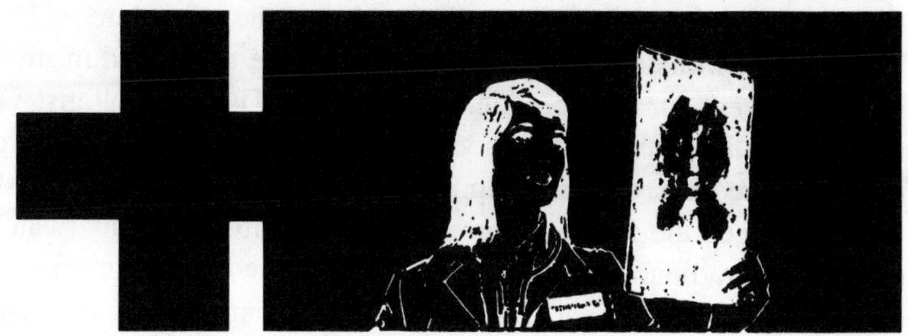

RADIOLOGIC TECHNOLOGY

Radiologic technology is the allied health profession concerned with the use of ionizing radiation, radioactive isotopes or sound waves for diagnostic and therapeutic purposes. There are four allied health careers in the field of radiologic technology: *radiographers* take radiographs (X-rays) of the internal structures of the body for diagnostic imaging purposes; *radiation therapy technologists* use prescribed doses of ionizing radiation to treat diseases, mainly cancer; *nuclear medicine technologists* work with radioactive materials for both diagnostic imaging and treatment; and *ultrasound technologists* operate non-ionizing equipment that utilizes sound waves to produce images. There occupations are generally supervised by the radiologist.

Diagnostic Radiologic Technologist or Radiographer

Also known as an *X-ray technologist,* the radiographer assists the radiologist in the use of X-ray equipment and the fluoroscopic screen in the diagnostic imaging of such medical problems as broken bones, ulcers, tumors, and other illnesses. The radiologist interprets the radiographs (X-rays) and may make a diagnosis based on the results. In using the radiographic equipment, the technologist positions the patient on the X-ray machine, determines proper voltage current and exposure time, takes the X-ray, and processes the X-ray film. The technologist pays careful attention to safety while handling the X-ray equipment. Lead shields and other protective devices are furnished to patients to protect them from excess exposure to radiation during the procedure.

Sometimes mobile X-ray equipment may have to be used in such places as emergency rooms, surgery, or at the patient's bedside. The technologist is also responsible for maintaining the equipment in good working order, except for major repairs, and for keeping radiograph records, ordering supplies, and possibly mixing processing solutions.

In the use of the fluoroscopic screen (a monitor that can "watch" a patient's internal organs), the radiographer prepares a contrast medium solution such as barium sulphate, administers it to the patient, positions the patient, and applies the correct radiation exposure. As the solution passes through the patient's body, the radiologist may watch the screen and detect diseases or injuries in the digestive tract, chest, heart, bones, or other areas.

Most radiographers work in hospitals, but there are also positions available in clinics, private physician's offices, the government, industry, public health facilities, laboratories, and in radiographic equipment sales.

Educational programs in radiography are available in hospitals, colleges and universities, vocational-technical schools, community and junior colleges, and in the military. Most training programs last twenty-four months, but some schools also offer bachelor's degree programs. The applicant to a training program must be a high school graduate or the equivalent.

Graduating from an educational program approved by the American Medical Association's Committee on Allied Health Education and Accreditation and successfully passing a qualifying examination are the requirements for certification as a radiographer.

Certification by the American Registry of Radiologic Technologists is a prerequisite for obtaining highly skilled and specialized positions. Many states also require radiographers to be licensed. Check with the state licensing division or contact the American Registry of Radiologic Technologists, 2600 Wayzata Boulevard, Minneapolis, Minnesota 55405, for further details on licensure.

Recommended high school courses include algebra, geometry, physics, chemistry, biology and computer science.

In addition to X-ray equipment, many radiographers are being trained to use sophisticated computer imaging machines such as the CT Scanner (computed tomographer) and the MRI (magnetic resonance imager). These machines provide detailed information about the body's anatomy using computer technology.

According to a recent survey by the University of Texas Medical Branch, starting annual salaries for radiographers average $17,500, while those with several years experience earn salaries in the mid-twenties. Radiographers with specialized training with the CT Scanner or MRI may receive additional compensation. With advanced education and training, radiographers may advance to managerial positions.

Below is a list of programs in radiography approved by the Committee on Allied Health Education and Accreditation of the American Medical Association. Although many of the education programs in radiography are offered by hospitals, there is a current trend for these programs to become affiliated with the more formalized and well-rounded teaching programs of educational institutions. Contact each school directly for entrance requirements, length of program and type of certificate or degree awarded.

SOURCES:

American Society of Radiologic Technologists
American Registry of Radiologic Technologists
Occupational Outlook Handbook

Radiographer Programs

ALABAMA

Radiographer Program
Northeast Alabama Regional Medical Center
400 E. 10th Street
Anniston, Alabama 36201

Radiographer Program
Carraway Methodist Medical Center
1600 North 26th Street
Birmingham, Alabama 35234

Radiographer Program
Jefferson State Junior College
Pinson Valley Parkway
2601 Carson
Birmingham, Alabama 35215-3098

Radiographer Program
The University of Alabama at Birmingham
University Station
Birmingham, Alabama 35294

Radiographer Program
Gadsden State Community College
Number One State College Blvd.
Gadsden, Alabama 35999

Radiographer Program
Wallace State Community College
P.O. Box 250
Hanceville, Alabama 35077-9080

Radiographer Program
Huntsville Cooperative School of Medical Tech.
101 Silvey Road
Huntsville, Alabama 35801

Radiographer Program
University of South Alabama
307 University Blvd.
Mobile, Alabama 36688

Radiographer Program
St. Margaret's Hospital
301 S. Ripley Street
P.O. Drawer 311
Montgomery, Alabama 36195-4701

Radiographer Program
DCH Regional Medical Center
809 University Blvd. E.
Tuscaloosa, Alabama 35403

Radiographer Program
Tuskegee University
Kresge Center
Tuskegee Institute, Alabama 36088

ARIZONA

Radiographer Program
Northern Arizona University
CU Box 4092
Flagstaff, Arizona 86011

Radiographer Program
Maricopa Technical Community College
108 N. 40th Street
Phoenix, Arizona 85034

Radiographer Program
Pima Community College
200 North Stone
Tucson, Arizona 85702

ARKANSAS

Radiographer Program
Southern Arkansas University-Eldorado Branch
300 South West Avenue
El Dorado, Arkansas 71730

Radiographer Program
Sparks Regional Medical Center
1311 South 'I' Street
Forth Smith, Arkansas 72901

Radiographer Program
St. Edward Mercy Medical Center
7301 Rogers Avenue
Fort Smith, Arkansas 72903

Radiographer Program
Helena Hospital
Highway 49 Bypass
Helena, Arkansas 72342

Radiographer Program
Garland County Community College
No. 1 College Drive
Hot Springs, Arkansas 71913

Radiographer Program
Baptist Medical Center
9601 1630 Exit 7
Little Rock, Arkansas 72205-7299

Radiographer Program
St. Vincent Infirmary
2 St. Vincent Circle
Little Rock, Arkansas 72205-5499

Radiographer Program
University of Arkansas for Medical Sciences
4301 West Markham
Little Rock, Arkansas 72205

Radiographer Program
Jefferson Regional Medical Center
1515 West 42nd Avenue
Pine Bluff, Arkansas 71603

Radiographer Program
Arkansas State University
P.O. Box 10
State University, Arkansas 72467

CALIFORNIA

Radiographer Program
Chaffey Community College
5885 Haven Avenue
Alta Loma, California 91701

Radiographer Program
Cabrillo College
6500 Soquel Drive
Aptos, California 95003

Radiographer Program
Bakersfield College
1801 Panorama Drive
Bakersfield, California 93305

Radiographer Program
St. Joseph Medical Center
Buena Vista & Alameda Sts.
Burbank, California 91505

Radiographer Program
Peninsula Hospital & Medical Center
1783 El Camino Real
Burlingame, California 94010

Radiographer Program
Orange Coast College
2701 Fairview Road
Costa Mesa, California 92628-0120

Radiographer Program
Cypress College
9200 Valley View Street
Cypress, California 90630

Radiographer Program
City of Hope National Medical Center
1500 East Duarte Road
Duarte, California 91010

Radiographer Program
Fresno City College
1101 E. University Avenue
Fresno, California 93741

Radiographer Program
Daniel Freeman Memorial Hospital
333 N. Prairie Avenue
Inglewood, California 90301

Radiographer Program
Loma Linda University
School of Allied Health Professions
Loma Linda, California 92350

Radiographer Program
Long Beach City College
4901 East Carson Street
Long Beach, California 90808

Radiographer Program
Foothill Community College
12345 El Monte Road
Los Altos Hills, California 94022

Radiographer Program
Childrens Hospital of Los Angeles
4650 Sunset Boulevard
Los Angeles, California 90027

Radiographer Program
King Drew Medical Center
1621 East 120th Street
Los Angeles, California 90059

Radiographer Program
Los Angeles City College
855 N. Vermont Avenue
Los Angeles, California 90029

Radiographer Program
Los Angeles County-USC Medical Center
1200 N. State Street
Los Angeles, California 90033

Radiographer Program
VA-Wadsworth Medical Center
Wilshire & Sawtelle Blvds.
Los Angeles, California 90073

Radiographer Program
St. Francis Medical Center
3630 E. Imperial Highway
Lynwood, California 90262

Radiographer Program
Yuba College
2088 N. Beale Road
Marysville, California 95901

Radiographer Program
Merced College
3600 "M"Street
Merced, California 95348-2898

Radiographer Program
California State University, Northridge
18111 Nordhoff Street
Northridge, California 91330

Radiographer Program
Merritt College
12500 Campus Drive
Oakland, California 94619

Radiographer Program
St. John's Regional Medical Center
333 North 'F' Street
Oxnard, California 93030

Radiographer Program
Huntington Memorial Hospital
100 Congress Street
Pasadena, California 91105

Radiographer Program
Pasadena City College
1570 E. Colorado Blvd.
Pasadena, California 91106

Radiographer Program
Canada College
4200 Farm Hill Blvd.
Redwood City, California 94061

Radiographer Program
Sutter Community Hospitals
1111 Howe Ave., Suite 600
Sacramento, California 95825

Radiographer Program
San Bernardino County Medical Center
780 East Gilbert Street
San Bernardino, California 92415

Radiographer Program
Naval School of Health Sciences
San Diego, California 92134-6000

Radiographer Program
San Diego Mesa College
7250 Mesa College Drive
San Diego, California 92111

Radiographer Program
City College of San Francisco
50 Phelan Avenue, E200
San Francisco, California 94112

Radiographer Program
Santa Barbara City College
721 Cliff Drive
Santa Barbara, California 93109

Radiographer Program
Santa Rosa Junior College
1501 Mendocino Avenue
Santa Rosa, California 95401

Radiographer Program
Sepulveda VA Medical Center
1611 Plummer Street
Sepulveda, California 91343

Radiographer Program
San Joaquin General Hospital
P.O. Box 1020
500 West Hospital Road
Stockton, California 95201

Radiographer Program
El Camino College
16007 Crenshaw Blvd.
Torrance, California 90509

Radiographer Program
LAC Harbor-UCLA Medical Center
1000 West Carson Street
Torrance, California 90509

Radiographer Program
Mt. San Antonio College
1100 N. Grand Avenue
Walnut, California 91789

COLORADO

Radiographer Program
Memorial Hospital
1400 E. Boulder Street
P.O. Box 1326
Colorado Springs, Colorado 80901

Radiographer Program
Community College of Denver-Auraria Campus
1068 Ninth Street, Box 250
Denver, Colorado 80204

Radiographer Program
Presbyterian Medical Center
1719 East 19th Avenue
Denver, Colorado 80218

Radiographer Program
St. Anthony Hospital
4231 West 16th
Denver, Colorado 80204

Radiographer Program
Mesa College
P.O. Box 2647
Grand Junction, Colorado 81502

Radiographer Program
Aims Community College
P.O. Box 69
Greeley, Colorado 80632

Radiographer Program
Pueblo Community College
900 West Orman Avenue
Pueblo, Colorado 81004

Radiographer Program
Lutheran Medical Center
8300 W. 38th Avenue
Wheat Ridge, Colorado 80033

CONNECTICUT

Radiographer Program
St. Vincent's Medical Center
2800 Main Street
Bridgeport, Connecticut 06606

Radiographer Program
Danbury Hospital
24 Hospital Avenue
Danbury, Connecticut 06810

Radiographer Program
Hartford Hospital
80 Seymour Street
Hartford, Connecticut 06115

Radiographer Program
Mount Sinai Hospital
500 Blue Hills Avenue
Hartford, Connecticut 06112

Radiographer Program
Manchester Memorial Hospital
71 Haynes Street
Manchester, Connecticut 06040

Radiographer Program
The Meriden-Wallingford Hospital
181 Cook Avenue
Meriden, Connecticut 06450

Radiographer Program
Middlesex Community College
100 Training Hill Road
Middletown, Connecticut 06457

Radiographer Program
New Britain General Hospital
100 Grand Street
New Britain, Connecticut 06050

Radiographer Program
South Central Community College
60 Sargent Drive
New Haven, Connecticut 06511

Radiographer Program
Lawrence & Memorial Hospitals
365 Montauk Avenue
New London, Connecticut 06320

Radiographer Program
Stamford Hospital
Shelburne Road
P.O. Box 9317
Stamford, Connecticut 06904-9317

Radiographer Program
Mattatuck Community College
750 Chase Parkway
Waterbury, Connecticut 06708

Radiographer Program
Windham Community Memorial Hospital
112 Mansfield Avenue
Willimantic, Connecticut 06226

DELAWARE

Radiographer Program
Medical Center of Delaware, Inc.
14th and Washington Streets
Wilmington, Delaware 19899

Radiographer Program
St. Francis Hospital, Inc.
Seventh & Clayton Streets
Wilmington, Delaware 19805

DISTRICT OF COLUMBIA

Radiographer Program
Howard University
2400 6th Street, N.W.
Washington, DC 20059

Radiographer Program
University of the District of Columbia
4200 Connecticut Ave., N.W.
Washington, DC 20008

Radiographer Program
Washington Hospital Center
110 Irving Street, N.W.
Washington, DC 20010

FLORIDA

Radiographer Program
Bethesda Kennedy Hospitals
2815 S. Seacrest Blvd.
Boynton Beach, Florida 33435

Radiographer Program
Manatee Community College
5840 26th Street West
P.O. Box 1849
Bradenton, Florida 33506

Radiographer Program
Brevard Community College
1519 Clearlake Road
Cocoa, Florida 32922

Radiographer Program
Halifax Hospital Medical Center
303 N C Morris Boulevard
P.O. Box 1990
Daytona Beach, Florida 32015

Radiographer Program
Broward Community College
225 East Las Olas Blvd.
Fort Lauderdale, Florida 33301

Radiographer Program
Lee Memorial Hospital
P.O. Drawer 2218
Fort Myers, Florida 33902

Radiographer Program
Indian River Community College
3209 Virginia Avenue
Fort Pierce, Florida 33450-9003

Radiographer Program
Santa Fe Community College
P.O. Box 1530
Gainesville, Florida 32602

Radiographer Program
Baptist Medical Center
800 Prudential Drive
Jacksonville, Florida 32207

Radiographer Program
St. Vincent's Medical Center
1800 Barns Street
P.O. Box 2982
Jacksonville, Florida 32203

Radiographer Program
University Hospital of Jacksonville
655 West 8th Street
Jacksonville, Florida 32209

Radiographer Program
Lakeland General Hospital
1324 Lakeland Hills Blvd.
Lakeland, Florida 33802

Radiographer Program
Jackson Memorial Medical Center
University of Miami
1611 N.W. 12th Avenue
Miami, Florida 33136

Radiographer Program
Miami-Dade Community College
11011 S.W. 104th Street
Miami, Florida 33176

Radiographer Program
Mt. Sinai Medical Center
4300 Alton Road
Miami Beach, Florida 33140

Radiographer Program
Marion City School of Rad. Technology
438 S.W. Third Street
Ocala, Florida 32670

Radiographer Program
Florida Hospital
601 E. Rollins Street
Orlando, Florida 32803

Radiographer Program
Orlando Regional Medical Center
1414 S. Kuhl Avenue
Orlando, Florida 32806

Radiographer Program
University of Central Florida
P.O. Box 25000
Orlando, Florida 32816

Radiographer Program
Baptist Hospital
1000 W. Moreno Street
Pensacola, Florida 32501

Radiographer Program
Sacred Heart Hospital
5151 N. 9th Avenue
Pensacola, Florida 32504

Radiographer Program
West Florida Medical Center
P.O. Box 18900
Pensacola, Florida 32523-8900

Radiographer Program
Medical Center Hospital
809 E. Marion Avenue
Punta Gorda, Florida 33950

Radiographer Program
Bayfront Medical Center, Inc.
701 6th Street, South
St. Petersburg, Florida 33701

Radiographer Program
St. Petersburg Junior College
P.O. Box 13489
St. Petersburg, Florida 33733

Radiographer Program
Tallahassee Community College
444 Appleyard Drive
Tallahassee, Florida 32304

Radiographer Program
Hillsborough Community College
P.O. Box 22127
Tampa, Florida 33630

Radiographer Program
St. Mary's Hospital
901 45th Street
West Palm Beach, Florida 33407

Radiographer Program
Polk Community College
999 Avenue H Northeast
Winter Haven, Florida 33881

GEORGIA

Radiographer Program
Albany Area Voc-Tech School
1021 Lowe Road
Albany, Georgia 31708

Radiographer Program
Crawford W. Long Memorial Hospital
35 Linden Avenue
Atlanta, Georgia 30365

Radiographer Program
Emory University
1300 Oxford Road
Atlanta, Georgia 30322

Radiographer Program
Georgia Baptist Medical Center
300 Boulevard Northeast
Atlanta, Georgia 30312

Radiographer Program
Grady Memorial Hospital
80 Butler Street S.E.
Atlanta, Georgia 30335

Radiographer Program
Medical College of Georgia
Office of the President, AA-31
Augusta, Georgia 30912-0450

Radiographer Program
University Hospital
1350 Walton Way
Augusta, Georgia 30910

Radiographer Program
Brunswick Junior College
Altama at Fourth Street
Brunswick, Georgia 31523

Radiographer Program
The Medical Center Hospital Authority
P.O. Box 951
Columbus, Georgia 31994-2299

Radiographer Program
Hamilton Medical Center
P.O. Box 1168
Dalton, Georgia 30720-1168

Radiographer Program
De Kalb General Hospital
2701 N. Decatur Road
Decatur, Georgia 30033

Radiographer Program
Troup County Area Voc-Tech School
Fort Drive
LaGrange, Georgia 30240

Radiographer Program
Medical Center of Central Georgia
777 Hemlock St., Box 137
Macon, Georgia 31206

Radiographer Program
Kennestone Hospital
737 Church Street
Marietta, Georgia 30060

Radiographer Program
Floyd Medical Center
Turner McCall Blvd.
Rome, Georgia 30161

Radiographer Program
Armstrong State College
11935 Abercorn Street
Savannah, Georgia 31419-1997

Radiographer Program
Thomas Area Voc-Tech School
P.O. Box 1578
Thomasville, Georgia 31799

Radiographer Program
Valdosta Area Voc-Tech School
Route 1, Box 202
Valdosta, Georgia 31602

Radiographer Program
Waycross-Ware Cty Area Voc-Tech School
1701 Carswell Avenue
Waycross, Georgia 31501

HAWAII

Radiographer Program
Kapiolani Community College
620 Pensacola Street
Honolulu, Hawaii 96814

IDAHO

Radiographer Program
Boise State University
1910 University Drive
Boise, Idaho 83725

Radiographer Program
Idaho State University
Campus Box 8310
Pocatello, Idaho 83209-0009

ILLINOIS

Radiographer Program
Northwest Community Hospital
800 W. Central Road
Arlington Heights, Illinois 60005

Radiographer Program
Belleville Area College
2500 Carlyle Road
Belleville, Illinois 6221-9989

Radiographer Program
Southern Illinois University
Anthony Hall
Carbondale, Illinois 62901

Radiographer Program
Kaskaskia Junior College
Shattuc Road
Centralia, Illinois 62801

Radiographer Program
Parkland College
2400 W. Bradley Avenue
Champaign, Illinois 61821

Radiographer Program
Cook County Hospital
1825 W. Harrison Street
Chicago, Illinois 60612

Radiographer Program
De Paul University
25 E. Jackson Blvd.
Chicago, Illinois 60604

Radiographer Program
Henrotin Hospital
111 W. Oak Street
Chicago, Illinois 60610

Radiographer Program
Malcolm X College
1900 W. Van Buren St.
Chicago, Illinois 60612

Radiographer Program
South Chicago Community Hospital
2320 East 93rd Street
Chicago, Illinois 60617

Radiographer Program
St. Joseph Hospital
2900 N. Lakeshore Drive
Chicago, Illinois 60657

Radiographer Program
University of Illinois at Chicago
1737 W. Polk Street
Chicago, Illinois 60680

Radiographer Program
Wilbur Wright College
3400 N. Austin Avenue
Chicago, Illinois 60634

Radiographer Program
Lake View Medical Center
812 N. Logan Avenue
Danville, Illinois 61832

Radiographer Program
Decatur Memorial Hospital
2300 N. Edward Street
Decatur, Illinois 62526

Radiographer Program
Oakton Community College
1600 E. Golf Road
Des Plaines, Illinois 60016

Radiographer Program
Sauk Valley College
RR - 5
Dixon, Illinois 61021

Radiographer Program
Illinois Central College
East Peoria, Illinois 61635

Radiographer Program
St. Joseph Hospital
77 N. Airlite Street
Elgin, Illinois 60120

Radiographer Program
St. Francis Hospital
355 Ridge Avenue
Evanston, Illinois 60202

Radiographer Program
Carl Sandburg College
2232 S. Lake Storey Road
P.O. Box 1407
Galesburg, Illinois 61402

Radiographer Program
College of Du Page
22nd St. & Lambert Road
Glen Ellyn, Illinois 60137

Radiographer Program
College of Lake County
19351 W. Washington St.
Grayslake, Illinois 60030

Radiographer Program
Hinsdale Hospital
120 N. Oak Street
Hinsdale, Illinois 60521

Radiographer Program
Kankakee Community College
P.O. Box 888
Kankakee, Illinois 60901

Radiographer Program
Mc Donough District Hospital
525 East Grant Street
Macomb, Illinois 61455

Radiographer Program
Kishwaukee College
Route 38 & Malta Road
Malta, Illinois 60150

Radiographer Program
Lutheran Hospital
501 Tenth Avenue
Moline, Illinois 61265

Radiographer Program
Moline Public Hospital
635 10th Avenue
Moline, Illinois 61265

Radiographer Program
Brokaw Hospital
Virginia & Franklin Ave.
Normal, Illinois 61761

Radiographer Program
Richland Memorial Hospital
800 E. Locust Street
Olney, Illinois 62450

Radiographer Program
Moraine Valley Community College
10900 S. 88th Avenue
Palos Hills, Illinois 60465

Radiographer Program
St. Francis Medical Center
530 N.E. Glen Oak Avenue
Peoria, Illinois 61637

Radiographer Program
Blessing Hospital
1005 Broadway Street
Quincy, Illinois 62301

Radiographer Program
St. Mary Hospital
1415 Vermont Street
Quincy, Illinois 62301

Radiographer Program
Triton College
2000 Fifth Avenue
River Grove, Illinois 60171

Radiographer Program
Franciscan Medical Center
2701 17th Street
Rock Island, Illinois 61282

Radiographer Program
Rockford Memorial Hospital
2400 N. Rockton Avenue
Rockford, Illinois 61103

Radiographer Program
Swedish American Hospital
1400 Charles Street
Rockford, Illinois 61108

Radiographer Program
Thornton Community College
15800 S. State Street
South Holland, Illinois 60473

Radiographer Program
Lincoln Land Community College
Shepherd Road
Springfield, Illinois 62708

Radiographer Program
Memorial Medical Center
800 North Rutledge
Springfield, Illinois 62781

INDIANA

Radiographer Program
Elkhart General Hospital
600 East Boulevard
P.O. Box 1329
Elkhart, Indiana 46514

Radiographer Program
University of Southern Indiana
8600 University Boulevard
Evansville, Indiana 47712

Radiographer Program
Welborn Memorial Baptist Hospital
401 S.E. Sixth Street
Evansville, Indiana 47713

Radiographer Program
Lutheran Hospital
3024 Fairfield Avenue
Fort Wayne, Indiana 46807

Radiographer Program
Parkview Memorial Hospital
2200 Randallia Drive
Fort Wayne, Indiana 46085

Radiographer Program
St. Joseph's Hosp. of Fort Wayne, Inc.
700 Broadway
Fort Wayne, Indiana 46802

Radiographer Program
Indiana University Northwest
1120 South Drive, FH302
Indianapolis, Indiana 46223

Radiographer Program
Hancock Memorial Hospital
P.O. Box 827
Greenfield, Indiana 46140

Radiographer Program
Community Hospital of Indianapolis, Inc.
1500 N Ritter Avenue
Indianapolis, Indiana 46219

Radiographer Program
Indiana University School of Medicine
1120 South Drive
Indianapolis, Indiana 46223

Radiographer Program
Indiana Vocational Technical College
One West 26th Street
P.O. Box 1763
Indianapolis, Indiana 46206-1763

Radiographer Program
Marian College
3200 Cold Spring Rd.
Indianapolis, Indiana 46222

Radiographer Program
St. Joseph Memorial Hospital
1907 W. Sycamore Street
Kokomo, Indiana 46901

Radiographer Program
King's Daughter's Hospital
112 Presbyterian Avenue
Madison, Indiana 47250

Radiographer Program
Ball Memorial Hosp. Association, Inc.
2401 University Avenue
Muncie, Indiana 47302

Radiographer Program
Ball State University
University Avenue
Muncie, Indiana 47306

Radiographer Program
Reid Memorial Hospital
1401 Chester Boulevard
Richmond, Indiana 47374

Radiographer Program
Memorial Hospital of South Bend
615 N. Michigan Street
South Bend, Indiana 46601

Radiographer Program
Indiana Voc-Technical College
7377 S. Dixie Bee Road
Terra Haute, Indiana 47802

Radiographer Program
Porter Memorial Hospital
814 La Porte Avenue
Valparaiso, Indiana 46383

Radiographer Program
Good Samaritan Hospital
520 South 7th Street
Vincennes, Indiana 47591

Radiographer Program
Northern Indiana School of Rad Tech Inc.
Purdue U - N Central Campus
Westville, Indiana 46360

IOWA

Radiographer Program
Scott Community College of EICCD
Belmont Road
Bettendorf, Iowa 52722

Radiographer Program
Mercy Hospital
701 Tenth Street, S.E.
Cedar Rapids, Iowa 52403

Radiographer Program
St. Luke's Methodist Hospital
1026 'A' Avenue Northeast
Cedar Rapids, Iowa 52402

Radiographer Program
Jennie Edmundson Memorial Hospital
933 E. Pierce Street
Council Bluffs, Iowa 51501

Radiographer Program
Iowa Methodist Medical Center
1200 Pleasant Street
Des Moines, Iowa 50308

Radiographer Program
Mercy Hospital Medical Center
6th & University
Des Moines, Iowa 50314

Radiographer Program
University of Iowa Hospitals and Clinics
State Health Affairs C107 GH
Iowa City, Iowa 52242-1059

Radiographer Program
St. Joseph Mercy Hospital
84 Beaumont Drive
Mason City, Iowa 50401

Radiographer Program
Indian Hills Community College
Grandview & Elm
Ottumwa, Iowa 52501

Radiographer Program
Marian Health Center
801 5th Street
Sioux City, Iowa 51101

Radiographer Program
Allen Memorial Hospital
1825 Logan Ave-Administration
Waterloo, Iowa 50613

Radiographer Program
Schoitz Medical Center
Kinball & Ridgeway
Waterloo, Iowa 50702

Radiographer Program
St. Francis Hospital
3421 West 9th Street
Waterloo, Iowa 50702

KANSAS

Radiographer Program
St. Catherine Hospital
608 N. 5th Street
Garden City, Kansas 67846

Radiographer Program
Fort Hays State University
600 Park Street
Hays, Kansas 67601

Radiographer Program
Hutchinson Community College
1300 N. Plum Street
Hutchinson, Kansas 67501

Radiographer Program
Bethany Medical Center
51 N. 12th Street
Kansas City, Kansas 66102

Radiographer Program
Providence-St. Margaret Health Center
8929 Parallel Parkway
Kansas City, Kansas 66112

Radiographer Program
University of Kansas Medical Center
39th & Rainbow Blvd.
Kansas City, Kansas 66103

Radiographer Program
Labette Community College
200 South 14th Street
Parsons, Kansas 67357

Radiographer Program
Washburn University of Topeka
1700 S.W. College Avenue
Topeka, Kansas 66621

Radiographer Program
St. Francis Regional Medical Center
929 North St. Francis Avenue
Wichita, Kansas 67214

Radiographer Program
St. Joseph Medical Center
3600 East Harry
Wichita, Kansas 67218

Radiographer Program
Wesley Medical Center
550 N. Hillside Avenue
Wichita, Kansas 67214

KENTUCKY

Radiographer Program
King's Daughter's Hospital
2201 Lexington Avenue
Ashland, Kentucky 41101

Radiographer Program
Bowling Green State Voc Tech School
1845 Loop Drive
P.O. Box 6000
Bowling Green, Kentucky 42101-6000

Radiographer Program
William Booth Memorial Hospital
7380 Turfway Road
Florence, Kentucky 41042

Radiographer Program
Northern Kentucky University
Administration Center, Rm. 817
Highland Heights, Kentucky 41076

Radiographer Program
Good Samaritan Hospital
310 S. Limestone Street
Lexington, Kentucky 40508

Radiographer Program
Lexington Community College
Cooper Drive
Lexington, Kentucky 40506

Radiographer Program
St. Joseph Hospital
1 St. Joseph Drive
Lexington, Kentucky 40504

Radiographer Program
University of Louisville
Administration Building
Louisville, Kentucky 40292

Radiographer Program
Madisonville Area Vocational School
P.O. Box 608
Madisonville, Kentucky 42431

Radiographer Program
Morehead State University
201 Howell-McDowell Admin. Bldg.
Morehead, Kentucky 40351

Radiographer Program
West Kentucky State Vo Tech School
P.O. Box 7408 Blandville Rd.
Paducah, Kentucky 42001

LOUISIANA

Radiographer Program
Rapides General Hospital
Box 30101, 211 Fourth St.
Alexandria, Louisiana 71301

Radiographer Program
Baton Rouge General Medical Center
3600 Florida Street
P.O. Box 2511
Baton Rouge, Louisiana 70821

Radiographer Program
Lallie Kemp Charity Hospital
P.O. Box 70, Hwy. 51 South
Independence, Louisiana 70443

Radiographer Program
Lafayette General Medical Center
1214 Coolidge Ave., Box 52009
Lafayette, Louisiana 70505

Radiographer Program
University Medical Center
2390 W. Congress
P.O. Box 4016-C
Lafayette, Louisiana 70502

Radiographer Program
McNeese State University
4100 Ryan Street
Lake Charles, Louisiana 70609

Radiographer Program
Northeast Louisiana University
Northeast Station
Monroe, Louisiana 71209-3000

Radiographer Program
Alton Ochsner Medical Foundation
1516 Jefferson Hwy
New Orleans, Louisiana 70121

Radiographer Program
Charity Hospital of Louisiana at New Orleans
1532 Tulane Avenue
New Orleans, Louisiana 70140

Radiographer Program
Delgado Community College
615 City Park Avenue
New Orleans, Louisiana 70119

Radiographer Program
Louisana State University Medical Center
1501 Kings Highway
Shreveport, Louisiana 71130-3932

Radiographer Program
Northwestern State University of Louisiana
College Avenue
Shreveport, Louisiana 71497-9998

MAINE

Radiographer Program
Eastern Maine Voc Tech Institute
354 Hogan Road
Bangor, Maine 04401

Radiographer Program
Central Maine Medical Center
300 Main Street
Lewiston, Maine 04240-0305

Radiographer Program
St. Mary's General Hospital
45 Golder Street
Lewiston, Maine 04240

Radiographer Program
Mercy Hospital
144 State Street
Portland, Maine 04101

Radiographer Program
Southern Maine Voc Tech Institute
Fort Road
South Portland, Maine 04106

Radiographer Program
Mid-Maine Medical Center-Thayer Unit
North Street
Waterville, Maine 04901

MARYLAND

Radiographer Program
Essex Community College-John Hopkins Hospital
7201 Rossville Boulevard
Baltimore, Maryland 21237

Radiographer Program
Francis Scott Key Medical Center
600 N. Wolfe Street
Baltimore, Maryland 21205

Radiographer Program
Greater Baltimore Medical Center
6701 N. Charles Street
Baltimore, Maryland 21204

Radiographer Program
Maryland General Hospital
827 Linden Avenue
Baltimore, Maryland 21201

Radiographer Program
Mercy Hospital, Inc.
301 St. Paul Place
Baltimore, Maryland 21202

Radiographer Program
Provident Hospital, Inc.
2600 Liberty Heights Avenue
Baltimore, Maryland 21215

Radiographer Program
Sinai Hospital of Baltimore, Inc.
Belvedere at Greenspring Aves.
Baltimore, Maryland 21215

Radiographer Program
South Baltimore General Hospital
3001 S. Hanover Street
Baltimore, Maryland 21230

Radiographer Program
The Johns Hopkins Hospital
600 N. Wolfe Street
Baltimore, Maryland 21205

Radiographer Program
Hood College
Rosemont Avenue
Frederick, Maryland 21701

Radiographer Program
Hagerstown Junior College
751 Robinwood Drive
Hagerstown, Maryland 21740

Radiographer Program
Prince George's Community College
301 Largo Road
Largo, Maryland 20772

Radiographer Program
Wor Wic Tech Community College
1202 Old Ocean City Road
Salisbury, Maryland 21801

Radiographer Program
Montgomery College
Takoma Ave. & Fenton St.
Takoma Park, Maryland 20912

Radiographer Program
Washington Adventist Hospital
7600 Carroll Avenue
Takoma Park, Maryland 20912

Radiographer Program
Chesapeake College
P.O. Box 8
Wye Mills, Maryland 21679

MASSACHUSETTS

Radiographer Program
Middlesex Community College
Springs Road
Bedford, Massachusetts 01730

Radiographer Program
North Shore Community College
3 Essex Street
Beverly, Massachusetts 01915

Radiographer Program
Bunker Hill Community College
Rutherford Avenue
Boston, Massachusetts 02129

Radiographer Program
Massachusetts General Hospital
Fruit Street
Boston, Massachusetts 02114

Radiographer Program
Northeastern University
360 Huntington Avenue
Boston, Massachusetts 02115

Radiographer Program
Mount Auburn Hospital
330 Mt. Auburn Street
Cambridge, Massachusetts 02238

Radiographer Program
Northern Essex Community College
100 Elliott Street
Haverhill, Massachusetts 01830

Radiographer Program
Holyoke Community College
303 Homestead Avenue
Holyoke, Massachusetts 01040

Radiographer Program
North Adams Regional Hospital
Hospital Avenue
North Adams, Massachusetts 02147

Radiographer Program
Salem Hospital
81 Highland Avenue
Salem, Massachusetts 01970

Radiographer Program
Springfield Tech Community College
1 Armory Square
Springfield, Massachusetts 01105

Radiographer Program
Goddard Memorial Hospital
909 Sumner Street
Stoughton, Massachusetts 02072

Radiographer Program
Massachusetts Bay Community College
50 Oakland Street
Wellesley Hills, Massachusetts 02181

Radiographer Program
Quinsigamond Community College
570 W. Boylston Street
Worcester, Massachusetts 01606

MICHIGAN

Radiographer Program
Washtenaw Community College
4800 Huron River
P.O. Box D-1
Ann Arbor, Michigan 48106

Radiographer Program
Kellogg Community College
450 North Avenue
Battle Creek, Michigan 49016

Radiographer Program
Delta College
University Center, Michigan 48710

adiographer Program
Lake Michigan College
2755 E. Napler Avenue
Benton Harbor, Michigan 49022

Radiographer Program
Ferris State College
901 S. State St., Starr 304
Big Rapids, Michigan 49307

Radiographer Program
Oakwood Hospital
18101 Oakwood Blvd.
Dearborn, Michigan 48124

Radiographer Program
Detroit Receiving Hospital
University Health Center
4201 St. Antoine
Detroit, Michigan 48201

Radiographer Program
Grace Hospital Division
18700 Meyers Road
Detroit, Michigan 48235

Radiographer Program
Harper-Grace Hospitals
3990 John R Street
Detroit, Michigan 48201-2097

Radiographer Program
Henry Ford Hospital
2799 W. Grand Blvd.
Detroit, Michigan 48202

Radiographer Program
Marygrove College
8425 W. McNichols Rd.
Detroit, Michigan 48221

Radiographer Program
Samaritan Health Center
5555 Connor Avenue
Detroit, Michigan 48213

Radiographer Program
St. John Hospital
22101 Moross Road
Detroit, Michigan 48236

Radiographer Program
Hurley Medical Center
Number One Hurley Plaza
Flint, Michigan 48502

Radiographer Program
St. Joseph Hospital
302 Kensington Avenue
Flint, Michigan 48502

Radiographer Program
Grand Rapids Junior College
143 Bostwick Ave., N.E.
Grand Rapids, Michigan 49503

Radiographer Program
Mid Michigan Community College
1375 S. Clare Avenue
Harrison, Michigan 48625

Radiographer Program
Jackson Community College
2111 Emmons Road
Jackson, Michigan 49201

Radiographer Program
Borgess Medical Center
1521 Gull Road
Kalamazoo, Michigan 49001

Radiographer Program
Bronson Methodist Hospital
252 E. Lovell Street
Kalamazoo, Michigan 49007

Radiographer Program
Lansing Community College
419 N. Capitol Avenue
Box 40010
Lansing, Michigan 48901-7211

Radiographer Program
Marquette General Hospital, Inc.
420 West Magnetic Street
Marquette, Michigan 49855

Radiographer Program
St. Joseph Hospital
15855 Nineteen Mile Rd.
Mt.Clemens, Michigan 48044

Radiographer Program
St. Joseph Mercy Hospital
900 Woodward Avenue
Pontiac, Michigan 48053

Radiographer Program
Port Huron Hospital
1001 Kearney Street
Port Huron, Michigan 48060

Radiographer Program
William Beaumont Hospital
3601 W. 13 Mile Road
Royal Oak, Michigan 48072

Radiographer Program
Providence Hospital
P.O. Box 2043
Southfield, Michigan 48037

Radiographer Program
Peoples Community Hospital Authority
33155 Annapolis Road
Wayne, Michigan 48184

Radiographer Program
Westland Medical Center
2345 Merriman Road
Westland, Michigan 48185

MINNESOTA

Radiographer Program
St Mary's Hospital
407 E. Third Street
Duluth, Minnesota 55805

Radiographer Program
St. Luke's Hospital
915 E. 1st. Street
Duluth, Minnesota 55805

Radiographer Program
Central Mesabi Medical Center
750 E. 34 Street
Hibbing, Minnesota 55746

Radiographer Program
Inver Hills Community College
8445 College Trail
Inver Grove Heights, Minnesota 55075

Radiographer Program
Abbott-Northwestern Hospital, Inc.
800 East 28th Street
Minneapolis, Minnesota 55407

Radiographer Program
Minneapolis VA Medical Center
54 St. & 48th Avenue S.
Minneapolis, Minnesota 55417

Radiographer Program
University of Minnesota Health Science Center
213 Morrill Hall
Minneapolis, Minnesota 55455

Radiographer Program
North Memorial Medical Center
3300 Oakdale North
Robbinsdale, Minnesota 55422

Radiographer Program
Mayo Clinic Foundation
200 First Street, S.W.
Rochester, Minnesota 55905

Radiographer Program
St. Cloud Hospital
1406 6th Avenue N.
St. Cloud, Minnesota 56301

Radiographer Program
Methodist Hospital
6500 Excelsior Blvd.
St. Louis Park, Minnesota 55426

Radiographer Program
Rice Memorial Hospital
301 Becker Avenue, S.W.
Willmar, Minnesota 56201

MISSISSIPPI

Radiographer Program
Itawamba Junior College
Fulton, Mississippi 38843

Radiographer Program
Mississippi Gulf Coast Junior College
Perkinston, Mississippi 39573

Radiographer Program
Hattiesburg Radiology Group
116 S. 25th Avenue
Hattiesburg, Mississippi 39401

Radiographer Program
Mississippi Baptist Medical Center
1225 N. State Street
Jackson, Mississippi 39202

Radiographer Program
University of Mississippi Medical Center
2500 N. State Street
Jackson, Mississippi 39216-4505

Radiographer Program
Jones County Community Hospital
Jefferson at 13th Ave., Box 607
Laurel, Mississippi 39440

Radiographer Program
Meridian Junior College
5000 Hwy 19 North
Meridian, Mississippi 39305

Radiographer Program
Mississippi Delta Junior College
Olive St., P.O. Box 668
Moorehead, Mississippi 38761

Radiographer Program
Copiah-Lincoln Junior College
P.O. Box 457
Wesson, Mississippi 39191

MISSOURI

Radiographer Program
St. Francis Medical Center
211 St. Francis Drive
Cape Girardeau, Missouri 63701

Radiographer Program
St. Louis County Hospital
601 S. Brentwood Blvd.
Clayton, Missouri 63105

Radiographer Program
University of Missouri-Columbia
105 Jesse Hall
Columbia, Missouri 65211

Radiographer Program
Mineral Area Osteopathic Hospital
1212 Weber Road
Farmington, Missouri 63640

Radiographer Program
Independence Sanitarium & Hospital
1509 W. Truman Road
Independence, Missouri 64050

Radiographer Program
Missouri Southern State College
Neuman & Duquesne Rds.
Joplin, Missouri 64801-1595

Radiographer Program
Avila College
11901 Wornall Rd.
Kansas City, Missouri 64145-9990

Radiographer Program
Baptist Medical Center
6601 Rockhill Road
Kansas City, Missouri 64131

Radiographer Program
Penn Valley Community College
3201 Southwest Trfwy.
Kansas City, Missouri 64111

Radiographer Program
Research Medical Center
2316 E. Meyer Boulevard
Kansas City, Missouri 64132

Radiographer Program
St. Luke's Hospital of Kansas City
Wornall Road at 44th
Kansas City, Missouri 64111

Radiographer Program
North Kansas City Memorial Hospital
2800 Hospital Drive
North Kansas City, Missouri 64116

Radiographer Program
Central Missouri
School of X-Ray Technology
1000 W 10th Street
Rolla, Missouri 65401

Radiographer Program
Lester E. Cox Medical Center
1423 N. Jefferson Street
Springfield, Missouri 65802

Radiographer Program
St. John's Regional Health Center
1234 East Cherokee
Springfield, Missouri 65802

Radiographer Program
Methodist Medical Center
8th & Faraon Streets
St. Joseph, Missouri 64501

Radiographer Program
Mallinckrodt Inst. of Rad-Washingtion University
510 S. Kingshighway Blvd.
St. Louis, Missouri 63110

Radiographer Program
St. John's Mercy Medical Center
615 S. New Ballas Road
St. Louis, Missouri 63141

Radiographer Program
St. Louis Comm. College at Forest Park
5600 Oakland Avenue
St. Louis, Missouri 63110

MONTANA

Radiographer Program
St. Vincent's Hospital
1233 N. 30th St. Box 35200
Billings, Montana 59101-5200

Radiographer Program
Columbus Hospital
500 15th Avenue S.
P.O. Box 5013
Great Falls, Montana 59403

Radiographer Program
Montana Deaconess Medical Center
1101 26th Street South
Great Falls, Montana 59405

Radiographer Program
St. Patrick Hospital
500 West Broadway
P.O. Bos 4587
Missoula, Montana 59806

NEBRASKA

Radiographer Program
Mary Lanning Memorial Hospital
715 North St. Joseph
Hastings, Nebraska 68901

Radiographer Program
Southeast Community College
8800 'O' Street
Lincoln, Nebraska 68520

Radiographer Program
Bergan Mercy Hospital
7500 Mercy Road
Omaha, Nebraska 68124

Radiographer Program
Immanuel Medical Center
6901 N. 72nd Street
Omaha, Nebraska 68122

Radiographer Program
St. Joseph Hospital
601 N. 30th Street
Omaha, Nebraska 68131

Radiographer Program
University of Nebraska Medical Center
42nd & Dewey Avenue
Omaha, Nebraska 68105

Radiographer Program
West Nebraska General Hospital
4021 Avenue 'B'
Scottsbluff, Nebraska 69361

NEVEDA

Radiographer Program
University of Nevada
4505 Maryland Pkwy
Las Vegas, Nevada 89154

Radiographer Program
Truckee Meadows Community College
7000 Dandini Boulevard
Reno, Nevada 89512

NEW HAMPSHIRE

Radiographer Program
New Hampshire Technical Institute
Institute Drive
Concord, New Hampshire 03301

NEW JERSEY

Radiographer Program
Atlantic City Medical Center
1925 Pacific Avenue
Atlantic City, New Jersey 08401

Radiographer Program
Hudson Area School of Rad Tech
29 E. 29th Street
Bayonne, New Jersey 07002

Radiographer Program
Clara Maass Memorial Hospital
1 Franklin Avenue
Belleville, New Jersey 07019

Radiographer Program
Bridgeton Hospital
Irving & Manheim Aves.
Bridgeton, New Jersey 08302

Radiographer Program
Cooper Hospital/University Medical Center
One Cooper Plaza
Camden, New Jersey 08103

Radiographer Program
West Jersey Hospital System
Mt. Ephraim & Atlantic Aves.
Camden, New Jersey 08104

Radiographer Program
Burdette Tomlin Memorial Hospital
Rt. 9 & Stone Harbor Blvd.
Cape May Courthouse, New Jersey 08210

Radiographer Program
Middlesex County College
155 Mill Road
P.O. Box 3050
Edison, New Jersey 08818-3050

Radiographer Program
Elizabeth General Medical Center
925 E. Jersey Street
Elizabeth, New Jersey 07201

Radiographer Program
Englewood Hospital Association
350 Engle Street
Englewood, New Jersey 07631

Radiographer Program
Hackensack Medical Center
30 Prospect Ave. 1 Conklin
Hackensack, New Jersey 07601

Radiographer Program
St. Barnabas Medical Center
94 Old Short Hills Rd.
Livingston, New Jersey 07039

Radiographer Program
Monmouth Medical Center
300 Second Avenue
Long Branch, New Jersey 07740

Radiographer Program
Fairleigh Dickinson University
285 Madison Avenue
Madison, New Jersey 07070

Radiographer Program
The Mountainside Hospital
Bay & Highland Aves.
Montclair, New Jersey 07042

Radiographer Program
Memorial Hospital of Burlington County
175 Madison Avenue
Mount Holly, New Jersey 08060

Radiographer Program
Essex County College
303 University Avenue
Newark, New Jersey 07102

Radiographer Program
St. Michael's Medical Center
268 Dr. Martin Luther King Jr. Blvd.
Newark, New Jersey 07102

Radiographer Program
University of Medical & Dental of New Jersey
Rutgers Medical School
100 Bergen Street
Newark, New Jersey 07103

Radiographer Program
Bergen Community College
400 Paramus Road
Paramus, New Jersey 07652

Radiographer Program
Passaic County Community College
College Boulevard
Paterson, New Jersey 07509

Radiographer Program
Muhlenberg Hospital
Park Ave. & Randolph Rd.
Plainfield, New Jersey 07061

Radiographer Program
Riverview Medical Center
35 Union Street
Red Bank, New Jersey 07701

Radiographer Program
The Valley Hospital
Linwood & N. Van Dien Aves.
Ridgewood, New Jersey 07451

Radiographer Program
Overlook Hospital
99 Beauvoir Ave at Sylvan Rd.
Summit, New Jersey 07901-0220

Radiographer Program
Helene Fuld Medical Center
750 Brunswick Avenue
Trenton, New Jersey 08638

Radiographer Program
Mercer County Community College
1200 Old Trenton Road
Trenton, New Jersey 08690

Radiographer Program
St. Francis Medical Center
601 Hamilton Avenue
Trenton, New Jersey 08629

NEW MEXICO

Radiographer Program
Univ. of New Mexico School of Medicine
Basic Medical Sciences Bldg.
Albuquerque, New Mexico 87131

Radiographer Program
University of Albuquerque
St. Joseph Place, N.W.
Albuquerque, New Mexico 87104-0021

Radiographer Program
Northern New Mexico Community College
P.O. Box 250
Espanola, New Mexico 87532

Radiographer Program
New Mexico State University
3 DAB
Las Cruces, New Mexico 88001

NEW YORK

Radiographer Program
Memorial Hospital
600 Northern Blvd.
Albany, New York 12204

Radiographer Program
Broome Community College
P.O. Box 1017
Binghamton, New York 13902

Radiographer Program
Hostos Community College
475 Grand Concourse
Bronx, New York 10451

Radiographer Program
Montefiore Hospital & Medical Center
111 E. 210th Street
Bronx, New York 10467

Radiographer Program
Long Island College Hospital
340 Henry Street
Brooklyn, New York 11201

Radiographer Program
Methodist Hospital of Brooklyn
506 6th Street
Brooklyn, New York 11215

Radiographer Program
New York City Technical College
300 Jay Street
Brooklyn, New York 11201

Radiographer Program
Millard Fillmore Hospital
3 Gates Circle
Buffalo, New York 14209

Radiographer Program
Trocaire College
110 Red Jacket Pkwy
Buffalo, New York 14220

Radiographer Program
Corning Hospital
176 Denison Parkway E
Corning, New York 14830

Radiographer Program
Arnot-Ogden Memorial Hospital
Roe Avenue
Elmira, New York 14905

Radiographer Program
St. Joseph's Memorial
555 E. Market Street
Elmira, New York 14902

Radiographer Program
Peninsula Hospital Center
51-15 Beach Channel Drive
Far Rockaway, New York 11691

Radiographer Program
Nassau Community College
Stewart Avenue
Garden City, New York 11530

Radiographer Program
The Community Hospital at Glen Cove
St. Andrews Lane
Glen Cove, New York 11542

Radiographer Program
Glens Falls Hospital
100 Park Street
Glens Falls, New York 12801

Radiographer Program
Long Island University
C. W. Post Campus
Northern Boulevard
Greenvale, New York 11548

Radiographer Program
St. James Mercy Hospital
411 Canisteo Street
Hornell, New York 14843

Radiographer Program
Tompkins Community Hospital
1205 Trumansburg Road
Ithaca, New York 14850

Radiographer Program
Catholic Medical Center
88-25 153rd Street
Jamaica, New York 11432

Radiographer Program
Women's Christian Association Hospital
207 Foote Avenue
Jamestown, New York 14701

Radiographer Program
Winthrop-University Hospital
259 First Street
Mineola, New York 11501

Radiographer Program
Bellevue Hospital Center
1st Avenue & 27th Street
New York, New York 10016

Radiographer Program
Northport VA Medical Center
Middleville Road
Northport, New York 11768

Radiographer Program
South Nassau Communities Hospital
2445 Oceanside Road
Oceanside, New York 11572

Radiographer Program
Champlain Valley Physicians Hosp Med Ctr.
Beekman Street
Plattsburgh, New York 12901

Radiographer Program
United Hospital
406 Boston Post Raod
Port Chester, New York 10573

Radiographer Program
Central Suffolk Hospital
1300 Roanoke Avenue
Riverhead, New York 11901

Radiographer Program
Monroe Community College
1000 E. Henrietta Road
Rochester, New York 14623

Radiographer Program
The Genesee Hospital
224 Alexander Street
Rochester, New York 14607

Radiographer Program
Mercy Hospital
1000 N. Village Avenue
Rockville Centre, New York 11570

Radiographer Program
North County Community College
20 Winona Ave., Box 89
Saranac Lake, New York 12983

Radiographer Program
SUNY Upstate Medical Center
155 Elizabeth Blackwell Street
Syracuse, New York 13210

Radiographer Program
Hudson Valley Community College
80 Vanderburgh Avenue
Troy, New York 12180

Radiographer Program
St. Elizabeth Hospital
2209 Genesee Street
Utica, New York 13501

Radiographer Program
St. Luke's Memorial Hospital Center
Champlin Avenue
P.O. Box 479
Utica, New York 13503-0479

Radiographer Program
Westchester Community College
75 Grasslands Road
Valhalla, New York 10595

NORTH CAROLINA

Radiographer Program
Asheville-Buncombe Technical College
340 Victoria Road
Asheville, North Carolina 28801

Radiographer Program
Sandhills Community College
Route 3, Box 182-C
Carthage, North Carolina 28327

Radiographer Program
University of North Carolina
103-C South Bldg. 005A
Chapel Hill, North Carolina 27514

Radiographer Program
Charlotte Memorial Hosp. & Medical Center
P.O. Box 32861
Charlotte, North Carolina 28232

Radiographer Program
Presbyterian Hospital
Box 33549 200 Hawthorne Lane
Charlotte, North Carolina 28233

Radiographer Program
Durham County General Hospital
3643 N. Roxboro Street
Durham, North Carolina 27704

Radiographer Program
Fayetteville Technical Institute
P.O. Box 35236
Fayetteville, North Carolina 28303-0236

Radiographer Program
Gaston Memorial Hospital, Inc.
2525 Court Drive
P.O. Box 1747
Gastonia, North Carolina 28054-1747

Radiographer Program
Moses H. Cone Memorial Hospital
1200 N. Elm Street
Greensboro, North Carolina 27401-1020

Radiographer Program
Pitt Community College
P.O. Drawer 7007 Hwy 11 S.
Greenville, North Carolina 27834-7007

Radiographer Program
Vance-Granville Community College
P.O. Box 917
Henderson, North Carolina 27536

Radiographer Program
Caldwell Community College & Tech Inst.
1000 Hickory Boulevard
Hudson, North Carolina 28638

Radiographer Program
Lenoir Memorial Hospital, Inc.
100 Airport Road
Kinston, North Carolina 28501

Radiographer Program
Carteret Technical College
3505 Arendell Street
Morehead City, North Carolina 28557

Radiographer Program
Wilkes General Hospital
P.O. Box 609
N. Wilkesboro, North Carolina 28659

Radiographer Program
Rex Hospital
4420 Lake Boone Trail
Raleigh, North Carolina 27607

Radiographer Program
Wake Technical College
9101 Fayetteville Road
Raleigh, North Carolina 27603

Radiographer Program
Rowan Technical College
P.O. Box 1595
Salisbury, North Carolina 28144

Radiographer Program
Cleveland Technical College
137 S. Post Road
Shelby, North Carolina 28150

Radiographer Program
Johnston Technical Institute
P.O. Box 2350
Smithfield, North Carolina 27577

Radiographer Program
Edgecombe Technical College
P.O. Box 550
Tarboro, North Carolina 27886

Radiographer Program
Forsyth Technical Institute
2100 Silas Creek Parkway
Winston-Salem, North Carolina 27103

NORTH DAKOTA

Radiographer Program
Medcenter One and Q & R Clinic
222 North 7th Street
Bismarck, North Dakota 58501

Radiographer Program
St. Alexius Medical Center
900 E Broadway
Box 1658
Bismarck, North Dakota 58501

Radiographer Program
St. Luke's Hospital
5th Street & Mills Avenue
Fargo, North Dakota 58122

Radiographer Program
United Hospital-Grand Forks Clinic
1000 S. Columbia Road
P.O. Box 6003
Grand Forks, North Dakota 58201

Radiographer Program
St. Joseph's Hospital
3rd St SE & Burdick Expressway
Minot, North Dakota 58701

Radiographer Program
Trinity Medical Center
Burdick Expressway at Main St.
Minot, North Dakota 58701

OHIO

Radiographer Program
Akron City Hospital
525 E. Market Street
Akron, Ohio 44309

Radiographer Program
Akron General Medical Center
400 Wabash Avenue
Akron, Ohio 44307

Radiographer Program
Children's Hospital Med. Center of Akron
281 Locust Street
Akron, Ohio 44308

Radiographer Program
St. Thomas Hospital Medical Center
444 North Main Street
Akron, Ohio 44310

Radiographer Program
Barberton Citizens Hospital
155 5th Street N.E.
Barberton, Ohio 44203

Radiographer Program
Aultman Hospital
2600 Sixth Street, S.W.
Canton, Ohio 44710

Radiographer Program
Timken Mercy Medical Center
1320 Timken Mercy Dr., N.W.
Canton, Ohio 44708

Radiographer Program
University of Cincinnati
Mail Location 63
Cincinnati, Ohio 45221-0063

Radiographer Program
Xavier University
3800 Victory Parkway
Cincinnati, Ohio 54207-1096

Radiographer Program
Cleveland Metropolitan General Hospital
3395 Scranton Road
Cleveland, Ohio 44109

Radiographer Program
Cuyahoga Community College
700 Carnegie Avenue
Cleveland, Ohio 44115

Radiographer Program
St. Alexis Hospital
5163 Broadway Avenue
Cleveland, Ohio 44127

Radiographer Program
University Hospitals of Cleveland
2074 Abington Road
Cleveland, Ohio 44106

Radiographer Program
Mt. Carmel Medical Center
793 W State Street
Columbus, Ohio 43222

Radiographer Program
Riverside Methodist Hospital
3535 Olentangy River Road
Columbus, Ohio 43214

Radiographer Program
The Ohio State University
190 N. Oval Mall
Columbus, Ohio 43210-1234

Radiographer Program
Sinclair Community College
444 W. Third Street
Dayton, Ohio 45402

Radiographer Program
Lorain County Community College
1005 North Abbee Road
Elyria, Ohio 44035

Radiographer Program
Euclid General Hospital
E. 185th & Lake Erie
Euclid, Ohio 44119

Radiographer Program
Marymount Hospital
12300 McCracken Road
Garfield Heights, Ohio 44125

Radiographer Program
Mercy Hospital
P.O. Box 418
Hamilton, Ohio 45012

Radiographer Program
Kettering College of Medical Arts
3535 Southern Boulevard
Kettering, Ohio 45429

Radiographer Program
Lancaster-Fairfield County Hospital
401 N Ewing Street
Lancaster, Ohio 43130

Radiographer Program
Lima Technical College
4240 Campus Drive
Lima, Ohio 45804

Radiographer Program
North Central Technical College
2441 Kenwood Circle
P.O. Box 698
Mansfield, Ohio 44901

Radiographer Program
Marietta Memorial Hospital
Ferguston Street
Marietta, Ohio 45750

Radiographer Program
Marion General Hospital
McKinley Park Drive
Marion, Ohio 43302

Radiographer Program
Hillcrest Hospital
6780 Mayfield Road
Mayfield Heights, Ohio 44124

Radiographer Program
Southwest General Hospital
18697 E. Bagley Road
Middleburg Heights, Ohio 44130

Radiographer Program
Middletown Regional Hospital
105 McKnight Drive
Middletown, Ohio 45044

Radiographer Program
Central Ohio Technical College
University Drive
Newark, Ohio 43055

Radiographer Program
Fisher-Titus Memorial Hospital
272 Benedict Avenue
Norwalk, Ohio 44857-2399

Radiographer Program
Shawnee State Community College
940 Second Street
Portsmouth, Ohio 45662

Radiographer Program
Robinson Memorial Hospital
6847 N. Chestnut Street
Ravenna, Ohio 44266

Radiographer Program
Richmond Heights General Hospital
27100 Chardon Road
Richmond Heights, Ohio 44143

Radiographer Program
Providence Hospital, Inc.
1912 Hayes Avenue
Sandusky, Ohio 44870

Radiographer Program
Community Hospital of Springfield & Clark City
2615 East High Street
Springfield, Ohio 45501

Radiographer Program
Jefferson Technical College
4000 Sunset Boulevard
Steubenville, Ohio 43952

Radiographer Program
Michael J. Owens Technical College
Caller-10,000 Oregon Road
Toledo, Ohio 43699-1947

Radiographer Program
St. Vincent Medical Center
2213 Cherry Street
Toledo, Ohio 43608

Radiographer Program
The Toledo Hospital
2142 North Cove Blvd.
Toledo, Ohio 43606

Radiographer Program
Trumbull Memorial Hospital
1350 E. Market Street
Warren, Ohio 44482

Radiographer Program
St. Elizabeth Hospital Medical Center
1044 Belmont Avenue
Youngstown, Ohio 44504

Radiographer Program
The Youngstown Hosp. Assoc-North Unit
345 Oak Hill Avenue
Youngstown, Ohio 44502

Radiographer Program
The Youngstown Hospital Association South Unit
345 Oak Hill Ave.
Youngstown, Ohio 44501

Radiographer Program
Muskingum Area Tech College
1555 Newark Road
Zanesville, Ohio 43701

OKLAHOMA

Radiographer Program
East Central Oklahoma State University
Ada, Oklahoma 74820

Radiographer Program
St. Mary's Hospital
305 S. Fifth Street
Enid, Oklahoma 73701

Radiographer Program
Comanche County Memorial Hospital
P.O. Box 129
Lawton, Oklahoma 73502

Radiographer Program
Rose State College
6420 S.E. 15th
Midwest City, Oklahoma 73110

Radiographer Program
Bacone College
Office of the President
Muskogee, Oklahoma 74403

Radiographer Program
Presbyterian Hospital
NE 13th St. at Lincoln Rd.
Oklahoma City, Oklahoma 73104

Radiographer Program
University of Oklahoma at Oklahoma City
P.O. Box 26901
Oklahoma City, Oklahoma 73190

Radiographer Program
Indian Meridian Area Voc Tech School
1313 S. Sangre Street
Stillwater, Oklahoma 74074

Radiographer Program
Tulsa City Area Voc Tech School-Dist-18
3420 S. Memorial Drive
Tulsa, Oklahoma 74145-1390

Radiographer Program
Tulsa Junior College
6111 E. Skelly Drive
Tulsa, Oklahoma 74135-6101

OREGON

Radiographer Program
Albany General Hospital
1046 W 6th Ave.
Albany, Oregon 97321

Radiographer Program
Oregon Institute of Technology
Oretech Branch PO
Klamath Falls, Oregon 97601

Radiographer Program
Portland Community College
12000 S.W. 49th Avenue
Portland, Oregon 97219

PENNSYLVANIA

Radiographer Program
Abington Memorial Hospital
1200 Old York Road
Abington, Pennsylvania 19001

Radiographer Program
Aliquippa Hospital
2500 Hospital Drive
Aliquippa, Pennsylvania 15001

Radiographer Program
Allentown Hospital Association
17th & Chew Streets
Allentown, Pennsylvania 18102

Radiographer Program
Altoona Hospital
7th & Howard Avenue
Altoona, Pennsylvania 16603

Radiographer Program
Mercy Hospital
2500 7th Avenue
Altoona, Pennsylvania 16603

Radiographer Program
Medical Center of Beaver City, Inc.
1000 Dutch Ridge Road
Beaver, Pennsylvania 15009

Radiographer Program
Northampton County Area Community College
3835 Green Pond Road
Bethlehem, Pennsylvania 18017

Radiographer Program
Bradford Hospital
116-156 Interstate Pkwy
Bradford, Pennsylvania 16701

Radiographer Program
Bryn Mawr Hospital
Bryn Mawr Avenue
Bryn Mawr, Pennsylvania 19010

Radiographer Program
Holy Spirit Hospital
North 21st Street
Camp Hill, Pennsylvania 17011

Radiographer Program
Carlisle Hospital
Box 310
Carlisle, Pennsylvania 17013

Radiographer Program
Crozer-Chester Medical Center
15th St. & Upland Avenue
Chester, Pennsylvania 19013

Radiographer Program
Sacred Heart Medical Center
Ninth & Wilson Streets
Chester, Pennsylvania 19013

Radiographer Program
Brandywine Hospital
201 Reeceville Road
Coatsville, Pennsylvania 19320

Radiographer Program
College Misericordia
Lake Street
Dallas, Pennsylvania 18612

Radiographer Program
Geisinger Medical Center
North Academy Avenue
Danville, Pennsylvania 17822

Radiographer Program
Doylestown Hospital
595 W. State Street
Doylestown, Pennsylvania 18901

Radiographer Program
Rolling Hill Hospital
60 E. Township Line Road
Elkins Park, Pennsylvania 19117

Radiographer Program
Gannon University
University Square
Erie, Pennsylvania 16541

Radiographer Program
Franklin Regional Medical Center
1 Spruce Street
Franklin, Pennsylvania 16323

Radiographer Program
Gwynedd-Mercy College
Sumneytown Pike
Gwynedd Valley, Pa 19437

Radiographer Program
Harrisburg Hospital
South Front Street
Harrisburg, Pennsylvania 17101

Radiographer Program
Polyclinic Medical Center
2601 N. Third Street
Harrisburg, Pennsylvania 17110

Radiographer Program
St. Joseph Medical Center
687 N. Church Street
Hazleton, Pennsylvania 18201

Radiographer Program
M.S. Hershey Medical Center Hospital
P.O. Box 850
500 University Drive
Hershey, Pennsylvania 17033

Radiographer Program
Monsour Medical Center
70 Lincoln Way East
Jeanette, Pennsylvania 15644

Radiographer Program
Conemaugh Valley Memorial Hospital
1086 Franklin Street
Johnstown, Pennsylvania 15905

Radiographer Program
Lee Hospital
320 Main Street
Johnstown, Pennsylvania 15901

Radiographer Program
Armstrong County Memorial Hospital
RR-8, Box 50
Kittanning, Pennsylvania 16201-8808

Radiographer Program
Lancaster General Hospital
555 North Duke Street
P.O. Box 3555
Lancaster, Pennsylvania 17603

Radiographer Program
St. Joseph Hospital & Health Care Center
250 College Avenue
P.O. Box 3509
Lancaster, Pennsylvania 17604

Radiographer Program
Robert Packer Hospital
Mansfield University
Mansfield, Pennsylvania 16933

Radiographer Program
RMC-Ohio Valley General Hospital
Heckel Road
Mc Kees Rocks, Pennsylvania 15136

Radiographer Program
Community College of Allegheny
Boyce Campus
595 Beatty Road
Monroeville, Pennsylvania 15146

Radiographer Program
Allegheny Valley Hospital
1301 Carlisle Street
Natrona Heights, Pennsylvania 15065

Radiographer Program
St. Francis Hospital of New Castle
Phillips & Mercer Street
New Castle, Pennsylvania 16101

Radiographer Program
The Pennsylvania State University
3550 Seventh Street Road
New Kensington, Pennsylvania 15068

Radiographer Program
Albert Einstein Medical Center-
Northern Division
York & Tabor Roads
Philadelphia, Pennsylvania 19141

Radiographer Program
Chestnut Hill Hospital
8835 Germantown Avenue
Philadelphia, Pennsylvania 19118

Radiographer Program
Community College of Philadelphia
1700 Spring Garden Street
Philadelphia, Pennsylvania 19130

Radiographer Program
Germantown Hospital & Medical Center
One Penn Boulevard
Philadelphia, Pennsylvania 19144

Radiographer Program
Hahnemann University
Broad & Vine Streets
Philadelphia, Pennsylvania 19102

Radiographer Program
Lankenau Hospital
Lancaster & City Line Avenues
Philadelphia, Pennsylvania 19151

Radiographer Program
Medical College of Pennsylvania
3300 Henry Avenue
Philadelphia, Pennsylvania 19129

Radiographer Program
Nazareth Hospital
2601 Holme Avenue
Philadelphia, Pennsylvania 19152

Radiographer Program
St. Joseph's Hospital
16th St. & Girard Avenue
Philadelphia, Pennsylvania 19130

Radiographer Program
Temple University Hospital
Broad St. & Montgomery Aves.
Philadelphia, Pennsylvania 19122

Radiographer Program
Thomas Jefferson University
Scott Bldg., 1020 Walnut St.
Philadelphia, Pennsylvania 19107

Radiographer Program
Montefiore Hospital
3459 Fifth Avenue
Pittsburgh, Pennsylvania 15213

Radiographer Program
Presbyterian-University Hospital
De Soto & O'Hara Streets
Pittsburgh, Pennsylvania 15213

Radiographer Program
Robert Morris College
Allegheny General Hospital
320 E. North Avenue
Pittsburgh, Pennsylvania 15212

Radiographer Program
Community General Hospital
145 N. Sixth Street
Reading, Pennsylvania 19601

Radiographer Program
Reading Hospital and Medical Center
Reading, Pennsylvania 19603

Radiographer Program
Saint Joseph Hospital
12th & Walnut Streets
Box 316
Reading, Pennsylvania 19603

Radiographer Program
Community Medical Center
1822 Mulberry Street
Scranton, Pennsylvania 18510

Radiographer Program
Scranton State General Hospital
205 Mulberry Street
Scranton, Pennsylvania 18501

Radiographer Program
Sewickley Valley Hospital
Blackburn Road
Sewickley, Pennsylvania 15143

Radiographer Program
Sharon General Hospital
740 E. State Street
Sharon, Pennsylvania 16146

Radiographer Program
Somerset Community Hospital
225 S. Center Avenue
Somerset, Pennsylvania 15501

Radiographer Program
Lyons Technical Institute, Inc.
67 Long Lane
Upper Darby, Pennsylvania 19082

Radiographer Program
Washington Hospital
155 Wilson Avenue
Washington, Pennsylvania 15301

Radiographer Program
Wilkes-Barre General Hospital
N. River & Auburn Streets
Wilkes-Barre, Pennsylvania 18764

Radiographer Program
Willamsport Area Community College
1005 W. Third Street
Williamsport, Pennsylvania 17701

Radiographer Program
York Hospital
1001 S. George St.
York, Pennsylvania 17405

PUERTO RICO

Radiographer Program
Universidad Central del Caribe
P.O. Box 935
Cayey, Puerto Rico 00634

Radiographer Program
University of Puerto Rico
GPO Box 5067
San Juan, Puerto Rico 00936

RHODE ISLAND

Radiographer Program
Community College of Rhode Island
Louisquisset Pike
Lincoln, Rhode Island 02865

SOUTH CAROLINA

Radiographer Program
Anderson Memorial Hospital
800 North Fant Street
Anderson, South Carolina 29621

Radiographer Program
Trident Technical College
P.O. Box 10367
Charleston, South Carolina 29411

Radiographer Program
Baptist Medical Center at Columbia
Taylor at Marion St.
Columbia, South Carolina 29220

Radiographer Program
Midlands Technical College
P.O. Box 2408
Columbia, South Carolina 29202

Radiographer Program
Florence-Darlington Tech College
P.O. Drawer F-8000
Florence, South Carolina 29501

Radiographer Program
Greenville Technical College
P.O. Box 5616-Station B
Greenville, South Carolina 29606-5616

Radiographer Program
Piedmont Technical College
P.O. Drawer 1467
Emerald Road
Greenwood, South Carolina 29646

Radiographer Program
Orangeburg-Calhoun Tech College
3250 St. Matthews Rd.
Orangeburg, South Carolina 29115

Radiographer Program
Piedmont Medical Center
222 S. Herlong Avenue
Rock Hill, South Carolina 29730

Radiographer Program
Spartanburg Technical College
P.O. Drawer 4386
Spartanburg, South Carolina 29305

SOUTH DAKOTA

Radiographer Program
St. Luke's Hospital
305 S. State Street
Aberdeen, South Dakota 57401

Radiographer Program
St. Joseph Hospital
5th & Foster
Mitchell, South Dakota 57301

Radiographer Program
Rapid City Regional Hospital, Inc.
353 Fairmont Boulevard
Rapid City, South Dakota 57709

Radiographer Program
McKennan Hospital
800 E. 21st Street
Sioux Falls, South Dakota 57101

Radiographer Program
Sioux Valley Hospital
1100 S. Euclid Avenue
P.O. Box 5039
Sioux Falls, South Dakota 57117-5039

Radiographer Program
Sacred Heart Hospital
501 Summit Street
Yankton, South Dakota 57078

TENNESSEE

Radiographer Program
Chattanooga State Tech Community College
4501 Amnicola Hwy
Chattanooga, Tennessee 37406

Radiographer Program
Columbia State Community College
P.O. Box 1315
Columbia, Tennessee 38401

Radiographer Program
East Tennessee State University
Box 24, 520 A
Johnson City, Tennessee 37614

Radiographer Program
Roane State Community College
Patton Lane
Harriman, Tennessee 37748

Radiographer Program
Jackson State Community College
P.O. Box 2467
Jackson, Tennessee 38302

Radiographer Program
East Tennessee Baptist Hospital
P.O. Box 1788
Knoxville, Tennessee 37901

Radiographer Program
University of Tennessee Memorial Hospital
1924 Alcoa Highway
Knoxville, Tennessee 37920

Radiographer Program
Blount Memorial Hospital
9000 New Walland Highway
Maryville, Tennessee 37801

Radiographer Program
Baptist Memorial Hospital
899 Madison Avenue
Memphis, Tennessee 38146

Radiographer Program
Methodist Hospital of Memphis
1265 Union Avenue
Memphis, Tennessee 38104

Radiographer Program
Shelby State Community College
1256 Union Avenue
P.O. Box 40568
Memphis, Tennessee 38174-0568

Radiographer Program
St. Joseph Hospital
220 Overton Ave. Box 178
Memphis, Tennessee 38105

Radiographer Program
Aquinas Junior College
4210 Harding Road
Nashville, Tennessee 37205

Radiographer Program
Metropolitan Nashville General Hospital
72 Hermitage Avenue
Nashville, Tennessee 37210

TEXAS

Radiographer Program
Hendrick Medical Center
19th & Hickory Streets
Abilene, Texas 79601

Radiographer Program
Amarillo College
P.O. Box 447
Amarillo, Texas 79178

Radiographer Program
Austin Community College
P.O. Box 2285
Austin, Texas 78768

Radiographer Program
San Jacinto Methodist Hospital
1101 Decker Drive
Baytown, Texas 77521

Radiographer Program
Lamar University
P.O. Box 10001
Beaumont, Texas 77710

Radiographer Program
The Baptist Hospital of SE Texas, Inc.
P.O. Drawer 1591
Beaumont, Texas 77704

Radiographer Program
Malone-Hogan Hospital
1601 W. 11th Place
Big Spring, Texas 79720

Radiographer Program
Texas Southmost College
80 Fort Brown
Brownsville, Texas 78520

Radiographer Program
Del Mar College
Baldwin & Ayers
Corpus Christi, Texas 78404

Radiographer Program
Baylor University Medical Center
3500 Gaston Avenue
Dallas, Texas 75246

Radiographer Program
El Centro College
Main & Lamar
Dallas, Texas 75202-3604

Radiographer Program
Parkland Memorial Hospital
5201 Harry Hines Blvd.
Dallas, Texas 75235

Radiographer Program
El Paso Community College
P.O. Box 20500
El Paso, Texas 79998

Radiographer Program
Academy of Health Sciences
Brooke Army Medical Center
Fort Sam Houston, Texas 78234-6200

Radiographer Program
All Saints Episcopal Hospital
1400 8th Avenue
P.O. Box 31
Forth Worth, Texas 76104-0031

Radiographer Program
Galveston College
The University of Texas
4015 Avenue Q
Galveston, Texas 77550

Radiographer Program
Houston Community College System
22 Waugh Drive
P.O. Box 7849
Houston, Texas 77270-7849

Radiographer Program
Memorial Hospital System
7777 SW Freeway
Houston, Texas 77074

Radiographer Program
University of Texas
School of Allied Health Sciences
P.O. Box 20036
Houston, Texas 77225

Radiographer Program
Tarrant County Junior College
828 Harwood Road
Hurst, Texas 76054

Radiographer Program
Laredo Junior College
West End Washington St.
Laredo, Texas 78040

Radiographer Program
The Good Shepard Hospital
621 N. Fifth Street
Longview, Texas 75601

Radiographer Program
Methodist Hospital
3615 19th Street
Lubbock, Texas 79410

Radiographer Program
South Plains College At Lubbock
1401 College Avenue
Levelland, Texas 79336

Radiographer Program
Angelina College
P.O. Box 1768
Lufkin, Texas 75901

Radiographer Program
Odessa College
201 W. University
Odessa, Texas 79764

Radiographer Program
San Jacinto College Central
8060 Spencer Hwy
P.O. Box 2007
Pasadena, Texas 77505-2007

Radiographer Program
Baptist Memorial Hospital System
111 Dallas Street
San Antonio, Texas 78286

Radiographer Program
St. Philip's College
2111 Nevada Street
San Antonio, Texas 78203

Radiographer Program
Wadley Regional Medical Center
1000 Pine Street
Texarkana, Texas 75501

Radiographer Program
Tyler Junior College
E. 5th Street, Box 9020
Tyler, Texas 75711

Radiographer Program
Citizens Memorial Hospital
2701 Hospital Drive
Victoria, Texas 77901

Radiographer Program
McLennan Community College
1400 College Drive
Waco, Texas 76708

Radiographer Program
Wharton County Junior College
911 Boling Highway
Wharton, Texas 77488

Radiographer Program
Midwestern State University
3400 Taft Boulevard
Wichita Falls, Texas 76308

Radiographer Program
School of Health Care Sciences, USAF
Sheppard AFB, Texas 76311-5465

UTAH

Radiographer Program
Weber State College
MS 1001
Ogden, Utah 84408

Radiographer Program
Utah Valley Hospital
1034 N. 5th West
Provo, Utah 84601

Radiographer Program
St. Mark's Hospital
1200 E. 3900 S.
Salt Lake City, Utah 84601

Radiographer Program
University of Utah
Park Building
Salt Lake City, Utah 84132

VERMONT

Radiographer Program
University of Vermont
349 Waterman Bldg.
Burlington, Vermont 05405

Radiographer Program
Rutland Regional Medical Center
160 Allen Street
Rutland, Vermont 05701

VIRGINIA

Radiographer Program
Northern Virginia Community College
8333 Little River Turnpike
Annandale, Virginia 22003

Radiographer Program
University of Virginia Medical Center
Box 148 M4
Charlottesville, Virginia 22908

Radiographer Program
Alleghany Regional Hospital
P.O. Box 627
Clifton Forge, Virginia 24422

Radiographer Program
The Memorial Hospital
142 S. Main Street
Danville, Virginia 24541

Radiographer Program
Rockingham Memorial Hospital
235 Cantrell Avenue
Harrisonburg, Virginia 22801

Radiographer Program
Central Virginia Community College
3506 Wards Road
Lynchburg, Virginia 24502

Radiographer Program
Newport News Public School
Riverside Hospital
500 J. Clyde Morris Blvd.
Newport News, Virginia 23601

Radiographer Program
DePaul Hospital
150 Kingsley Lane
Norfolk, Virginia 23505

Radiographer Program
Norfolk General Hospital
600 Gresham Drive
Norfolk, Virginia 23507

Radiographer Program
Petersburg General Hospital
801 S. Adams Street
Petersburg, Virginia 23803

Radiographer Program
Maryview Hospital
3636 High Street
Portsmouth, Virginia 23707

Radiographer Program
Naval School of Health Sciences
Naval Hospital
Bethesda Detachmen
Portsmouth, Virginia 23708-5000

Radiographer Program
Southwest Virginia Community College
P.O. Box SVCC
Richlands, Virginia 24641-1510

Radiographer Program
Medical College of Virginia
Virginia Commonwealth University
910 West Franklin Street
Richmond, Virginia 23284

Radiographer Program
St. Mary's Hospital
5801 Bremo Road
Richmond, Virginia 23226

Radiographer Program
Roanoke Memorial Hospital
P.O. Box 13367
Roanoke, Virginia 24033

Radiographer Program
Virginia Western Community College
3095 Colonial Ave., S.W.
Roanoke, Virginia 24038

Radiographer Program
Tidewater Community College
Portsmouth, Virginia 23703

Radiographer Program
Winchester Medical Center, Inc.
South Stewart Street
Winchester, Virginia 22601

WASHINGTON

Radiographer Program
Bellevue Community College
P.O. Box 92700
Bellevue, Washington 98009-2037

Radiographer Program
Holy Family Hospital
N. 5633 Lidgerwood Ave.
Spokane, Washington 92207

Radiographer Program
Tacoma Community College
5900 S. 12th Street
Tacoma, Washington 98465

Radiographer Program
Wenatchee Valley College
1300 Fifth Street
Wenatchee, Washington 98801

Radiographer Program
Yakima Valley College
P.O. Box 1647
Yakima, Washington 98907

WEST VIRGINIA

Radiographer Program
Bluefield State College
Rock Street
Bluefield, West Virginia 24701

Radiographer Program
University of Charleston
2300 McCorkle Ave., S.E.
Charleston, West Virginia 25304

Radiographer Program
United Hospital Center
3 Hospital Plaza
Clarksburg, West Virginia 26301

Radiographer Program
St. Mary's Hospital
2900 1st Avenue
Huntington, West Virginia 25702

Radiographer Program
West Virginia University Hospital
Medical Center Drive
P.O. Box 6401
Morgantown, West Virginia 26506-6401

Radiographer Program
Camden Clark Memorial Hospital
800 Garfield Avenue
Parkersburg, West Virginia 26101

Radiographer Program
Ohio Valley Medical Center, Inc.
2000 Eoff Street
Wheeling, West Virginia 26003

Radiographer Program
Wheeling Hospital, Inc.
Medical Park
Wheeling, West Virginia 26003

WISCONSIN

Radiographer Program
Beliot Memorial Hospital
1969 W. Hart Road
Beliot, Wisconsin 53511

Radiographer Program
Luther Hospital
1221 Whipple Street
Eau Claire, Wisconsin 54702-4105

Radiographer Program
VTAE District One Tech Institute
620 W. Clairemont Avenue
Eau Claire, Wisconsin 54701

Radiographer Program
Bellin Memorial Hospital
744 S. Webster Avenue
Green Bay, Wisconsin 54305

Radiographer Program
St. Catherine's Hospital
3556 7th Avenue
Kenosha, Wisconsin 53140

Radiographer Program
Western Wisconsin Technical Institute
304 N. 6th Street
P.O. Box 908
La Crosse, Wisconsin 54602-0908

Radiographer Program
Madison General Hospital
School of Radiologic Technology
202 S. Park Street
Madison, Wisconsin 53715

Radiographer Program
St. Mary's Hospital Medical Center
707 S. Mills Street
Madison, Wisconsin 53715

Radiographer Program
St. Anges Hospital
430 E. Division Street
Fond du Lac, Wisconsin 54935

Radiographer Program
University Hospital School of Rad Tech
600 Highland Avenue
Madison, Wisconsin 53792

Radiographer Program
St. Joseph's Hospital
6121 St. Joseph's Avenue
Marshfield, Wisconsin 54449

Radiographer Program
Clement J. Zablocki VA Medical Center
5000 W. National Avenue
Milwaukee, Wisconsin 53193

Radiographer Program
Columbia Hospital
2025 E. Newport Avenue
Milwaukee, Wisconsin 53211

Radiographer Program
Family Hospital
2711 W. Wells Street
Milwaukee, Wisconsin 53208

Radiographer Program
Good Samaritan Medical Center
Deaconess Hospital Campus
2200 W. Kilbourn Avenue
Milwaukee, Wisconsin 53233

Radiographer Program
Milwaukee Area Technical College
1015 N. Sixth Street
Milwaukee, Wisconsin 53203

Radiographer Program
Milwaukee Area Technical College
1015 N. Sixth Street
Milwaukee, Wisconsin 53203

Radiographer Program
Milwaukee County Medical Complex
8700 West Wisconsin Avenue
Milwaukee, Wisconsin 53226

Radiographer Program
St. Luke's Hospital
2900 W. Oklahoma Ave.
Milwaukee, Wisconsin 53215

Radiographer Program
St. Mary's Hospital
2323 N. Lake Drive
P.O. Box 503
Milwaukee, Wisconsin 53201

Radiographer Program
St. Michael Hospital
2400 W. Villard Avenue
Milwaukee, Wisconsin 53209

Radiographer Program
Theda Clark Regional Medical Center
130 Second Street
Neenah, Wisconsin 54956

Radiographer Program
Mercy Medical Center
631 Hazel Street
Oshkosh, Wisconsin 54902

Radiographer Program
St. Luke's Memorial Hospital
1320 S. Wisconsin Avenue
Racine, Wisconsin 53403

Radiographer Program
St. Mary's Medical Center
3801 Spring Street
Racine, Wisconsin 53405

Radiographer Program
North Central Technical Institute
1000 Campus Drive
Wausau, Wisconsin 54401

WYOMING

Radiographer Program
Casper College
125 College Drive
Casper, Wyoming 82601

Radiographer Program
Laramie County Community College
1400 E. College Drive
Cheyenne, Wyoming 82007

Radiographer Program
West Park Hospital
707 Sheridan Avenue
Cody, Wyoming 82414

Radiographer Program
Western Wyoming College
2500 College Drive
P.O. Box 428
Rock Springs, Wyoming 82901

Radiation Therapy Technologist

As part of the cancer treatment team, which may include physicians, nurses, radiologists, oncologists (physicians who specialize in treating cancer), and clinical physicists, the *radiation therapy technologist* uses radiation producing equipment to treat, mainly, cancer patients. Radiation therapy may be used separately or in combination with surgery or drug therapy (chemotherapy). After positioning the patient and the equipment, the technologist is directed by the radiologist to administer prescribed concentrations of X-rays or other forms of ionizing radiation to the diseased areas of the patient's body. Different levels of radiation, including alpha, beta, gamma, neutron, and X-rays are used, depending upon the treatment required. The technologist sets the controls for a specific intensity and exposure time, and monitors these controls throughout the duration of the treatment. Throughout the procedure the technologist is responsible for the safety of the patient and the other medical personnel. The technologist also assists in the preparation and handling of the radioactive materials used in therapy, keeps records of all treatments, and maintains equipment. Radiation therapy technologists work mainly in cancer treatment centers or large hospitals.

There are currently two types of approved educational programs in radiation therapy technology. Admission into the twelve month program generally requires that the applicant be either a graduate of an approved radiologic technology program or a registered nurse. Other health professionals wishing to apply to these programs should contact the program director for specific requirements. Admission into the twenty-four month program requires that the applicant be a high school graduate or equivalent, with an acceptable background in basic sciences and mathematics. Graduates of approved educational programs in radiation therapy technology may become certified by the American Registry of Radiologic Technologists. Certification is granted to radiation therapy technologists after graduating from a radiation therapy program accredited by the American Medical Association's Committee on Allied Health Education and Accreditation, and successfully passing a qualifying examination. Some states require radiation therapy technologists to be licensed. For additional information on certification, contact the American Registry of Radiologic Technologists, 2600 Wayzata Boulevard, Minneapolis, Minnesota 55405.

With advanced education and/or work experience, radiation therapy technologists may move into managerial positions.

Recommended high school subjects include algebra, geometry, physics, chemistry, biology and computer science.

According to a recent survey conducted by the University of Texas Medical Branch, starting salaries for certified radiation therapy technologists averaged $19,000, while those with experience earned approximately $26,000.

Listed below are college, university and hospital based programs approved by the American Medical Association's Committee on Health, Education and Accreditation. Contact the program directly for entrance requirements, length of program and type of certificate/degree awarded.

For more information as a radiation therapy technologist, write to the American Society of Radiologic Technologists, 15000 Central Avenue, S.E., Albuquerque, New Mexico 87123.

SOURCES:

American Society of Radiologic Technologists
American Registry of Radiologic Technologists
Occupational Outlook Handbook

Radiation Therapy Technologist Programs

ALABAMA

Radiation Therapy Technologist Program
The University of Alabama at Birmingham
University Station
Birmingham, Alabama 35294

Radiation Therapy Technologist Program
Mobile Infirmary Medical Center
P.O. Box 2144
Mobile, Alabama 36652

ARIZONA

Radiation Therapy Technologist Program
University Medical Center
1501 N. Campbell Avenue
Tucson, Arizona 85724

ARKANSAS

Radiation Therapy Technologist Program
CARTI-School of Radiation Therapy Tech
P.O. Box 5210
Little Rock, Arkansas 72215

CALIFORNIA

Radiation Therapy Technologist Program
Orange Coast College
2701 Fairview Road
Costa Mesa, California 92628-0120

Radiation Therapy Technologist Program
City of Hope National Medical Center
1500 East Duarte Road
Duarte, California 91010

Radiation Therapy Technologist Program
Loma Linda University
School of Allied Health Professions
Loma Linda, California 92350

Radiation Therapy Technologist Program
Foothill Community College
12345 El Monte Road
Los Altos Hills, California 94022

Radiation Therapy Technologist Program
Los Angeles County-USC Medical Center
1200 N. State Street
Los Angeles, California 90033

Radiation Therapy Technologist Program
Radiological Associates of Sacramento
1800 'I' Street
Sacramento, California 95814

Radiation Therapy Technologist Program
University of California Medical Center, San Diego
225 W. Dickinson, H-910
San Diego, California 92103

Radiation Therapy Technologist Program
City College of San Francisco
50 Phelan Avenue
San Francisco, Califronia 94112

Radiation Therapy Technologist Program
Cancer Foundation of Santa Barbara
300 W. Pueblo Street
P.O. Box 837
Santa Barbara, California 93105

COLORADO

Radiation Therapy Technologist Program
Community College of Denver-Auraria Campus
1068 Ninth Street, Box 250
Denver, Colorado 80204

CONNECTICUT

Radiation Therapy Technologist Program
South Central Community College
60 Sargent Drive
New Haven, Connecticut 06511

DISTRICT OF COLUMBIA

Radiation Therapy Technologist Program
George Washington University Medical Center
2121 Eye Street, N.W., Suite 800
Washington, DC 20037

Radiation Therapy Technologist Program
Howard University
2400 6th Street, N.W.
Washington, DC 20059

FLORIDA

Radiation Therapy Technologist Program
Halifax Hospital Medical Center
303 N C Morris Boulevard
P.O. Box 1990
Daytona Beach, Florida 32015

Radiation Therapy Technologist Program
Broward Community College
225 East Las Olas Blvd.
Fort Lauderdale, Florida 33301

Radiation Therapy Technologist Program
St. Vincent's Medical Center
1800 Barrs Street
P.O. Box 2982
Jacksonville, Florida 32203

Radiation Therapy Technologist Program
Jackson Memorial Medical Center
University of Miami
1611 N.W. 12th Avenue
Miami, Florida 33136

Radiation Therapy Technologist Program
Hillsborough Community College
P.O. Box 22127
Tampa, Florida 33630

GEORGIA

Radiation Therapy Technologist Program
Grady Memorial Hospital
80 Butler Street S.E.
Atlanta, Georgia 30335

Radiation Therapy Technologist Program
St. Joseph Hospital
5665 Peachtree-Dunwoody Rd. N.E.
Atlanta, Georgia 30342

Radiation Therapy Technologist Program
Medical College of Georgia
Office of the President, AA-31
Augusta, Georgia 30912-0450

IDAHO

Radiation Therapy Technologist Program
St. Luke's Regional Medical Center
190 East Bannock
Boise, Idaho 83712

ILLINOIS

Radiation Therapy Technologist Program
Chicago State University
95th & King Drive
Chicago, Illinois 60628

Radiation Therapy Technologist Program
Michael Reese Hospital & Medical Center
29th South Ellis
Chicago, Illinois 60616

Radiation Therapy Technologist Program
St. Joseph Hospital
77 North Airlite Street
Elgin, Illinois 60120

Radiation Therapy Technologist Program
National College of Education
2840 Sheridan Road
Evanston, Illinois 60201

Radiation Therapy Technologist Program
Edward Hines Jr. VA Hospital
Fifth Ave. & Roosevelt Road
Hines, Illinois 60141

Radiation Therapy Technologist Program
Swedish American Hospital
1400 Charles Street
Rockford, Illinois 61108

INDIANA

Radiation Therapy Technologist Program
Memorial Hospital
615 N. Michigan Avenue
South Bend, Indiana 46601

Radiation Therapy Technologist Program
Deaconess Hospital, Inc.
600 Mary Street
Evansville, Indiana 47747

Radiation Therapy Technologist Program
Indiana University School of Medicine
1120 South Drive
Indianapolis, Indiana 46223

IOWA

Radiation Therapy Technologist Program
University of IA Hospitals and Clinics
State Health Affairs C107 GH
Iowa City, Iowa 52242-1059

KANSAS

Radiation Therapy Technologist Program
Washburn University of Topeka
1700 College
Topeka, Kansas 66621

Radiation Therapy Technologist Program
University of Kansas Medical Center
39th & Rainbow Blvd.
Kansas City, Kansas 66103

KENTUCKY

Radiation Therapy Technologist Program
University of Kentucky
103 Administration Bldg.
Lexington, Kentucky 40506-0032

Radiation Therapy Technologist Program
St. Anthony Hospital
1313 St. Anthony Place
Louisville, Kentucky 40204

LOUISIANA

Radiation Therapy Technologist Program
Mercy Hospital
301 N. Jefferson Davis Pkwy.
New Orleans, Louisiana 70119

MAINE

Radiation Therapy Technologist Program
Southern Maine Voc Tech Institute
Fort Road
South Portland, Maine 04106

MARYLAND

Radiation Therapy Technologist Program
Essex Community College-John Hopkins Hospital
7201 Rossville Boulevard
Baltimore, Maryland 21237

MASSACHUSETTS

Radiation Therapy Technologist Program
Middlesex Community College
Springs Road
Bedford, Massachusetts 01730

Radiation Therapy Technologist Program
Catherine Labourne College
2120 Dorchester Avenue
Boston, Massachusetts 02124

Radiation Therapy Technologist Program
Springfield Tech Community College
1 Armory Square
Springfield, Massachusetts 01105

MICHIGAN

Radiation Therapy Technologist Program
University of Michigan Hospitals
1405 East Ann Street
Ann Arbor, Michigan 48109

Radiation Therapy Technologist Program
Henry Ford Hospital
2799 W. Grand Boulevard
Detroit, Michigan 48202

Radiation Therapy Technologist Program
Wayne State University
1142 Mackenzie Hall
Detroit, Michigan 48202

Radiation Therapy Technologist Program
Lansing Community College
419 N. Capitol Ave., Box 40010
Lansing, Michigan 48901-7211

MINNESOTA

Radiation Therapy Technologist Program
University of Minnesota Health Science Center
213 Morrill Hall
Minneapolis, Minnesota 55455

Radiation Therapy Technologist Program
Mayo Clinic Foundation
200 First Street, S.W.
Rochester, Minnesota 55905

MISSOURI

Radiation Therapy Technologist Program
St. Luke's Hospital of Kansas City
Wornall Road at 4th
Kansas City, Missouri 64111

Radiation Therapy Technologist Program
Mallinckrodt Inst. of Rad-Washingtion University
510 S. Kingshighway Blvd.
St. Louis, Missouri 63110

NEBRASKA

Radiation Therapy Technologist Program
University of Nebraska Medical Center
42 & Dewey Avenue
Omaha, Nebraska 68105

NEW JERSEY

Radiation Therapy Technologist Program
Cooper Hospital University Medical Center
One Cooper Plaza
Camden, New Jersey 08103

Radiation Therapy Technologist Program
St. Barnabas Medical Center
94 Old Short Hills Rd.
Livingston, New Jersey 07039

NEW YORK

Radiation Therapy Technologist Program
Montefiore Hospital & Medical Center
111 E. 210th Street
Bronx, New York 10467

Radiation Therapy Technologist Program
Erie Community College
121 Ellicott Street
Buffalo, New York 14202

Radiation Therapy Technologist Program
Nassau Community College
Stewart Avenue
Garden City, New York 11530

Radiation Therapy Technologist Program
Memorial Sloan Kettering Cancer Center
1275 York Avenue
New York, New York 10021

Radiation Therapy Technologist Program
New York University Medical Center
550 First Avenue
New York, New York 10016

Radiation Therapy Technologist Program
The University of Rochester Cancer Center
Box 647, 601 Elmwood Ave.
Rochester, New York 14642

Radiation Therapy Technologist Program
SUNY Upstate Medical Center
155 Elizabeth Blackwell St.
Syracuse, New York 13210

NORTH CAROLINA

Radiation Therapy Technologist Program
North Carolina Memorial Hospital
Manning Drive
Chapel Hill, North Carolina 27514

OHIO

Radiation Therapy Technologist Program
Aultman Hospital
2600 Sixth Street, S.W.
Canton, Ohio 44710

Radiation Therapy Technologist Program
University of Cincinnati
Mail Location 63
Cincinnati, Ohio 45221-0063

Radiation Therapy Technologist Program
Cleveland Clinic Foundation
9500 Euclid Avenue
Cleveland, Ohio 44106

Radiation Therapy Technologist Program
Michael J. Owens Technical College
Caller-10,000 Oregon Road
Toledo, Ohio 43699-1947

OKLAHOMA

Radiation Therapy Technologist Program
University of Oklahoma at Oklahoma City
P.O. Box 26901
Oklahoma City, Oklahoma 73190

OREGON

Radiation Therapy Technologist Program
Oregon Health Sciences University
3181 S.W. Sam Jackson Pk. Rd.
Portland, Oregon 97201

PENNSYLVANIA

Radiation Therapy Technologist Program
Mercy Hospital
2500 Seventh Avenue
Altoona, Pennsylvania 16603

Radiation Therapy Technologist Program
Geisinger Medical Center
North Academy Avenue
Danville, Pennsylvania 17822

Radiation Therapy Technologist Program
Gwynedd-Mercy College
Sumneytown Pike
Gwynedd Valley, Pennsylvania 19437

Radiation Therapy Technologist Program
Community College of Allegheny
County-Allegheny Campus
808 Ridge Avenue
Pittsburgh, Pennsylvania 15212

RHODE ISLAND

Radiation Therapy Technologist Program
Rhode Island Hospital
593 Eddy Street
Providence, Rhode Island 02902

SOUTH CAROLINA

Radiation Therapy Technologist Program
Medical University of South Carolina
171 Ashley Avenue
Charleston, South Carolina 29425

TENNESSEE

Radiation Therapy Technologist Program
Baptist Memorial Hospital
899 Madison Avenue
Memphis, Tennessee 38146

Radiation Therapy Technologist Program
Vanderbilt University Medical Center
21st & Garland
Nashville, Tennessee 37232

TEXAS

Radiation Therapy Technologist Program
Amarillo College
P.O. Box 447
Amarillo, Texas 79178

Radiation Therapy Technologist Program
Allen Shivers Radiation Therapy Center
2600 E. Martin Luther King Blvd.
Austin, Texas 78702

Radiation Therapy Technologist Program
Baylor University Medical Center
3500 Gaston Avenue
Dallas, Texas 75246

Radiation Therapy Technologist Program
El Paso Community College
P.O. Box 20500
El Paso, Texas 79998

Radiation Therapy Technologist Program
Moncrief Radiation Center
1450 8th Avenue
Fort Worth, Texas 76104

Radiation Therapy Technologist Program
Galveston College
The University of Texas
4015 Avenue Q
Galveston, Texas 77550

Radiation Therapy Technologist Program
M.D. Anderson Hospital & Tumor Institute
6723 Bertner Avenue
Houston, Texas 77030

Radiation Therapy Technologist Program
Methodist Hospital
3615 19th Street
Lubbock, Texas 79410

Radiation Therapy Technologist Program
Cancer Therapy & Research Center
4450 Medical Drive
San Antonio, Texas 78229

VIRGINIA

Radiation Therapy Technologist Program
Norfolk General Hospital
600 Gresham Drive
Norfolk, Virginia 23507

Radiation Therapy Program
Norfolk General Hospital
600 Gresham Drive
Norfolk, Virginia 23507

Radiation Therapy Technologist Program
Medical College of Virginia
Virginia Commonwealth University
910 West Franklin Street
Richmond, Virginia 23284

Radiation Therapy Technologist Program
Roanoke Memorial Hospital
P.O. Box 13367
Roanoke, Virginia 24033

WASHINGTON

Radiation Therapy Technologist Program
Laboratory of Pathology of Seattle, Inc.
747 Summit Avenue
Seattle, Washington 98104

WEST VIRGINIA

Radiation Therapy Technologist Program
West Virginia University Hospital
Medical Center Drive
P.O. Box 6401
Morgantown, West Virginia 26506-6401

WISCONSIN

Radiation Therapy Technologist Program
University of Wisconsin-Madison
Bascom Hall
Madison, Wisconsin 53706

Radiation Therapy Technologist Program
Medical College of Wisconsin
8700 Watertown Plank Road
Milwaukee, Wisconsin 53226

Radiation Therapy Technologist Program
St. Joseph's Hospital
5000 W. Chambers Street
Milwaukee, Wisconsin 53210

UTAH

Radiation Therapy Technologist Program
Weber State College
M S 1001
Ogden, Utah 84408

Radiation Therapy Technologist Program
LDS Hospital
325 8th Avenue
Salt Lake City, Utah 84143

Radiation Therapy Technologist Program
University of Utah
Park Building
Salt Lake City, Utah 84132

VERMONT

Radiation Therapy Technologist Program
University of Vermont
349 Waterman Bldg.
Burlington, Vermont 05405

VIRGINIA

Radiation Therapy Technologist Program
University of Virginia Medical Center
Box 148 M4
Charlottesville, Virginia 22908

Nuclear Medicine Technology

Nuclear medicine technology is the allied health specialty concerned with the use of radioactive materials for diagnostic purposes.

One of two such diagnostic procedures is organ imaging, where a radioactive material (a radiopharmaceutical) is administered orally or intravenously to a patient. The radiopharmaceutical accumulates in a specific tissue or an organ, such as the brain, liver, kidney, etc., or a lump, and emits radiation that can be detected as a "picture" on a scanner video screen. Often the video screens are connected to a computer which can sort and process large amounts of data.

Some common types of nuclear medicine tests include scans of the bones, liver, lungs, and heart. Using adjusted prescribed dosages of radiation, nuclear medicine technologists perform nuclear medicine tests for children, adults and the elderly.

The second diagnostic procedure involves radioactive analysis of biologic specimens, such as blood or urine collected from a patient. The specimen is mixed with radioactive materials to measure presence and amounts of hormones, drugs, blood constituents and other components.

A third use of radioactive material in nuclear medicine technology is the therapeutic application to patients in treatment of specific diseased organs or tissues, without exposing normal tissues to radiation. For example, radioactive iodine may be administered to a patient who has a thyroid condition. The thyroid will trap the iodine and control the disease without giving excessive radiation to normal tissue.

The allied health career that employs nuclear medicine technology is the *nuclear medicine technologist.*

Nuclear Medicine Technologist

Under supervision of a radiologist, the *nuclear medicine technologist* assists with the administration and detection of radioactive materials in diagnosis and therapy. The technologist verifies patients' records, prepares and administers the radiopharmaceutical in prescribed dosages, positions the patient for imaging procedures, and operates the nuclear instruments. The technologist prepares the results and presents them to the radiologist. In therapy, the nuclear medicine technologist administers radioactive materials to treat specific diseases, and is responsible for the protection of the patient and medical personnel from excessive radiation.

The technologist is careful about radiation safety and quality control. He or she keeps inventory of the radiopharmaceuticals and is responsible for their safe storage and use and for the disposal of radioactive waste. Although mainly employed in large hospitals, nuclear medicine technologists also work in small community hospitals, laboratories, and research centers.

There are two types of approved educational programs in nuclear medicine technology. Admission into the twelve-month certificate program generally requires that the applicant be either a graduate of an approved radiologic program, a registered nurse, or medical laboratory technologist. Other health professionals wishing to apply to these programs should contact the program director for specific requirements. Admission into the twenty-four month program requires a high school degree, or equivalent, plus two to three years of postsecondary education, with emphasis on science and mathematics. Bachelor degrees are also available in some institutions.

Certification is offered by two organizations; the American Registry of Radiologic Technologists, and the Nuclear Medicine Technology Certification Board. Certification with one of these is a job prerequisite in almost all nuclear medicine departments. Certification as a RT (N) is granted to nuclear medicine technologists after graduating from a nuclear medicine technology program accredited by the Committee on Allied Health Education and Accreditation of the American Medical Association, and successfully passing a qualifying examination. The Nuclear Medicine Technology Certification Board also requires clinical experience as a certification requirement. Many states require that nuclear medicine technologists be licensed. For more information on licensure contact the state's licensing division. Certification information is available from the American Registry of Radiologic Technologists, 2600 Wayzata Boulevard, Minneapolis, Minnesota 55405, or the Nuclear Medicine Technology Certification Board, 136 Madison Ave., New York, New York 10016.

Recommended high school courses include English, mathematics, chemistry, biology, physiology, and physics.

According to a recent survey, starting salaries for nuclear medicine technologists averaged $20,000 a year and over $26,000 a year for experienced technologists. Nuclear medicine technologists working for the federal government earn approximately $22,000.

Below is a list of nuclear medicine technology educational programs, accredited by the Committee on Allied Health Education and Accreditation of the American Medical Association.

For more information on a career in nuclear medicine technology, contact the American Society of Radiologic Technologists, 15000 Central Avenue, S.E., Albuquerque, New Mexico, 87123, or the Society of Nuclear Medicine, 136 Madison Avenue, New York, New York 10016.

SOURCES:

American Society of Radiologic Technologists
American Registry of Radiologic Technologists
Society of Nuclear Medicine
Nuclear Medicine Technology Certification Board
Occupational Outlook Handbook

Nuclear Medicine Technologist Programs

ALABAMA

Nuclear Medicine Technologist Program
The University of Alabama at Birmingham
University Station
Birmingham, Alabama 35294

ARIZONA

Nuclear Medicine Technologist Program
University Medical Center
1501 N. Campbell Avenue
Tucson, Arizona 85724

ARKANSAS

Nuclear Medicine Technologist Program
St. Vincent Infirmary
2 St. Vincent Circle
Little Rock, Arkansas 72205-5499

CALIFORNIA

Nuclear Medicine Technologist Program
Loma Linda University
School of Allied Health Professions
Loma Linda, California 92350

Nuclear Medicine Technologist Program
King Drew Medical Center
12021 S. Wilmington Ave.
Los Angeles, California 90059

Nuclear Medicine Technologist Program
Los Angeles City College
855 N. Vermont Avenue
Los Angeles, California 90029

Nuclear Medicine Technologist Program
Los Angeles County-USC Medical Center
1200 N. State Street
Los Angeles, California 90033

Nuclear Medicine Technologist Program
VA-Wadsworth Medical Center
Wilshire & Sawtelle Blvds.
Los Angeles, California 90073

Nuclear Medicine Technologist Program
Sutter Community Hospitals
1111 Howe Ave., Suite 600
Sacramento, California 95825

Nuclear Medicine Technologist Program
University of CA Davis Medical Center
2315 Stockton Boulevard
Sacramento, California 95817

Nuclear Medicine Technologist Program
University of California, San Francisco
Parnassus and 3rd Aves.
San Francisco, California 94143

Nuclear Medicine Technologist Program
Cancer Foundation of Santa Barbara
300 W. Pueblo Street
P.O. Box 837
Santa Barbara, California 93105

COLORADO

Nuclear Medicine Technologist Program
Penrose Hospitals
2215 N. Cascade Avenue
P.O. Box 7021
Colorado Springs, Colorado 80933

Nuclear Medicine Technologist Program
Community College of Denver-Auraruia Campus
1068 Ninth St., Box 250
Denver, Colorado 80204

Nuclear Medicine Technologist Program
St. Anthony Hospital
4231 West 16th Avenue
Denver, Colorado 80204

CONNECTICUT

Nuclear Medicine Technologist Program
St. Vincent's Medical Center
2800 Main Street
Bridgeport, Connecticut 06606

Nuclear Medicine Technologist Program
Quinnipiac College
Mt. Carmel Avenue
Hamden, Connecticut 06518

Nuclear Medicine Technologist Program
South Central Community College
60 Sargent Drive
New Haven, Connecticut 06511

DELAWARE

Nuclear Medicine Technologist Program
Delaware Technical and Community College
P.O. Box 610
Georgetown, Delaware 19947

DISTRICT OF COLUMBIA

Nuclear Medicine Technologist Program
George Washington University Medical Center
2121 Eye St., NW, Suite 800
Washington, DC 20037

FLORIDA

Nuclear Medicine Technologist Program
Santa Fe Community College
P.O. Box 1530
Gainesville, Florida 32602

Nuclear Medicine Technologist Program
Jackson Memorial Medical Center
University of Miami
1611 N.W. 12th Avenue
Miami, Florida 33136

Nuclear Medicine Technologist Program
Mt. Sinai Medical Center
4300 Alton Road
Miami Beach, Florida 33140

Nuclear Medicine Technologist Program
Hillsborough Community College
P.O. Box 22127
Tampa, Florida 33630

GEORGIA

Nuclear Medicine Technologist Program
Medical College of Georgia
Office of the President, AA-31
Augusta, Georgia 30912-0450

ILLINOIS

Nuclear Medicine Technologist Program
Illinois Masonic Medical Center
836 W. Wellington Avenue
Chicago, Illinois 60657

Nuclear Medicine Technologist Program
Northwestern Memorial Hospital
250 E. Superior Street
Chicago, Illinois 60611

Nuclear Medicine Technologist Program
College of Du Page
22nd St. & Lambert Road
Glen Ellyn, Illinois 60137

Nuclear Medicine Technologist Program
Edward Hines Jr. VA Hospital
Fifth Ave. & Roosevelt Rd.
Hines, Illinois 60141

Nuclear Medicine Technologist Program
Christ Hospital
4440 W. 95th Street
Oak Lawn, Illinois 60453

Nuclear Medicine Technologist Program
St. Francis Medical Center
530 N.E. Glen Oak Avenue
Peoria, Illinois 61637

Nuclear Medicine Technologist Program
Triton College
2000 Fifth Avenue
River Grove, Illinois 60171

INDIANA

Nuclear Medicine Technologist Program
Our Lady of Mercy Hospital
US Highway 30
Dyer, Indiana 46311

Nuclear Medicine Technologist Program
Indiana University School of Medicine
1120 South Drive
Indianapolis, Indiana 46223

Nuclear Medicine Technologist Program
St. Anthony Hospital
301 W. Homer Street
Michigan City, Indiana 46360

Nuclear Medicine Technologist Program
Ball State University
University Avenue
Muncie, Indiana 47306

IOWA

Nuclear Medicine Technologist Program
The University of Iowa
101 Jessup Hall
Iowa City, Iowa 52242

KANSAS

Nuclear Medicine Technologist Program
University of Kansas Medical Center
39th & Rainbow Blvd.
Kansas City, Kansas 66103

Nuclear Medicine Technologist Program
Wesley Medical Center
550 N. Hillside Avenue
Wichita, Kansas 67214

KENTUCKY

Nuclear Medicine Technologist Program
Lexington Community College
Cooper Drive
Lexington, Kentucky 40506

Nuclear Medicine Technologist Program
University of Louisville
Administration Bldg.
Louisville, Kentucky 40292

LOUISIANA

Nuclear Medicine Technologist Program
Alton Ochsner Medical Foundation
1516 Jefferson Hwy.
New Orleans, Louisiana 70121

Nuclear Medicine Technologist Program
Charity Hospital of Louisiana at New Orleans
1532 Tulane Avenue
New Orleans, Louisiana 70140

Nuclear Medicine Technologist Program
Veterans Administration Medical Center
510 East Stoner Avenue
Shreveport, Louisiana 71130

MARYLAND

Nuclear Medicine Technologist Program
Essex Community College-John Hopkins Hospital
7201 Rossville Boulevard
Baltimore, Maryland 21237

Nuclear Medicine Technologist Program
Naval School of Health Sciences
Building 141
Bethesda, Maryland 20814-5033

Nuclear Medicine Technologist Program
Prince George's Community College
301 Largo Road
Largo, Maryland 20772

MASSACHUSETTS

Nuclear Medicine Technologist Program
Bunker Hill Community College
Rutherford Avenue
Boston, Massachusetts 02129

Nuclear Medicine Technologist Program
Massachusetts College of Pharmacy & Allied Health
179 Longwood Avenue
Boston, Massachusetts 02115

Nuclear Medicine Technologist Program
Newton-Wellesley Hospital
2014 Washington Street
Newton, Massachusetts 02162

Nuclear Medicine Technologist Program
Salem State College
352 Lafayette Street
Salem, Massachusetts 01970

Nuclear Medicine Technologist Program
Springfield Tech Community College
1 Armory Square
Springfield, Massachusetts 01105

Nuclear Medicine Technologist Program
Goddard Memorial Hospital
909 Sumner Street
Stoughton, Massachusetts 02072

Nuclear Medicine Technologist Program
Worcester State College
University of Massachusetts Medical Center
55 Lake Avenue North
Worcester, Massachusetts 01605

MICHIGAN

Nuclear Medicine Technologist Program
Ferris State College
901 S. State St., Starr 304
Big Rapids, Michigan 49307

Nuclear Medicine Technologist Program
Detroit-Macomb Hospital Corp.
7815 E. Jefferson Avenue
Detroit, Michigan 48214

Nuclear Medicine Technologist Program
Henry Ford Hospital
2799 W. Grand Blvd.
Detroit, MI 48202

Nuclear Medicine Technologist Program
University of Detroit
4001 W. McNichols Road
Detroit, Michigan 48221

Nuclear Medicine Technologist Program
William Beaumont Hospital
3601 W. 13 Mile Road
Royal Oak, Michigan 48072

MINNESOTA

Nuclear Medicine Technologist Program
Mayo Clinic Foundation
200 First Street, S.W.
Rochester, Minnesota 55905

Nuclear Medicine Technologist Program
St. Mary's College
Terrance Heights
P.O. Box 30
Winona, Minnesota 55987

MISSISSIPPI

Nuclear Medicine Technologist Program
University of Mississippi Medical Center
2500 N. State Street
Jackson, Mississippi 39216-4505

MISSOURI

Nuclear Medicine Technologist Program
St. Francis Medical Center
211 St. Francis Drive
Cape Girardeau, Missouri 63701

Nuclear Medicine Technologist Program
University of Missouri-Columbia
105 Jesse Hall
Columbia, Missouri 65211

Nuclear Medicine Technologist Program
Research Medical Center
2316 E. Meyer Boulevard
Kansas City, Missouri 64132

Nuclear Medicine Technologist Program
St. Luke's Hospital of Kansas City
Wornall Road at 44th
Kansas City, Missouri 64111

Nuclear Medicine Technologist Program
Mallinckrodt Inst. of Rad-Washington University
510 S. Kingshighway Blvd.
St. Louis, Missouri 63110

Nuclear Medicine Technologist Program
St. John's Mercy Medical Center
615 S. New Ballas Road
St. Louis, Missouri 63141

Nuclear Medicine Technologist Program
St. Louis University
3556 Caroline
St. Louis, Missouri 63014

NEBRASKA

Nuclear Medicine Technologist Program
University of Nebraska Medical Center
42nd & Dewey Avenue
Omaha, Nebraska 68105

NEVADA

Nuclear Medicine Technologist Program
University of Nevada
4505 Maryland Pkwy
Las Vegas, Nevada 89154

NEW JERSEY

Nuclear Medicine Technologist Program
Atlantic City Medical Center
1925 Pacific Avenue
Atlantic City, New Jersey 08401

Nuclear Medicine Technologist Program
John F. Kennedy Medical Center
98 James Street
Edison, New Jersey 08818-3059

Nuclear Medicine Technologist Program
St. Barnabas Medical Center
94 Old Short Hills Rd.
Livingston, New Jersey 07039

Nuclear Medicine Technologist Program
Robert Wood Johnson-University Hospital
180 Somerset Street
New Brunswick, New Jersey 08901

Nuclear Medicine Technologist Program
Gloucester County College
Deptford Township
Sewell, New Jersey 08080

Nuclear Medicine Technologist Program
Overlook Hospital
99 Beauvoir Ave at Sylvan Rd.
Summit, New Jersey 07901-0220

NEW MEXICO

Nuclear Medicine Technologist Program
University of New Mexico Hospital
2211 Lomas Blvd. N.E.
Albuquerque, New Mexico 87131

NEW YORK

Nuclear Medicine Technologist Program
Einstein College of Medicine of Yeshiva University
Eastchester Rd. & Morris Park
Bronx, New York 10461

Nuclear Medicine Technologist Program
Bronx Community College of CUNY
University Ave. & West 181 St.
Bronx, New York 10453

Nuclear Medicine Technologist Program
SUNY at Buffalo
501 Capen Hall
Buffalo, New York 14260

Nuclear Medicine Technologist Program
New York University Medical Center
550 First Avenue
New York, New York 10016

Nuclear Medicine Technologist Program
St. Vincent's Hospital & Medical Center of NY
153 West 11th Street
New York, New York 10011

Nuclear Medicine Technologist Program
The Institute of Allied Medical Professions
145 West 58th Street
New York, New York 10019

Nuclear Medicine Technologist Program
Northport VA Medical Center
Middleville Road
Northport, New York 11768

Nuclear Medicine Technologist Program
Manhattan College
Manhattan College Pkwy
Riverdale, New York 10471

Nuclear Medicine Technologist Program
Rochester Institute of Technology
1 Lomb Memorial Drive
P.O. Box 9887
Rochester, New York 14623-0887

Nuclear Medicine Technologist Program
Wagner College
631 Howard Avenue
Staten Island, New York 10301

Nuclear Medicine Technologist Program
SUNY Upstate Medical Center
155 Elizabeth Blackwell Street
Syracuse, New York 13210

NORTH CAROLINA

Nuclear Medicine Technologist Program
North Carolina Memorial Hospital
Manning Drive
Chapel Hill, North Carolina 27514

Nuclear Medicine Technologist Program
Caldwell Community College & Tech Inst.
1000 Hickory Boulevard
Hudson, North Carolina 28638

Nuclear Medicine Technologist Program
Forsyth Technical Institute
2100 Silas Creek Parkway
Winston-Salem, North Carolina 27103

OHIO

Nuclear Medicine Technologist Program
Aultman Hospital
2600 Sixth Street, S.W.
Canton, Ohio 44710

Nuclear Medicine Technologist Program
University of Cincinnati
Mail Location 63
Cincinnati, Ohio 45221-0063

Nuclear Medicine Technologist Program
Ohio State University Hospitals
450 W. 10th Avenue
Columbus, Ohio 43210

Nuclear Medicine Technologist Program
Riverside Methodist Hospital
3535 Olentangy River Road
Columbus, Ohio 43214

Nuclear Medicine Technologist Program
Miami Valley Hospital
1 Wyoming Street
Dayton, Ohio 45409

Nuclear Medicine Technologist Program
Findlay College
1000 N. Main Street
Findlay, Ohio 45840

Nuclear Medicine Technologist Program
St. Elizabeth Hospital Medical Center
1044 Belmont Avenue
Youngstown, Ohio 44504

OKLAHOMA

Nuclear Medicine Technologist Program
University of Oklahoma at Oklahoma City
P.O. Box 26901
Oklahoma City, Oklahoma 73190

OREGON

Nuclear Medicine Technologist Program
Veterans Administration Medical Center
P.O. Box 1034
Portland, Oregon 97207

PENNSYLVANIA

Nuclear Medicine Technologist Program
Cedar Crest College
30th & Walnut Streets
Allentown, Pennsylvania 18104

Nuclear Medicine Technologist Program
Geisinger Medical Center
North Academy Avenue
Danville, Pennsylvania 17822

Nuclear Medicine Technologist Program
Gwynedd-Mercy College
Sumneytown Pike
Gwynedd Valley, Pennsylvania 19437

Nuclear Medicine Technologist Program
Southcentral Pennsylvania Consortium for Nuclear Medicine Technology Training
South Front Street
Harrisburg, Pennsylvania 17101

Nuclear Medicine Technologist Program
Lancaster General Hospital
555 North Duke Street
P.O. Box 3555
Lancaster, Pennsylvania 17603

Nuclear Medicine Technologist Program
Temple University Hospital
Broad St. & Montgomery Aves.
Philadelphia, Pennsylvania 19122

Nuclear Medicine Technologist Program
Community College of Allegheny County
Allegheny Campus
808 Ridge Avenue
Pittsburgh, Pennsylvania 15212

Nuclear Medicine Technologist Program
York Hospital
1001 S. George St.
York, Pennsylvania 17405

PUERTO RICO

Nuclear Medicine Technologist Program
University of Puerto Rico
GPO Box 5067
San Juan, Puerto Rico 00936

RHODE ISLAND

Nuclear Medicine Technologist Program
Rhode Island Hospital
593 Eddy Street
Providence, Rhode Island 02903

SOUTH CAROLINA

Nuclear Medicine Technologist Program
Medical University of South Carolina
171 Ashley Avenue
Charleston, South Carolina 29425

Nuclear Medicine Technologist Program
Midlands Technical College
P.O. Box 2408
Columbia, South Carolina 29202

TENNESSEE

Nuclear Medicine Technologist Program
Chattanooga State Tech Community College
4501 Amnicola Hwy
Chattanooga, Tennessee 37406

Nuclear Medicine Technologist Program
UTN Memorial Hospital & Research Center
1924 Alcoa Hwy
Knoxville, Tennessee 37920

Nuclear Medicine Technologist Program
Baptist Memorial Hospital
899 Madison Avenue
Memphis, Tennessee 38146

Nuclear Medicine Technologist Program
Methodist Hospital of Memphis
1265 Union Avenue
Memphis, Tennessee 38104

Nuclear Medicine Technologist Program
Regional Medical Center at Memphis
842 Jefferson Avenue
Memphis, Tennessee 38103

Nuclear Medicine Technologist Program
Vanderbilt University Medical Center
21st & Garland
Nashville, Tennesse 37232

TEXAS

Nuclear Medicine Technologist Program
Galveston College
The University of Texas
4015 Avenue Q
Galveston, Texas 77550

Nuclear Medicine Technologist Program
Baylor College of Medicine
One Baylor Plaza
Houston, Texas 77030

Nuclear Medicine Technologist Program
Houston Community College System
22 Waugh Drive
P.O. Box 7849
Houston, Texas 77270-7849

Nuclear Medicine Technologist Program
Incarnate Word College
4301 Broadway
San Antonio, Texas 78209

Nuclear Medicine Technologist Program
McLennan Community College
1400 College Drive
Waco, Texas 76708

UTAH

Nuclear Medicine Technologist Program
Weber State College
M S 1001
Ogden, Utah 84408

VERMONT

Nuclear Medicine Technologist Program
University of Vermont
349 Waterman Bldg.
Burlington, Vermont 05405

VIRGINIA

Nuclear Medicine Technologist Program
University of Virginia Medical Center
Box 148 M4
Charlottesville, Virginia 22908

Nuclear Medicine Technologist Program
Medical College of Virginia
Virginia Commonwealth University
910 West Franklin Street
Richmond, Virginia 23284

Nuclear Medicine Technologist Program
St. Mary's Hospital
5801 Bremo Road
Richmond, Virginia 23226

Nuclear Medicine Technologist Program
Roanoke Memorial Hospitals
P.O. Box 13367
Roanoke, Virginia 24033

WASHINGTON

Nuclear Medicine Technologist Program
Seattle University
12th & East Columbia
Seattle, Washington 98122

WEST VIRGINIA

Nuclear Medicine Technologist Program
West Virginia State College
P.O. Box 200
Institute, West Virginia 25112

Nuclear Medicine Technologist Program
West Virginia University Hospital
Medical Center Drive
P.O. Box 6401
Morgantown, West Virginia 26506-6401

Nuclear Medicine Technologist Program
Wheeling College
316 Washington Avenue
Wheeling, West Virginia 26003

WISCONSIN

Nuclear Medicine Technologist Program
St. Joseph's Hospital
611 St. Joseph's Avenue
Marshfield, Wisconsin 54449

Nuclear Medicine Technologist Program
Family Hospital
2711 W. Wells Street
Milwaukee, Wisconsin 53208

Nuclear Medicine Technologist Program
Milwaukee County Medical Complex
8700 West Wisconsin Avenue
Milwaukee, Wisconsin 53226

Nuclear Medicine Technologist Program
St. Luke's Hospital
2900 W. Oklahoma Ave.
Milwaukee, Wisconsin 53215

Nuclear Medicine Technologist Program
St. Mary's Hospital
2323 N. Lake Drive
P.O. Box 503
Milwaukee, Wisconsin 53201

Diagnostic Ultrasound

Diagnostic ultrasound is the relatively new medical technique that uses high frequency sound waves (ultrasound) for diagnostic purposes. By transmitting ultrasound through various parts of the body, images are created on video screens that show the shape and composition of organs, tissues, and other bodily masses such as fluid accumulations. These images are then used by a licensed physician (one who has been trained to interpret ultrasound images) to diagnose disease, injury, or other physical conditions. Unlike X-rays (which used radiation to create images on film) ultrasound is noninvasive (it does not invade healthy tissue), and to date has not demonstrated any known biological effects. The technical practitioner of diagnostic ultrasound is the *diagnostic medical sonographer.*

Diagnostic Medical Sonographer

Also called an *ultrasound technologist,* the diagnostic medical sonographer works under the direction of a physician to provide quality imaging techniques in ultrasound diagnoses. The sonographer may perform a variety of studies, including the examination of the contour and inner structures of the brain (neurosonology); examination of the heart and its structures (echocardiography); examination of the soft tissue structures of the abdomen such as the liver, spleen, kidneys and pancreas; examination of the female anatomy and of pregnant females (gynecology and obstetrics); and the examination of the eyes (ophthalmology). The diagnostic medical sonographer is well knowledgeable of the human anatomy.

The medical sonographer is responsible for the personal comfort of the patient in his or her care. The sonographer prepares the patient for the examination, explains the procedure, scans the patient with the ultrasound equipment, and provides the physician with the final results. He or she may also perform clerical duties such as keeping records of the patients and of the imaging films. The medical sonographer should be capable of working with little supervision within the rules set by the physician or department head.

Diagnostic medical sonographers work in all health facilities that utilize ultrasound devices - mainly large hospitals and medical centers. A few are employed in smaller rural hospitals, private physician practices, public health services, industry, and sales.

Training programs in diagnostic ultrasound are offered by universities, radiological institutes, and hospitals. Classes are usually small to allow hands-on experience of the complex ultrasound equipment. Programs are usually one year in length and require that the applicant have previously completed two years of college education in an accredited allied health program or have had at least two years of an equivalent combination of education and work experience in allied health.

Satisfactory completion of specific educational and clinical experience requirements qualifies the candidate to take the registry examination and if successfully passed, apply for registration as a Registered Diagnostic Medical Sonographer (RDMS) with the American Registry of Diagnostic Medical Sonographers. The registry examination consists of two parts: the first is a prerequisite ultrasound physics examination; and the second, an examination in at least one ultrasound specialty; Abdomen, Obstetrics and Gynecology. Neurosonology, Adult Echocardiography, Pediatric Echocardiography, or Ophthalmology. An individual may specialize in more than one. The registry credential of Registered Vascular Technologist (RVT) is also available after successfully passing the Vascular Physics and Vascular Technology examinations.

The following is a summary of the educational and clinical prerequisites needed to take the registry examinations:

(1) Graduation from a training program in diagnostic ultrasound, accredited by the American Medical Association's Committee on Allied Health Education and Accreditation (CAHEA), or (2) Completion of a two year patient related allied health occupation such as diagnostic medical sonographer, registered nurse, radiologic technologist, respiratory therapist, physical therapist, occupational therapist or medical technologist and 12 months clinical experience in diagnostic ultrasound, or (3) Completion of a bachelor's degree in ultrasound or radiology (minor must be in ultrasound) and at least 12 months clinical experience in diagnostic ultrasound, or (4) Completion of a two-year college degree, plus 24 months clinical experience in diagnostic ultrasound.

For more information on registration requirements contact the American Registry for Diagnostic Medical Sonographers, 32 E. Hollister St., Cincinnati, Ohio 45219.

Recommended high school subjects for a career in ultrasound technology are physics, chemistry, biology and mathematics.

According to a recent survey provided by the Society of Diagnostic Medical Sonographers, full time diagnostic medical sonographers earn salaries ranging from $21,500 to $27,700 annually, with average salaries equalling approximately $24,000. Many factors, however, effect salary levels including education, experience, and geographic location.

Below is a list of currently existing educational programs in diagnostic ultrasound provided by the Society of Diagnostic Medical Sonographers. The Society of Diagnostic Medical Sonographers does not accredit programs but does recommend that students first investigate programs accredited by the Committee on Allied Health Education and Accreditation (CAHEA) of The American Medical Association. Programs that are CAHEA approved are noted by an asterisk (*).

For further information on a career as a diagnostic medical sonographer, contact the Society of Diagnostic Medical Sonographers, 1222 S. Greenville Ave, Suite 434, Dallas, Texas 75243.

SOURCE:

Society of Diagnostic Medical Sonographers

Diagnostic Ultrasound Programs

ALABAMA

School of Diagnostic Ultrasound
Providence Hospital
1504 Springhill Avenue
Mobile, Alabama 36610

CALIFORNIA

Diagnostic Ultrasound Technology Program
Foothill College
12345 El Monte Road
Los Altos, California 94022

Department of Diagnostic Ultrasound
Grossmont College
8800 Grossmont College Drive
El Cajon, California 92020

Department of Diagnostic Ultrasound (*)
Loma Linda University
11234 Anderson Street
Loma Linda, California 92354

Department of Diagnostic Ultrasound
Orange Coast College
2701 Fairview Road
Costa Mesa, California 92628-0120

Division of Diagnostic Ultrasound
University of California San Diego Medical Center
225 Dickinson Street
San Diego, California 92103-9981

COLORADO

Ultrasound Department (*)
Penrose Hospital
P.O. Box 7021
Colorado Springs, Colorado 80933

Diagnostic Sonography Training Program
University of Colorado Health Sciences Center
C-277, Denver Metro
Denver, Colorado 80262

CONNECTICUT

Dept. of Radiologic Sciences (*)
Quinnipiac College, School of Allied Health and Natural Sciences
Mt. Carmel Avenue
Hamden, Connecticut 06518

Diagnostic Ultrasound Training Program
St. Vincent's Medical Center
2800 Main Street
Bridgeport, Connecticut 06606

School of Ultrasonography
Yale New Haven Hospital
20 York Street
New Haven, Connecticut 06511

FLORIDA

School of Ultrasound Technology
Mt. Sinai Medical Center
4300 Alton Road
Miami Beach, Florida 33140

Diagnostic Medical Sonography (*)
University of Miami-Jackson Memorial Hospital
1611 N.W. 12th Avenue
Miami, Florida 33136

GEORGIA

Diagnostic Medical Sonography Program (*)
Medical College of Georgia
School of Radiologic Technologies
Augusta, Georgia 30912

ILLINOIS

Program in Diagnostic Medical Ultrasound (*)
Department of Radiology Ultrasound Div.
University of Illinois Hospital
1740 W. Taylor Street, Suite 2461
Chicago, Illinois 60612

IOWA

Diagnostic Ultrasonography Program
Department of Radiology
University of Iowa Hospitals and Clinics
Department of Radiology
Iowa City, Iowa 52242

LOUISIANA

School of Diagnostic Ultrasound
Charity Hospital of Louisiana
1532 Tulane Avenue
New Orleans, Louisiana 70140

Program in Diagnostic Medical Sonography (*)
Alton Ochsner Medical Foundation
1516 Jefferson Highway
New Orleans, Louisiana 70121

MARYLAND

Ultrasound Technology Program (*)
Maryland Institute of Ultrasound Technology
P.O. Box 161
Riderwood, Maryland 21139

MASSACHUSETTS

Diagnostic Medical Sonography Program (*)
Middlesex Community College
Springs Road
Bedford, Massachusetts 01730

MICHIGAN

Diagnostic Ultrasound Program (*)
School of Ultrasound Technology
Henry Ford Hospital
2799 W. Grand Blvd.
Detroit, Michigan 48202

Department of Diagnostic Medical Sonography (*)
Oakland Community College
Diagnostic Medical Sonography
S.E. Campus System-22322 Rutland Drive
Southfield, Michigan 48075

MISSOURI

Department of Diagnostic Medical Sonography (*)
St. Louis Community College at Forest Park
5600 Oakland Avenue
St. Louis, Missouri 63110

NEW JERSEY

Diagnostic Medical Ultrasonography Program (*)
St. Barnabas Medical Center
Short Hills Road
Livingston, New Jersey 07039

NEW MEXICO

Department of Medical Sonography
The University of New Mexico School of Medicine
Mexico Allied Health Center
Albuquerque, New Mexico 87131

NEW YORK

Radiologic Sciences & Technology Program (*)
Downstate Medical Center
450 Clarkson Avenue
Brooklyn, New York 11203

Diagnostic Ultrasound Technology Program (*)
New York University Medical Center
550 1st Avenue
New York, New York 10016

Diagnostic Medical Sonography Program (*)
Rochester Institute of Technology
Box 9887
Rochester, New York 14623

Diagnostic Ultrasound Program
Ultrasound Diagnostic School
30 East 23rd Street
New York, New York 10010

OHIO

School of Diagnostic Medical Ultrasound (*)
Aultman Hospital
2600 6th Street, S.W.
Canton, Ohio 44710

School of Diagnostic Medical Sonography
Cleveland Clinic Foundation
9500 Euclid Avenue
Cleveland, Ohio 44106

Diagnostic Ultrasound Technology Program
Kettering College of Medical Arts
3737 Southern Boulevard
Kettering, Ohio

School of Diagnostic Medical Ultrasound (*)
Mt. Sinai Medical Center
1800 105th Street
Cleveland, Ohio 44106

OKLAHOMA

Dept. of Radiologic Technology (*)
University of Oklahoma
College of Allied Health
P.O. Box 26901
Oklahoma City, Oklahoma 73190

PENNSYLVANIA

Diagnostic Medical Sonography Program (*)
Thomas Jefferson University, College of Allied Health Science
Division of Diagnostic Ultrasound
1020 Locust Street
Philadelphia, Pennsylvania 19107

TENNESSEE

Dept. of Radiology-Ultrasound Section (*)
Vanderbilt University Medical Center
Nashville, Tennessee 37232

TEXAS

Diagnostic Ultrasound Program
El Centro College
Main & Lamar
Dallas, Texas 75202

UTAH

Department of Diagnostic Ultrasound (*)
Weber State College
Ogden, Utah 84408

WASHINGTON

Diagnostic Ultrasound Division (*)
Seattle University
Seattle, Washington 98122

Echocardiographic Technology Program
Spokane Community College
N. 1810 Greene Street
Spokane, Washington 99207

WEST VIRGINIA

Department of Radiology
West Virginia University Hospitals, Inc.
Morgantown, West Virginia 26506

WISCONSIN

Department of Diagnostic Medical Ultrasound
District One Technical Institute-Eau Claire
620 West Clairemont Avenue
Eau Claire, Wisconsin 54701

Department of Diagnostic Ultrasound (*)
St. Francis Hospital School of Diagnostic Ultrasound
3237 S. 16th Street
Milwaukee, Wisconsin 53215

School of Diagnostic Ultrasonography (*)
St. Luke's Hospital
2900 Oklahoma Avenue
Milwaukee, Wisconsin 53215

School of Diagnostic Medical Sonography
University of Wisconsin Hospital and Clinics
600 Highland Avenue
Madison, Wisconsin 53792

CANADA

Diagnostic Medical Sonography
Royal Alexandra Hospital
10240 Kinsway
Edmonton, Alberta, Canada T5H 3V9

Diagnostic Ultrasound Program
Dept. of Radiology
University of Alberta Hospital
8440 112th Street
Edmonton, Alberta, Canada T5H 2B7

Diagnostic Ultrasound Program
British Columbia Institute of Technology
3700 Willingdon
Vancouver, BC, Canada V5G 3H2

Diagnostic Ultrasound Program
Health Science Centre
700 William Avenue
Winnipeg, Manitoba, Canada

Diagnostic Ultrasound Program
College of Trades and Technology
P.O. Box 1693
St. John's, Newfoundland, Canada A1C 5P7

Diagnostic Ultrasound Program
Toronto Institute of Medical Technology
222 St. Patrick Street
Toronto, Ontario, Canada M5T 1V4

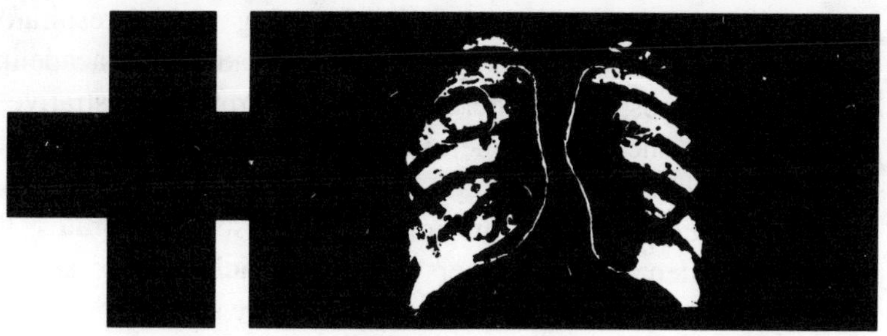

RESPIRATORY THERAPY

Respiratory therapy is the healthcare specialty employed to treat seriously ill patients with heart and lung (cardiopulmonary) problems. Under medical direction, respiratory therapy procedures involve the prevention, diagnosis, treatment, control, and rehabilitation of breathing disorders such as asthma and emphysema, and also in the emergency care of cardiac failure, cerebral thrombosis, hemorrhage, embolism, and shock.

Respiratory therapy is of immediate and crucial importance in the treatment of acute respiratory conditions arising from head injury, drowning, or drug poisoning. If breathing is not restored in three to five minutes, brain damage will likely occur. Death will occur if breathing is not restored in nine minutes. Respiratory therapy is also concerned with the medical problems associated with cigarette smoking and air pollution. There are three career classifications in this field; *respiratory therapist*, *respiratory therapy technician*, and *respiratory therapy aide*.

Respiratory Therapist

Under the direction of a physician, the *respiratory therapist* administers respiratory care treatments to patients with cardiopulmonary disorders. The respiratory therapist may also supervise technicians and aides, make recommendations for respiratory therapy, and evaluate patients' progress. In both emergency and temporary care the therapist is able to administer gas, aerosol, and humidity therapies, and intermittent positive-pressure breathing treatments, as well as cardiopulmonary resuscitation, long term continuous artificial ventilation, and other special therapeutic procedures.

Other responsibilities of a respiratory therapist often include providing instruction in breathing exercises, operating and maintaining special respiratory equipment such as mechanical ventilators and oxygen tents. With additional academic training and/or work experience, the respiratory therapist may perform administrative, teaching and research duties, and advance from general care to the care of patients with difficult or unusual diagnostic problems.

Most respiratory therapists are employed in hospital respiratory therapy, anesthesiology, or pulmonary departments. Others work in physicians' offices, nursing homes, industries, or contracting firms that provide respiratory care services. A small, but expanding group of respiratory therapists are employed by home healthcare agencies, providing at-home instruction to patients and their families.

Admittance into educational programs, accredited by the American Medical Association's Committee on Allied Health Education and Accreditation or holding a Letter of Review by the Joint Review Committee for Respiratory Therapy Education, requires a high school diploma or the equivalent. Formal training programs are offered by colleges and universities, community and junior colleges, vocational technical schools, trade schools, hospitals and the Armed Forces, and award either an associate or bachelor's degree for a two or four year program.

Graduation from an approved educational program, and completion of specific experience requirements qualifies the candidate to take the national examinations, and if successful, to become certified by the National Board for Respiratory Care as a registered respiratory therapist (RRT). Some states require respiratory therapists to be licensed, and often use the National Board's entry level exam for this purpose. For more details on certification requirements, write to the National Board for Respiratory Care, 11015 West 75th Terrace, Shawnee Mission, Kansas 66214. High school students interested in a career in respiratory therapy are advised to take courses in health, biology, mathematics, and physics.

According to a 1987 salary survey compiled by the American Association for Respiratory Care, staff respiratory therapists in non-supervisory positions earned salaries ranging from $7,200 to nearly $45,000 a year, with average salaries equalling $21,600.

Below is a list of formal training programs provided by the Joint Review Committee for Respiratory Therapy Education. Contact the schools directly for length of program and award granted.

KEY:

(1) Accreditation by the American Medical Association's Committee on Allied Health Education and Accreditation.

(2) A Letter of Review from the Joint Review Committee for Respiratory Therapy Education is held by this program.

(Graduates of both categories are eligible to take the national certifying examinations.)

SOURCES:

American Association for Respiratory Care
Joint Review Committee for Respiratory Therapy Education
National Board for Respiratory Care
Occupational Outlook Handbook

Respiratory Therapist Programs

ALABAMA

Respiratory Therapist Program (1)
University of Alabama in Birmingham
School of Community & Allied Health
Regional Technical Institute, No. 219
University Station
Birmingham, Alabama 35294

Respiratory Therapist Program (1)
George C. Wallace Community College
Dothan, Alabama 36303

Respiratory Therapist Program (1)
Wallace State Community College
Post Office Box 250
Hanceville, Alabama 35077

Respiratory Therapist Program (1)
University of South Alabama
Mobile, Alabama 36688

ARIZONA

Respiratory Therapist Program (1)
Maricopa Technical Community College
108 North 40th Street
Phoenix, Arizona 85034

Respiratory Therapist Program (1)
Biosystems, Inc.
1701 S. 52nd Street
Tempe, Arizona 85282

Respiratory Therapist Program (1)
Pima Community College
2202 West Anklam Road
Tucson, Arizona 85709

ARKANSAS

Respiratory Therapist Program (1)
University of Arkansas for Medical Science
College of Health Related Professions
4301 W. Markham, Slot 619
Little Rock, Arkansas 72205

CALIFORNIA

Respiratory Therapist Program (1)
Orange Coast College
2701 Fairview Road
Post Office Box 5005
Costa Mesa, California 92628-0120

Respiratory Therapist Program (1)
Grossmont College
8800 Grossmont College Drive
El Cajon, California 92020

Respiratory Therapist Program (1)
Ohlone College
43600 Mission Boulevard
Freemont, California 94539

Respiratory Therapist Program (1)
Fresno City College
1101 East University
Fresno, California 93741

Respiratory Therapist Program (1)
Loma Linda University
School of Allied Health Professions
Loma Linda, California 92350

Respiratory Therapist Program (1)
Long Beach City College
4901 East Carson Street
Long Beach, California 90808

Respiratory Therapist Program (1)
University of California at L.A.
Santa Monica College
10833 LeConte
Los Angeles, California 90024

Respiratory Therapist Program (1)
Foothill College
12345 El Monte Road
Los Altos Hills, California 94022

Respiratory Therapist Program (1)
East Los Angeles College
1301 Brooklyn Avenue
Monterey Park, California 91754

Respiratory Therapist Program (1)
Napa Valley College
2277 Napa Vallejo Highway
Napa, California 94558

Respiratory Therapist Program (1)
Napa Valley College
2277 Napa Vallejo Highway
Napa, California 94558

Respiratory Therapist Program (1)
Butte College
Route One, Box 183A
Oroville, California 95938

Respiratory Therapist Program (1)
College of the Desert
43-500 Monterey Avenue
Palm Desert, California 92260

Respiratory Therapist Program (1)
American River College
4700 College Oak Drive
Sacramento, California 95841

Respiratory Therapist Program (1)
Skyline College
3300 College Drive
San Bruno, California 94066

Respiratory Therapist Program (1)
California College of San Diego, CA.
1810 State Street
San Diego, California 92101

Respiratory Therapist Program (1)
El Camino College
16007 Crenshaw Boulevard
Torrance, California 90506

Respiratory Therapist Program (1)
Los Angeles Valley College
5800 Fulton Avenue
Van Nuys, California 91401

Respiratory Therapist Program (1)
Victor Valley College
P.O. Drawer 00
Victorville, California 92392

Respiratory Therapist Program (1)
Mt. San Antonio College
1100 North Grand Avenue
Walnut, California 91789

Respiratory Therapist Program (1)
Rio Hondo College
3600 Workman Mill Road
Whittier, California 90608

Respiratory Therapist Program (1)
Crafton Hills College
11711 Sand Canyon Road
Yucaipa, California 92399

COLORADO

Respiratory Therapist Program (1)
Pueblo Community College
900 West Orman Avenue
Pueblo, Colorado 81004

Respiratory Therapist Program (1)
Front Range Community College
North Campus
3645 West 112th Avenue
Westminster, Colorado 80030

CONNECTICUT

Respiratory Therapist Program (1)
Sacred Heart University
St. Vincent's Consortium
5229 Park Avenue
Bridgeport, Connecticut 06606

Respiratory Therapist Program (1)
Quinnipiac College
Mount Carmel Avenue
Hamden, Connecticut 06518

Respiratory Therapist Program (1)
Manchester Community College
60 Bidwell Street
Manchester, Connecticut 06040

Respiratory Therapist Program (1)
Norwalk Hospital
24 Maple Street
Norwalk, Connecticut 06856

Respiratory Therapist Program (1)
University of Hartford
200 Bloomfield Avenue
West Hartford, Connecticut 06117

DELAWARE

Respiratory Therapist Program (1)
Delaware Technical and Community College
Allied Health Department
Wilmington Campus
333 Shipley Street
Wilmington, Delaware 19801

DISTRICT OF COLUMBIA

Respiratory Therapist Program (1)
University of the District of Columbia
4100 Connecticut Avenue, Northwest
Washington, D.C. 20008

FLORIDA

Respiratory Therapist Program (1)
Manatee Junior College
P.O. Box 1849
Bradenton, Florida 33506

Respiratory Therapist Program (1)
Daytona Beach Community College
Post Office Box 1111
Daytona Beach, Florida 32015

Respiratory Therapist Program (1)
Broward Community College
Allied Health Center Campus
3501 Southwest Davie Road
Fort Lauderdale, Florida 33314

Respiratory Therapist Program (1)
Edison Community College
College Parkway
Fort Myers, Florida 33907

Respiratory Therapist Program (1)
Santa Fe Community College
P.O. Box 1530
Gainesville, Florida 32601

Respiratory Therapist Program (1)
Flagler Career Institute
3225 University Blvd., South
Jacksonville, Florida 32216

Respiratory Therapist Program (1)
Florida Junior College at Jacksonville
North Campus
4501 Copper Road
Jacksonville, Florida 32118

Respiratory Therapist Program (1)
Flagler Career Institute
2125 Biscayne Boulevard
Miami, Florida 33137

Respiratory Therapist Program (1)
Miami-Dade Community College
Medical Center Campus
950 Northwest 20th Street
Miami, Florida 33127

Respiratory Therapist Program (1)
University of Central Florida
Department of Cardiopulmonary Sciences
Post Office Box 25000
Orlando, Florida 32816-0994

Respiratory Therapist Program (1)
Valencia Community College
P.O. Box 3028
Orlando, Florida 32802

Respiratory Therapist Program (1)
Pensacola Junior College
Warrington Campus
555 West Highway 98
Pensacola, Florida 32507

Respiratory Therapist Program (1)
St. Petersburg Junior College
6605 Fifth Avenue, North
St. Petersburg, Florida 33710

Respiratory Therapist Program (2)
Florida Agricultural and Mechanical University
School of Allied Health Sciences
Ware-Rhaney Building
Tallahassee, Florida 32307

Respiratory Therapist Program (1)
Tallahassee Community College
444 Appleyard Drive
Tallahassee, Florida 32301

GEORGIA

Respiratory Therapist Program (1)
Georgia State University
University Plaza
Atlanta, Georgia 30303

Respiratory Therapist Program (1)
Medical College of Georgia
1120 15th Street
Augusta, Georgia 30902

Respiratory Therapist Program (1)
Columbus College
Algonquin Drive
Columbus, Georgia 31993-2399

Respiratory Therapist Program (1)
Armstrong State College
11935 Abercorn Street
Savannah, Georgia 31406

HAWAII

Respiratory Therapist Program (1)
Kapiolani Community College
University of Hawaii
620 Pensacola Street
Honolulu, Hawaii 96814

IDAHO

Respiratory Therapist Program (1)
Boise State University
1910 University Drive
Boise, Idaho 83725

ILLINOIS

Respiratory Therapist Program (1)
Southern Illinois University at Carbondale
School of Technical Careers
Division of Allied Health & Public Service
Allied Health Career Specialties
Carbondale, Illinois 62901

Respiratory Therapist Program (1)
Parkland College
2400 West Bradley
Champaign, Illinois 61820

Respiratory Therapist Program (1)
Malcolm X College
1900 West Van Buren Street
Chicago, Illinois 60612

Respiratory Therapist Program (1)
Northwestern University Medical School
303 East Chicago Avenue
Chicago, Illinois 60611

Respiratory Therapist Program (1)
University of Chicago Hospitals & Clinics
5841 South Maryland Avenue, Box 170
Chicago, Illinois 60637

Respiratory Therapist Program (2)
Illinois Central College
East Peoria, Illinois 61635

Respiratory Therapist Program (1)
Black Hawk College
6600 34th Avenue
Moline, Illinois 61265

Respiratory Therapist Program (1)
Moraine Valley Community College
10900 South 88th Avenue
Palos Hills, Illinois 60465

Respiratory Therapist Program (1)
Triton College
2000 North Fifth Avenue
River Grove, Illinois 60171

Respiratory Therapist Program (1)
Rock Valley College
3301 North Mulford Road
Rockford, Illinois 61111

Respiratory Therapist Program (1)
Lincoln Land Community College
Shepard Road
Springfield, Illinois 62708

INDIANA

Respiratory Therapist Program (1)
University of Southern Indiana
8600 University Boulevard
Evansville, Indiana 47712

Respiratory Therapist Program (1)
Indiana Vocational Technical College
3800 North Anthony Boulevard
Fort Wayne, Indiana 46805

Respiratory Therapist Program (1)
Indiana University
Northwest Campus
3400 North Broadway
Gary, Indiana 46408

Respiratory Therapist Program (1)
Indiana University School of Medicine
Division of Allied Health Sciences
120 Coleman Hall
1140 West Michigan Street
Indianapolis, Indiana 46223

Respiratory Therapist Program (1)
Marian College
3200 Cold Springs Road
Indianapolis, Indiana 46222

Respiratory Therapist Program (1)
Ball State University
Department of Physiology and Health Science
Muncie, Indiana 47306

Respiratory Therapist Program (1)
Vincennes University
1002 North First Street
Vincennes, Indiana 47591

IOWA

Respiratory Therapist Program (1)
Des Moines Area Community College
2006 Ankeny Boulevard
Ankeny, Iowa 50021

Respiratory Therapist Program (1)
Kirkwood Community College
6301 Kirkwood Boulevard Southwest
Post Office Box 2068
Cedar Rapids, Iowa 52406

KANSAS

Respiratory Therapist Program (1)
University of Kansas
College of Health Sciences and Hospital
School of Allied Health
39th and Rainbow Boulevard
Kansas City, Kansas 66103

Respiratory Therapist Program (2)
Seward County Community College
Box 1137
Liberal, Kansas 67901

Respiratory Therapist Program (1)
Labette Community College
200 South 14th
Parsons, Kansas 67357

Respiratory Therapist Program (2)
Washburn University
School of Applied and Continuing Education
Topeka, Kansas 66621

Respiratory Therapist Program (1)
Wichita State University
College of Health Related Professions
Box 43
Wichita, Kansas 67208

KENTUCKY

Respiratory Therapist Program (1)
Lexington Community College
University of Kentucky
Oswald Building, Cooper Drive
Lexington, Kentucky 40506-0235

Respiratory Therapist Program (1)
Jefferson Community College
University of Kentucky
109 E. Broadway
Louisville, Kentucky 40202

Respiratory Therapist Program (1)
University of Louisville
Carmichael Building
525 East Madison Street
Louisville, Kentucky 40292

Respiratory Therapist Program (1)
Madisonville Community College
University Drive
Madisonville, Kentucky 42431

LOUISIANA

Respiratory Therapist Program (1)
Alton Ochsner Medical Foundation
1516 Jefferson Highway
New Orleans, Louisiana 70121

Respiratory Therapist Program (1)
Delgado Junior College
615 City Park Avenue
New Orleans, Louisiana 70119

Respiratory Therapist Program (1)
Louisiana State University Medical Center
School of Allied Health Professions
Department of Cardiopulmonary Science
1732 Canal Street, Suite 265
New Orleans, Louisiana 70112

MAINE

Respiratory Therapist Program (1)
Southern Maine Vocational-Technical Institute
2 Fort Road
South Portland, Maine 04106

MARYLAND

Respiratory Therapist Program (1)
Community College of Baltimore
2901 Liberty Heights Avenue
Baltimore, Maryland 21215

Respiratory Therapist Program (1)
Allegany Community College
Willow Brook Road
Post Office Box 1695
Cumberland, Maryland 21502

Respiratory Therapist Program (1)
Prince George's Community College
301 Largo Road
Largo, Maryland 20771

Respiratory Therapist Program (2)
Salisbury State College
College and Camden Avenue
Salisbury, Maryland 21801

Respiratory Therapist Program (1)
Columbia Union College
7600 Flower Avenue
Takoma Park, Maryland 20912

MASSACHUSETTS

Respiratory Therapist Program (1)
North Shore Community College
3 Essex Street
Beverly, Massachusetts 01915

Respiratory Therapist Program (1)
Catherine LaBoure College
2120 Dorchester Avenue
Boston, Massachusetts 02124

Respiratory Therapist Program (1)
Newbury Junior College
921 Boylston Street
Boston, Massachusetts 02115

Respiratory Therapist Program (1)
Northeastern University
College of Pharmacy and Allied Health Professions
360 Huntington Avenue
Boston, Massachusetts 02115

Respiratory Therapist Program (1)
Massasoit Community College
1 Massasoit Boulevard
Brockton, Massachusetts 02402

Respiratory Therapist Program (1)
Northern Essex Community College
101 Elliott Street
Haverhill, Massachusetts 01830

Respiratory Therapist Program (1)
Springfield Technical Community College
One Armory Square
Springfield, Massachusetts 01105

Respiratory Therapist Program (1)
Quinsigamond Community College
670 West Boylston Street
Worcester, Massachusetts 01606

MICHIGAN

Respiratory Therapist Program (1)
Washtenaw Community College
Post Office Box D-1
4800 East Huron River Drive
Ann Arbor, Michigan 48106

Respiratory Therapist Program (1)
Ferris State College
School of Allied Health
401 Spathelf Center
Big Rapids, Michigan 49307

Respiratory Therapist Program (1)
Oakland Community College
2480 Opdyke Road
Bloomfield, Michigan 48013

Respiratory Therapist Program (1)
Henry Ford Community College
22586 Ann Arbor Trail
Dearborn Heights, Michigan 48127

Respiratory Therapist Program (2)
Marygrove College
8425 W. McNichols Road
Detroit, Michigan 48221

Respiratory Therapist Program (1)
Mercy College of Detroit
8200 West Outer Drive
Detroit, Michigan 48219

Respiratory Therapist Program (1)
Charles Stewart Mott Community College
1401 East Court Street
Flint, Michigan 48502

Respiratory Therapist Program (1)
Kalamazoo Valley Community College
6767 West O" Avenue"
Kalamazoo, Michigan 49009

Respiratory Therapist Program (1)
Lansing Community College
Post Office Box 40010
Lansing, Michigan 48901

Respiratory Therapist Program (1)
Monroe County Community College
1555 South Raisinville Road
Monroe, Michigan 48161

Respiratory Therapist Program (1)
Macomb Community College
Detroit-Macomb Hospitals Association
44575 Garfield Road
Mt. Clemens, Michigan 48044

Respiratory Therapist Program (2)
Muskegon Community College
221 South Quarterline Road
Muskegon, Michigan 49442

Respiratory Therapist Program (1)
North Central Michigan College
1515 Howard Street
Petoskey, Michigan 49770

Respiratory Therapist Program (1)
Delta College
University Center, Michigan 48710

MINNESOTA

Respiratory Therapist Program (2)
East Grand Forks Area Vocational Technical Institute
Highway 220 North
East Grand Forks, Minnesota 56721

Respiratory Therapist Program (1)
St. Mary's Junior College
2500 South Sixth Street
Minneapolis, Minnesota 55454

Respiratory Therapist Program (1)
Rochester Community College
Mayo Foundation
East Highway 14
Rochester, Minnesota 55904

Respiratory Therapist Program (1)
St. Paul Technical Vocational Institute
235 Marshall Avenue
St. Paul, Minnesota 55102

MISSISSIPPI

Respiratory Therapist Program (1)
Itawamba Junior College
Fulton, Mississippi 38843

Respiratory Therapist Program (1)
University of Mississippi Medical Center
School of Health Related Professions
2500 North State Street
Jackson, Mississippi 39216

Respiratory Therapist Program (1)
Hinds Junior College
Raymond, Mississippi 39154

Respiratory Therapist Program (1)
Northwest Mississippi Junior College
DeSoto Center
Southaven, Mississippi 38671

MISSOURI

Respiratory Therapist Program (1)
University of Missouri-Columbia
School of Health Related Professions
200 Clark Hall
Columbia, Missouri 65211

Respiratory Therapist Program (1)
Kansas City College Alliance for Respiratory Therapy Education
Avila College
Division of Allied Health
11901 Wornall Road
Kansas City, Missouri 64145

Respiratory Therapist Program (1)
Southwest Missouri State University
1900 South National Avenue
Springfield, Missouri 65804

Respiratory Therapist Program (1)
St. Louis Community College at Forest Park
5600 Oakland Avenue
St. Louis, Missouri 63110

MONTANA

Respiratory Therapist Program (2)
Great Falls Vocational Technical Center
2100 16 Avenue South
Great Falls, Montana 59405

NEBRASKA

Respiratory Therapist Program (1)
Southeast Community College
8800 "O" Street
Lincoln, Nebraska 68520

Respiratory Therapist Program (1)
College of Saint Mary
1901 South 72nd Street
Omaha, Nebraska 68124

Respiratory Therapist Program (1)
Creighton University
School of Pharmacy & Allied Health Sciences
2500 California Street
Omaha, Nebraska 68178

Respiratory Therapist Program (1)
Immanuel Medical Center-Midland
Lutheran College
6901 North 72nd Street
Omaha, Nebraska 68122

NEVADA

Respiratory Therapist Program (1)
Clark County Community College
3200 East Cheyenne Avenue
North Las Vegas, Nevada 89030

NEW HAMPSHIRE

Respiratory Therapist Program (1)
New Hampshire Vocational Technical College
Hanover Street Extension
Claremont, New Hampshire 03743

NEW JERSEY

Respiratory Therapist Program (1)
Brookdale Community College
765 Newman Springs Road
Lincroft, New Jersey 07738

Respiratory Therapist Program (1)
Fairleigh Dickinson University
Florham-Madison Campus
285 Madison Avenue
Madison, New Jersey 07940

Respiratory Therapist Program (1)
Atlantic Community College
Black Horse Pike
Mays Landing, New Jersey 08330

Respiratory Therapist Program (1)
Bergen Community College
400 Paramus Road
Paramus, New Jersey 07652

Respiratory Therapist Program (1)
Union County College
1776 Raritan Road
Scotch Plains, New Jersey 07076

NEW YORK

Respiratory Therapist Program (1)
Long Island University
University Plaza
Brooklyn, New York 11201

Respiratory Therapist Program (1)
Erie Community College
Main and Youngs Road
Buffalo, New York 14221

Respiratory Therapist Program (1)
Nassau Community College
Stewart Avenue
Garden City, New York 11530

Respiratory Therapist Program (1)
Borough of Manhattan Community College
199 Chambers Street
New York, New York 10007

Respiratory Therapist Program (1)
New York City Health and Hospitals Corporation
Office of Training and Development
125 Worth Street
New York, New York 10013

Respiratory Therapist Program (1)
New York University Medical Center
Bellevue Hospital
550 First Avenue
New York, New York 10016

Respiratory Therapist Program (1)
State University of New York-Stony Brook
School of Allied Health Professions
Health Sciences Center
Stony Brook, New York 11794

Respiratory Therapist Program (1)
Rockland Community College
145 College Road
Suffern, New York 10901

Respiratory Therapist Program (1)
Onondaga Community College
Route 173
Syracuse, New York 13215

Respiratory Therapist Program (1)
State University of New York
Upstate Medical Center
750 East Adams Street
Syracuse, New York 13210

Respiratory Therapist Program (1)
Hudson Valley Community College
80 Vandenburgh Avenue
Troy, New York 12180

Respiratory Therapist Program (1)
Westchester Community College
75 Grasslands Road
Valhalla, New York 10595

NORTH CAROLINA

Respiratory Therapist Program (1)
Stanley Technical College
Route 4, Box 55
Albemarle, North Carolina 28234

Respiratory Therapist Program (1)
Sandhills Community College
Route 3, Box 182-C
Carthage, North Carolina 28327

Respiratory Therapist Program (1)
Central Piedmont Community College
P.O. Box 35009
Charlotte, North Carolina 28235

Respiratory Therapist Program (1)
Durham Technical Institute
Post Office Drawer 11307
1637 Lawson Street
Durham, North Carolina 27703

Respiratory Therapist Program (1)
Fayetteville Technical Institute
2201 Hull Road
Fayetteville, North Carolina 28303

Respiratory Therapist Program (2)
Pitt Community College
Post Office Drawer 7007
Greenville, North Carolina 27834

Respiratory Therapist Program (1)
Carteret Technical College
3505 Arendell Street
Morehead City, North Carolina 28557

Respiratory Therapist Program (1)
Forsyth Technical Institute
2100 Silas Creek Parkway
Winston-Salem, North Carolina 27103

NORTH DAKOTA

Respiratory Therapist Program (1)
North Dakota School of Respiratory Therapy
St. Alexius Hospital
Post Office Box 1658
Bismarck, North Dakota 58502

OHIO

Respiratory Therapist Program (1)
University of Akron
302 E. Buchtel Avenue
Akron, Ohio 44325

Respiratory Therapist Program (1)
Cincinnati Technical College
3520 Central Parkway
Cincinnati, Ohio 45223

Respiratory Therapist Program (1)
Columbus Technical Institute
550 East Spring Street
Columbus, Ohio 43216

Respiratory Therapist Program (1)
Ohio State University
1583 Perry Street
Columbus, Ohio 43210

Respiratory Therapist Program (1)
Sinclair Community College
444 West Third Street
Dayton, Ohio 45402

Respiratory Therapist Program (1)
Kettering College of Medical Arts
3737 Southern Boulevard
Kettering, Ohio 45429

Respiratory Therapist Program (2)
Lima Technical College
4240 Campus Drive
Lima, Ohio 45804

Respiratory Therapist Program (2)
North Central Technical College
2441 Kenwood Circle
Mansfield, Ohio 44901-0698

Respiratory Therapist Program (1)
Lakeland Community College
Mentor, Ohio 44060

Respiratory Therapist Program (1)
College of Mt. St. Joseph on the Ohio
5701 Delhi Road
Mt. St. Joseph, Ohio 45051

Respiratory Therapist Program (1)
Cuyahoga Community College
11000 Pleasant Valley Road
Parma, Ohio 44130

Respiratory Therapist Program (1)
Shawnee State Community College
940 Second Street
Portsmouth, Ohio 45662

Respiratory Therapist Program (1)
University of Toledo
Community and Technical College
2801 West Bancroft Street
Toledo, Ohio 43606

Respiratory Therapist Program (2)
Jefferson Technical College
4000 Sunset Boulevard
Steubenville, Ohio 43952

Respiratory Therapist Program (1)
Youngstown State University
410 Wick Avenue
Youngstown, Ohio 44555

OKLAHOMA

Respiratory Therapist Program (1)
Rose State College
6420 Southeast 15th Street
Midwest City, Oklahoma 73110

Respiratory Therapist Program (1)
Tulsa Junior College
909 South Boston
Tulsa, Oklahoma 74119

OREGON

Respiratory Therapist Program (1)
Lane Community College
4000 East 30th Avenue
Eugene, Oregon 97405

Respiratory Therapist Program (1)
Mt. Hood Community College
26000 Southeast Stark Street
Gresham, Oregon 97030

Respiratory Therapist Program (1)
Rogue Community College
3345 Redwood Highway
Grants Pass, Oregon 97526

PENNSYLVANIA

Respiratory Therapist Program (1)
Gannon University
Perry Square
Erie, Pennsylvania 16541

Respiratory Therapist Program (1)
Gwynedd Mercy College
Gwynedd Valley, Pennsylvania 19437

Respiratory Therapist Program (1)
Harrisburg Area Community College
3300 Cameron Street Road
Harrisburg, Pennsylvania 17110

Respiratory Therapist Program (1)
University of Pittsburgh at Johnstown
Johnstown, Pennsylvania 15904

Respiratory Therapist Program (1)
Mansfield University of Pennsylvania
Mansfield, Pennsylvania 16933

Respiratory Therapist Program (1)
Millersville University of Pennsylvania
Millersville, Pennsylvania 17551

Respiratory Therapist Program (1)
Community College of Allegheny County
Allegheny Campus
808 Ridge Avenue
Pittsburgh, Pennsylvania 15212

Respiratory Therapist Program (1)
Indiana University of Pennsylvania
Western Pennsylvania Hospital
4800 Friendship Avenue
Pittsburgh, Pennsylvania 15224

Respiratory Therapist Program (1)
Community College of Philadelphia
1700 Spring Garden Street
Philadelphia, Pennsylvania 19130

Respiratory Therapist Program (1)
Hahnemann School of Allied Health Professions
230 North Broad Street
Philadelphia, Pennsylvania 19102

Respiratory Therapist Program (1)
Delaware County Community College
Crozer-Chester Medical Center
15th Street and Upland Avenue
Upland, Chester, Pennsylvania 19013

Respiratory Therapist Program (1)
York College of Pennsylvania
York, Pennsylvania 17403-3426

Respiratory Therapist Program (1)
West Chester University
West Chester, Pennsylvania 19383

PUERTO RICO

Respiratory Therapist Program (2)
Universidad Metropolitana
Post Office Box CUM
Rio Piedras, Puerto Rico 00928

RHODE ISLAND

Respiratory Therapist Program (1)
Roger Williams College
Rhode Island Hospital
Old Ferry Road
Bristol, Rhode Island 02809

Respiratory Therapist Program (2)
Community College of Rhode Island
Flanagan Campus
1762 Louisquisset Pike
Lincoln, Rhode Island 02865

SOUTH CAROLINA

Respiratory Therapist Program (1)
Trident Technical College
Post Office Box 10367
Charleston, South Carolina 29411

Respiratory Therapist Program (1)
Midlands Technical College
Post Office Box 2408
Columbia, South Carolina 29202

Respiratory Therapist Program (1)
Greenville Technical College
P.O. Box 5616, Station B
Greenville, South Carolina 29606

SOUTH DAKOTA

Respiratory Therapist Program (1)
Dakota State College
Madison, South Dakota 57042

Respiratory Therapist Program (1)
Mount Marty College
West Fifth Street
Yankton, South Dakota 57078

TENNESSEE

Respiratory Therapist Program (1)
Chattanooga State Technical Community College
4501 Amnicola Highway
Chattanooga, Tennessee 37406

Respiratory Therapist Program (1)
Columbia State Community College
P.O. Box 1315 - Highway 99 West
Columbia, Tennessee 38401

Respiratory Therapist Program (1)
Roane State Community College
Patton Lane
Harriman, Tennessee 37748

Respiratory Therapist Program (1)
Jackson State Community College
Post Office Box 2467
Jackson, Tennessee 38302-2467

Respiratory Therapist Program (1)
Christian Brothers College
650 East Parkway South
Memphis, Tennessee 38104

TEXAS

Respiratory Therapist Program (1)
Alvin Community College
3110 Mustang Road
Alvin, Texas 77511

Respiratory Therapist Program (1)
Amarillo College
P.O. Box 447
Amarillo, Texas 79178

Respiratory Therapist Program (1)
Lamar University
College of Health and Behavioral Sciences
Post Office Box 100096
Beaumont, Texas 77710

Respiratory Therapist Program (1)
Texas Southmost College
83 Fort Brown
Brownsville, Texas 78520

Respiratory Therapist Program (1)
Del Mar College
Baldwin and Ayers
Corpus Christi, Texas 78404

Respiratory Therapist Program (1)
El Centro College
Main and Lamar Streets
Dallas, Texas 75202

Respiratory Therapist Program (1)
El Paso Community College
P.O. Box 20500
El Paso, Texas 79998

Respiratory Therapist Program (1)
University of Texas Medical Branch
Galveston College
4015 Avenue Q
Galveston, Texas 77550

Respiratory Therapist Program (1)
Houston Community College
Division of Health Careers Education
3100 Shenadoah
Houston, Texas 77021

Respiratory Therapist Program (1)
Texas Southern University
3201 Wheeler Street
Houston, Texas 77004

Respiratory Therapist Program (1)
University of Texas Health Science Center
School of Allied Health Sciences
P.O. Box 20708
Houston, Texas 77030

Respiratory Therapist Program (1)
Tarrant County Junior College
Northeast Campus
828 Harwood Road
Hurst, Texas 76053

Respiratory Therapist Program (1)
South Plains College at Lubbock
1302 Main Street
Lubbock, Texas 79401

Respiratory Therapist Program (1)
Midland College
3600 North Garfield
Midland, Texas 79701

Respiratory Therapist Program (1)
Odessa College
201 West University
Odessa, Texas 79762

Respiratory Therapist Program (1)
San Jacinto College
8060 Spencer Highway
Pasadena, Texas 77505

Respiratory Therapist Program (1)
Southwest Texas State University
San Marcos, Texas 78666

Respiratory Therapist Program (1)
Temple Junior College
2600 South First Street
Temple, Texas 76501

Respiratory Therapist Program (1)
Tyler Junior College
Post Office Box 9020
Tyler, Texas 75711

UTAH

Respiratory Therapist Program (1)
Weber State College
Box 1102
3750 Harrison Boulevard
Ogden, Utah 84408

VIRGINIA

Respiratory Therapist Program (1)
Northern Virginia Community College
8333 Little River Turnpike
Annandale, Virginia 23003

Respiratory Therapist Program (1)
Piedmont Virginia Community College
Route 6, Box 1A
Charlottesville, Virginia 22901

Respiratory Therapist Program (1)
J. Sargeant Reynolds Community College
Post Office Box 12084
Richmond, Virginia 23241

Respiratory Therapist Program (1)
Community Hospital of Roanoke Valley
College of Health Sciences
Post Office 12946
Roanoke, Virginia 24029

Respiratory Therapist Program (1)
Tidewater Community College
Virginia Beach Campus
1700 College Crescent
Virginia Beach, Virginia 23456

Respiratory Therapist Program (1)
Shenandoah College
Winchester Memorial Hospital
Post Office Box 3340
Winchester, Virginia 22601

WASHINGTON

Respiratory Therapist Program (1)
Highline Community College
Midway, Washington 98031-0424

Respiratory Therapist Program (1)
Spokane Community College
North 1810 Greene Street
Spokane, Washington 99207

Respiratory Therapist Program (1)
Tacoma Community College
5900 South 12th Street
Tacoma, Washington 98465

Respiratory Therapist Program (1)
Walla Walla Community College
500 Tausick Way
Walla Walla, Washington 99362

WEST VIRGINIA

Respiratory Therapist Program (1)
University of Charleston
College of Health Sciences
2300 Mac Corkle Avenue, S.E.
Charleston, West Virginia 25304

Respiratory Therapist Program (1)
Wheeling College
316 Washington Avenue
Wheeling, West Virginia 26003

Respiratory Therapist Program (1)
West Virginia Northern Community College
College Square
Wheeling, West Virginia 26003

WISCONSIN

Respiratory Therapist Program (1)
Madison Area Technical College
211 North Carroll
Madison, Wisconsin 53703

Respiratory Therapist Program (1)
Mid-State Technical Institute
110 West Third Street
Post Office Box 50
Marshfield, Wisconsin 54449

Respiratory Therapist Program (1)
Milwaukee Area Technical College
1015 North Sixth Street
Milwaukee, Wisconsin 53203

Respiratory Therapy Technician

The *respiratory therapy technician* is often supervised by the respiratory therapist and is responsible for the majority of bedside patient care. The technician carries out most of the non-critical respiratory treatments, such as administering oxygen and other gases, delivering breathing treatments, and setting up and operating equipment. He or she also cleans, sterilizes, and maintains the respiratory therapy equipment, and keeps medical records of patient's therapies.

Training to become a respiratory therapy technician involves completion of high school and a 10 - 15 month certificate educational program. The educational programs are generally offered by hospitals and community and junior colleges. Certification by examination is available from the National Board for Respiratory Care after graduation from an approved respiratory therapy technician program. After successfully meeting all requirements, the respiratory therapy technician may use the title, "Certified Respiratory Therapy Technician (CRTT)".

According to a 1987 salary survey compiled by the American Association for Respiratory Care, staff respiratory therapy technicians with no supervisory responsibilities earned salaries ranging from $7,800 to $34,000 annually, with average salaries equalling $18,000.

Below is a list of educational programs for respiratory therapy technicians provided by the Joint Review Committee for Respiratory Therapy Education.

KEY:

(1) Accredited by the American Medical Association Committee on Allied Health Education and Accreditation.

(2) Program holds a Letter of Review from the Joint Review Committee for Respiratory Therapy Education.

(Graduates of catagories (1) and (2) are eligible to take the national certifying examinations.)

SOURCES:

American Association for Respiratory Care
Joint Review Committee for Respiratory Therapy Education
National Board for Respiratory Care
Occupational Outlook Handbook

Respiratory Therapy Technician Programs

ARIZONA

Respiratory Therapy Technician Program (1)
Arizona College of Medical-Dental Careers
4020 North 19th Avenue
Phoenix, Arizona 85015

Respiratory Therapy Technician Program (1)
Maricopa Technical Community College
108 North 40th Street
Phoenix, Arizona 85034

Respiratory Therapy Technician Program (1)
Long Medical Institute
4126 North Black Canyon Highway
Phoenix, Arizona 85020

Respiratory Therapy Technician Program (1)
Biosystems, Inc.
1701 S. 52nd Street
Tempe, Arizona 85282

Respiratory Therapy Technician Program (1)
Arizona College of Medical & Dental Careers
3975 North Tucson Blvd.
Tucson, Arizona 85719

ARKANSAS

Respiratory Therapy Technician Program (1)
Pulaski Vo-Tech
3000 West Scenic Drive
North Little Rock, Arkansas 72118

Respiratory Therapy Technician Program (1)
Arkansas Valley Vocational Technical School
P.O. Box 506
Ozark, Arkansas 72949

CALIFORNIA

Respiratory Therapy Technician Program (2)
Southland College of Medical & Dental Careers
15610 Crenshaw Boulevard
Gardena, California 90249

Respiratory Therapy Technician Program (1)
Hacienda La Puente Unified School District
La Puente Valley Adult Schools
Valley Vocational Center
1110 Fickewirth Avenue
La Puente, California 91744

Respiratory Therapy Technician Program (1)
California Paramedical and Technical College
3745 Long Beach Boulevard
Long Beach, California 90807

Respiratory Therapy Technician Program (1)
Modesto Junior College
Post Office Box 4065
Modesto, California 95352

Respiratory Therapy Technician Program (1)
Valley College of Medical & Dental Careers
4150 Lankershim Boulevard
North Hollywood, California 91602

Respiratory Therapy Technician Program (1)
California College for Respiratory Therapy
1810 State Street
San Diego, California 92101

Respiratory Therapy Technician Program (1)
Simi Valley Adult School
3150 School Street
Simi Valley, California 93065

Respiratory Therapy Technician Program (1)
San Joaquin Valley College of Medical and Dental Careers
4706 W. Mineral King, Suite K
Visalia, California 93291

Respiratory Therapy Technician Program (1)
Mt. San Antonio College
1100 North Grand Avenue
Walnut, California 91789

Respiratory Therapy Technician Program (1)
Crafton Hills College
11711 Sand Canyon Road
Yucaipa, California 92399

COLORADO

Respiratory Therapy Technician Program (1)
T. H. Pickens Technical Center
Aurora Public Schools
500 Buckley Road
Aurora, Colorado 80011

CONNECTICUT

Respiratory Therapy Technician Program (1)
Bridgeport Hospital
267 Grant Street
Post Office Box 5000
Bridgeport, Connecticut 06610

Respiratory Therapy Technician Program (1)
Saint Francis Hospital & Medical Center
114 Woodland Street
Hartford, Connecticut 06105

FLORIDA

Respiratory Therapy Technician Program (1)
Boca Raton Community Hospital, Inc.
800 Meadows Road
Boca Raton, Florida 33432

Respiratory Therapy Technician Program (1)
Brevard Community College
1519 Clearlake Road
Cocoa, Florida 32922

Respiratory Therapy Technician Program (1)
Daytona Beach Community College
Post Office Box 1111
Daytona Beach, Florida 32015

Respiratory Therapy Technician Program (1)
Broward Community College
3501 Southwest Davie Road
Fort Lauderdale, Florida 33314

Respiratory Therapy Technician Program (1)
Flagler Career Institute
3225 University Blvd., South
Jacksonville, Florida 32216

Respiratory Therapy Technician Program (1)
Flagler Career Institute
2125 Biscayne Boulevard
Miami, Florida 33137

Respiratory Therapy Technician Program (1)
Miami-Dade Community College
Medical Center Campus
950 Northwest 20th Street
Miami, Florida 33127

Respiratory Therapy Technician Program (1)
Gulf Coast Community College
5230 West U.S. Highway 98
Panama City, Florida 32401

Respiratory Therapy Technician Program (1)
Pensacola Junior College
Warrington Campus
5555 West Highway 98
Pensacola, Florida 32507

Respiratory Therapy Technician Program (1)
Seminole Community College
Highway 17
92 South
Sanford, Florida 32771

Respiratory Therapy Technician Program (1)
Sarasota County Vo-Tech Adult Center
4748 Beneva Road
Sarasota, Florida 33581

Respiratory Therapy Technician Program (1)
St. Petersburg Vocational Technical Institute
901 34th Street South
St. Petersburg, Florida 33711-2298

Respiratory Therapy Technician Program (1)
Erwin Vocational Technical Center
2010 E. Hillsborough Avenue
Tampa, Florida 33610

GEORGIA

Respiratory Therapy Technician Program (1)
Athens Area Vocational Technical School
U.S. Highway 29, North
Athens, Georgia 30610

Respiratory Therapy Technician Program (1)
Georgia State University
University Plaza
Atlanta, Georgia 30303

Respiratory Therapy Technician Program (1)
August Area Technical School
Health Occupations Education
Lawton B. Evans Campus
1399 Walton Way
Augusta, Georgia 30902

Respiratory Therapy Technician Program (2)
Gwinnett Area Technical School
1250 Atkinson Road
P.O. Box 1505
Lawrenceville, Georgia 30246

Respiratory Therapy Technician Program (1)
Thomas Area Vocational Technical College
Post Office Box 1578
Thomasville, Georgia 31792

HAWAII

Respiratory Therapy Technician Program (1)
Kapiolani Community College
University of Hawaii
620 Pensacola Street
Honolulu, Hawaii 96814

IDAHO

Respiratory Therapy Technician Program (1)
Respiratory Therapy Technician School of Idaho
1717 Arlington
Caldwell, Idaho 83605

ILLINOIS

Respiratory Therapy Technician Program (1)
Belleville Area Junior College
2500 Caryle Road
Belleville, Illinois 62221

Respiratory Therapy Technician Program (1)
Marion Adult Education and Career Training Center, Inc.
128 South Paulina Street
Chicago, Illinois 60612

Respiratory Therapy Technician Program (1)
South Chicago Community Hospital
2320 East 93rd Street
Chicago, Illinois 60617

Respiratory Therapy Technician Program (2)
Illinois Central College
East Peoria, Illinois 61635

Respiratory Therapy Technician Program (1)
College of DuPage
22nd Street and Lambert Road
Glen Ellyn, Illinois 60137

Respiratory Therapy Technician Program (1)
Kankakee Community College
Box 888
Kankakee, Illinois 60901

Respiratory Therapy Technician Program (1)
Black Hawk College
6600 34th Avenue
Moline, Illinois 61265

Respiratory Therapy Technician Program (1)
Rock Valley College
3301 North Mulford Road
Rockford, Illinois 61111

Respiratory Therapy Technician Program (1)
St. John's Hospital
800 East Carpenter
Springfield, Illinois 62769

Respiratory Therapy Technician Program (1)
Victory Memorial Hospital
1324 North Sheridan Road
Waukegan, Illinois 60085

INDIANA

Respiratory Therapy Technician Program (1)
Indiana Vocational Technical College
3116 Canterbury Court
P.O. Box 46
Bloomington, Indiana 47402

Respiratory Therapy Technician Program (1)
Indiana Vocational Technical College
3800 North Anthony
Fort Wayne, Indiana 46805

Respiratory Therapy Technician Program (1)
Indiana Vocational Technical College
Northwest Technical Institute
1440 East 35th Avenue
Gary, Indiana 46409

Respiratory Therapy Technician Program (1)
Indiana Vocational Technical College
One West 26th Street
P.O. Box 1763
Indianapolis, Indiana 46202-1763

Respiratory Therapy Technician Program (1)
Indiana Vocational Technical College
3208 Ross Road
P.O. Box 6299
Lafayette, Indiana 47903

IOWA

Respiratory Therapy Technician Program (1)
Northeast Iowa Technical Institute
R.R. 1
Peosta, Iowa 52068

Respiratory Therapy Technician Program (1)
Hawkeye Institute of Technology
1501 E. Orange Road
P.O. Box 8015
Waterloo, Iowa 50704

KANSAS

Respiratory Therapy Technician Program (1)
Bethany Medical Center
51 North 12th Street
Kansas City, Kansas 66102

Respiratory Therapy Technician Program (2)
Seward County Community College
Box 1137
Liberal, Kansas 67901

Respiratory Therapy Technician Program (1)
Labette Community College
200 South 24th
Parsons, Kansas 67357

Respiratory Therapy Technician Program (2)
Washburn University
School of Applied and Continuing Education
Topeka, Kansas 66621

KENTUCKY

Respiratory Therapy Technician Program (1)
Bowling Green State Vocational Technical School
1845 Loop Drive
Bowling Green, Kentucky 42101

Respiratory Therapy Technician Program (1)
Madisonville State Vocational Technical School
Health Occupations Annex
701 North Laffoon Street
Madisonville, Kentucky 42431

Respiratory Therapy Technician Program (1)
West Kentucky State Vocational Technical School
Post Office Box 7408, Blandville Road
Paducah, Kentucky 42001

LOUISIANA

Respiratory Therapy Technician Program (1)
Baton Rouge General Medical Center
3600 Florida Boulevard
P.O. Box 2511
Baton Rouge, Louisiana 70806

Respiratory Therapy Technician Program (1)
Bossier Parish Community College
2719 Airline Drive
Bossier City, Louisiana 71111

Respiratory Therapy Technician Program (1)
Louisiana State University at Eunice
P.O. Box 1129
Eunice, Louisiana 70535

Respiratory Therapy Technician Program (1)
Jefferson Parish West Bank Vocational Technical School
475 Manhattan Boulevard
Harvey, Louisiana 70058

Respiratory Therapy Technician Program (1)
Alton Ochsner Medical Foundation
1516 Jefferson Highway
New Orleans, Louisiana 70121

Respiratory Therapy Technician Program (1)
Delgado Junior College
615 City Park Avenue
New Orleans, Louisiana 70119

Respiratory Therapy Technician Program (1)
Nichols State University
Thibodaux, Louisiana 70301

MAINE

Respiratory Therapy Technician Program (1)
Kennebec Valley Vocational Technical Institute
Gilman Street
Waterville, Maine 04901

MARYLAND

Respiratory Therapy Technician Program (2)
Community College of Baltimore
2901 Liberty Heights Avenue
Baltimore, Maryland 21215

Respiratory Therapy Technician Program (1)
Essex Community College
201 Rosville Boulevard
Baltimore, Maryland 21237

MASSACHUSETTS

Respiratory Therapy Technician Program (1)
Newbury College, Inc.
921 Boylston Street
Boston, Massachusetts 02115

Respiratory Therapy Technician Program (1)
Northern Essex Community College
100 Elliott Street
Haverhill, Massachusetts 01830

MIGHIGAN

Respiratory Therapy Technician Program (1)
Saint John Hospital
22101 Moross Road
Detroit, Michigan 48236

Respiratory Therapy Technician Program (1)
Kalamazoo Valley Community College
6767 West "O" Avenue
Kalamazoo, Michigan 49009

Respiratory Therapy Technician Program (1)
Lansing Community College
Post Office Box 40010
Lansing, Michigan 48901

Respiratory Therapy Technician Program (1)
Monroe County Community College
1555 South Raisinville Road
Monroe, Michigan 48161

Respiratory Therapy Technician Program (1)
Macomb Community College
44575 Garfield Road
Mt. Clemens, Michigan 48044

Respiratory Therapy Technician Program (1)
Muskegon Community College
221 South Quarterline Road
Muskegon, Michigan 49442

Respiratory Therapy Technician Program (1)
Delta College
University Center, Michigan 48710

MINNESOTA

Respiratory Therapy Technician Program (2)
East Grand Forks Area Vocational Technical Institute
Highway 220 North
East Grand Forks, Minnesota 56721

Respiratory Therapy Technician Program (1)
St. Paul Technical Vocational Institute
235 Marshall Avenue
St. Paul, Minnesota 55102

MISSISSIPPI

Respiratory Therapy Technician Program (1)
Northeast Mississippi Junior College
Cunningham Boulevard
Booneville, Mississippi 38829

Respiratory Therapy Technician Program (1)
Itawamba Junior College
Fulton, Mississippi 38843

Respiratory Therapy Technician Program (1)
Mississippi Gulf Coast Junior College
Jackson County Campus
P.O. Box 100
Gautier, Mississippi 39553

Respiratory Therapy Technician Program (1)
Pearl River Junior College
Forrest County Branch
Route 6, Box 406
Hattiesburg, Mississippi 39401

Respiratory Therapy Technician Program (1)
Hinds Junior College-Jackson Branch
Nursing Allied Health Center
1750 Chadwick Drive
Jackson, Mississippi 39204

Respiratory Therapy Technician Program (1)
University of Mississippi Medical Center
School of Health Related Professions
2500 North State Street
Jackson, Mississippi 39216

Respiratory Therapy Technician Program (1)
Meridian Junior College
5500 Highway 19 North
Meridian, Mississippi 39301

MISSOURI

Respiratory Therapy Technician Program (1)
Cape Girardeau Area Vocational Technical School
301 North Clark Avenue
Cape Girardeau, Missouri 63701

Respiratory Therapy Technician Program (1)
Columbia Public Schools
Health Occupations Center
600 Strawn Road
Columbia, Missouri 65201

Respiratory Therapy Technician Program (1)
Hannibal Area Vocational Technical School
4500 McMasters Avenue
Hannibal, Missouri 63401

Respiratory Therapy Technician Program (1)
State Fair Community College
1900 Clarendon Road
Sedalia, Missouri 65301

Respiratory Therapy Technician Program (1)
School District of Springfield R-12
Graff Area Vocational Technical Center
815 North Sherman
Springfield, Missouri 65802

Respiratory Therapy Technician Program (1)
St. Louis Community College at Forest Park
5600 Oakland Avenue
St. Louis, Missouri 63110

MONTANA

Respiratory Therapy Technician Program (1)
Great Falls Vocational Technical Center
2100 16 Avenue South
Great Falls, Montana 59405

Respiratory Therapy Technician Program (1)
Missoula Technical Center
909 South Avenue West
Missoula, Montana 59801

NEBRASKA

Respiratory Therapy Technician Program (1)
Southeast Community College
8800 O" Street"
Lincoln, Nebraska 68520

Respiratory Therapy Technician Program (1)
Metropolitan Technical College
P.O. Box 3777
Omaha, Nebraska 68103

NEVEDA

Respiratory Therapy Technician Program (1)
Clark County Community College
3200 East Cheyenne Avenue
North Las Vegas, Nevada 89030

NEW JERSEY

Respiratory Therapy Technician Program (1)
Saint Barnabas Medical Center
Old Short Hills Road
Livingston, New Jersey 07039

Respiratory Therapy Technician Program (1)
Atlantic Community College
Black Horse Pike
Mays Landings, New Jersey 08330

Respiratory Therapy Technician Program (1)
Passaic County Community College
College Boulevard
Paterson, New Jersey 07509

Respiratory Therapy Technician Program (1)
Gloucester County College
Tanyard Road
Deptford Township
Sewell, New Jersey 08080

NEW MEXICO

Respiratory Therapy Technician Program (1)
Albuquerque Technical-Vocational Institute
525 Buena Vista Southeast
Albuquerque, New Mexico 87106

NEW YORK

Respiratory Therapy Technician Program (1)
United Health Services School of Respiratory Therapy
33-57 Harrison Street
Johnson City, New York 13790

Respiratory Therapy Technician Program (1)
New York City Health & Hospitals Corporation
346 Broadway, Room 1136
New York, New York 10013

Respiratory Therapy Technician Program (1)
Onondaga Community College
Route 173
Syracuse, New York 13215

Respiratory Therapy Technician Program (1)
Mohawk Valley Community College
1101 Sherman Drive
Utica, New York 13501

NORTH CAROLINA

Respiratory Therapy Technician Program (1)
Stanly Technical College
Route 4, Box 5
Albemarle, North Carolina 28001

Respiratory Therapy Technician Program (1)
Durham Technical Institute
Post Office Box 11307
Durham, North Carolina 27703

Respiratory Therapy Technician Program (1)
Carteret Technical College
3505 Arendale Street
Morehead City, North Carolina 28557

Respiratory Therapy Technician Program (1)
Forsyth Technical Institute
2100 Silas Creek Parkway
Winston-Salem, North Carolina 27103

NORTH DAKOTA

Respiratory Therapy Technician Program (1)
St. Luke's Hospitals
Fifth at Mills Avenue
Fargo, North Dakota 58122

OHIO

Respiratory Therapy Technician Program (1)
Stark Technical College
600 Frank Avenue, N.W.
Canton, Ohio 44720

Respiratory Therapy Technician Program (1)
Cincinnati Technical College
3520 Central Parkway
Cincinnati, Ohio 45223

Respiratory Therapy Technician Program (1)
Columbus Technical Institute
550 East Spring Street
Columbus, Ohio 43215

Respiratory Therapy Technician Program (1)
Lima Technical College
4240 Campus Drive
Lima, Ohio 45804

Respiratory Therapy Technician Program (1)
Cuyahoga Community College
11000 Pleasant Valley Road
Parma, Ohio 44130

Respiratory Therapy Technician Program (1)
Shawnee State Community College
940 Second Street
Portsmouth, Ohio 45662

Respiratory Therapy Technician Program (1)
University of Toledo
Community and Technical College
2801 West Bancroft Street
Toledo, Ohio 43606

Respiratory Therapy Technician Program (1)
Mid-East Ohio Vocational School
400 Richards Road
Zanesville, Ohio 43701

OKLAHOMA

Respiratory Therapy Technician Program (1)
Francis Tuttle Vo-Tech Center
12777 North Rockwell
Oklahoma City, Oklahoma 73142

Respiratory Therapy Technician Program (1)
Rose State College
6420 Southeast 15th Street
Midwest City, Oklahoma 73110

Respiratory Therapy Technician Program (1)
Tulsa Junior College
909 South Boston
Tulsa, Oklahoma 74119

OREGON

Respiratory Therapy Technician Program (1)
Rogue Community College
3345 Redwood Highway
Grants Pass, Oregon 97526

PENNSYLVANIA

Respiratory Therapy Technician Program (1)
Thiel College
College Avenue
Greenville, Pennsylvania 16125

Respiratory Therapy Technician Program (1)
Gwynedd Mercy College
Gwynedd Valley, Pennsylvania 19437

Respiratory Therapy Technician Program (1)
Harrisburg Area Community College
3300 Cameron Street Road
Harrisburg, Pennsylvania 17110

Respiratory Therapy Technician Program (1)
Luzerne County Community College
Middle Road & Prospect Street
Naticoke, Pennsylvania 18634

Respiratory Therapy Technician Program (1)
James Martin School
Adult Vocational Training Center
Richmond and Ontario Streets
Philadelphia, Pennsylvania 19134

Respiratory Therapy Technician Program (1)
Community College of Allegheny County
Allegheny Campus
808 Ridge Avenue
Pittsburgh, Pennsylvania 15212

Respiratory Therapy Technician Program (1)
St. Francis Medical Center
45th Street off Penn Avenue
Pittsburgh, Pennsylvania 15201

Respiratory Therapy Technician Program (1)
Lehigh County Community College
2370 Main Street
Schnecksville, Pennsylvania 18078

Respiratory Therapy Technician Program (1)
York College of Pennsylvania
York, Pennsylvania 17403-3426

SOUTH CAROLINA

Respiratory Therapy Technician Program (1)
Midlands Technical College
Post Office Box 2408
Columbia, South Carolina 29200

Respiratory Therapy Technician Program (1)
Florence-Darlington Technical College
P.O. Drawer 8000
Florence, South Carolina 29501

Respiratory Therapy Technician Program (1)
Greenville Technical College
P.O. Box 5616, Station B
Greenville, South Carolina 29606

Respiratory Therapy Technician Program (1)
Piedmont Technical College
Post Office Drawer 1467
Greenwood, South Carolina 29646

Respiratory Therapy Technician Program (1)
Orangeburg-Calhoun Technical College
P.O. Drawer 1767
Highway 601, North
Orangeburg, South Carolina 29115

Respiratory Therapy Technician Program (1)
Spartanburg Technical College
Drawer 4386
Spartanburg, South Carolina 29305

SOUTH DAKOTA

Respiratory Therapy Technician Program (1)
Dakota State College
Madison, South Dakota 57042

Respiratory Therapy Technician Program (1)
Mount Marty College
West Fifth Street
Yankton, South Dakota 57078

TENNESSEE

Respiratory Therapy Technician Program (1)
East Tennessee State University
Paramedical Center
1000 West E Street
Elizabethton, Tennessee 37643

Respiratory Therapy Technician Program (1)
Volunteer State Community College
Nashville Pike
Gallatin, Tennessee 37066

Respiratory Therapy Technician Program (1)
Memphis Area Vocational-Technical School
620 Mosby Avenue
Memphis, Tennessee 38105

TEXAS

Respiratory Therapy Technician Program (1)
Alvin Community College
3110 Mustang Road
Alvin, Texas 77511

Respiratory Therapy Technician Program (1)
Lamar University
Post Office Box 10096
Beaumont, Texas 77710

Respiratory Therapy Technician Program (1)
Texas Southmost College
80 Fort Brown
Brownsville, Texas 78520

Respiratory Therapy Technician Program (1)
Del Mar College
Baldwin and Ayers
Corpus Christi, Texas 78404

Respiratory Therapy Technician Program (1)
El Centro College
Main and Lamar Streets
Dallas, Texas 75202

Respiratory Therapy Technician Program (1)
Academy of Health Sciences
Brooke Army Medical Center
Department of Medicine
Fort Sam
Houston, Texas 78234-6200

Respiratory Therapy Technician Program (1)
Houston Community College
3100 Shenandoah
Houston, Texas 77021

Respiratory Therapy Technician Program (1)
University of Texas Health Science Center at Houston
P.O. Box 20708
Houston, Texas 77030

Respiratory Therapy Technician Program (2)
North Harris County College District
East Campus
20,000 Kingwood Drive
Kingwood, Texas 77339

Respiratory Therapy Technician Program (1)
South Plains College at Lubbock
1302 Main Street
Lubbock, Texas 79401

Respiratory Therapy Technician Program (1)
Midland College
3600 North Garfield
Midland, Texas 79701

Respiratory Therapy Technician Program (1)
Odessa College
201 West University
Odessa, Texas 79762

Respiratory Therapy Technician Program (1)
San Jacinto College
8060 Spencer Highway
Pasadena, Texas 77505

Respiratory Therapy Technician Program (1)
St. Philip's College
2111 Nevada Street
San Antonio, Texas 78203

Respiratory Therapy Technician Program (1)
Southwest Texas State University
San Marcos, Texas 78666

Respiratory Therapy Technician Program (1)
Tyler Junior College
Post Office Box 9020
Tyler, Texas 75711

Respiratory Therapy Technician Program (1)
Victoria College
2200 East Red River
Victoria, Texas 77901

Respiratory Therapy Technician Program (1)
McLennan Community College
1400 College Drive
Waco, Texas 76708

UTAH

Respiratory Therapy Technician Program (1)
Weber State College
Box 1102
3750 Harrison Boulevard
Ogden, Utah 84408

VIRGINIA

Respiratory Therapy Technician Program (1)
Mountain Empire Community College
Drawer 700
Big Stone Gap, Virginia 24219

Respiratory Therapy Technician Program (1)
Central Virginia Community College
Fort Hill Station
P.O. Box 4098
Lynchburg, Virginia 24502

Respiratory Therapy Technician Program (1)
Southwest Virginia Community College
Box SVCC
Richlands, Virginia 24641

Respiratory Therapy Technician Program (1)
J. Sargeant Reynolds Community College
P.O. Box 12084
Richmond, Virginia 23241

Respiratory Therapy Technician Program (1)
Tidewater Community College
1700 College Crescent
Virginia Beach, Virginia 23456

Respiratory Therapy Technician Program (1)
Shenandoah College
Winchester Medical Center
Post Office Box 3340
Winchester, Virginia 22601

WASHINGTON

Respiratory Therapy Technician Program (1)
Skagit Valley College
2405 College Way
Mount Vernon, Washington 98273

Respiratory Therapy Technician Program (1)
Seattle Central Community College
1701 Broadway, 2BE3210
Seattle, Washington 98122

Respiratory Therapy Technician Program (1)
Tacoma Community College
5900 South 12th Street
Building "19"
Tacoma, Washington 98465

WISCONSIN

Respiratory Therapy Technician Program (1)
Fox Valley Technical Institute
1825 West Bluemound Drive
Appleton, Wisconsin 54913

Respiratory Therapy Technician Program (1)
Northeast Wisconsin Technical Institute
2740 West Mason Street
Post Office Box 19042
Green Bay, Wisconsin 54307-9042

Respiratory Therapy Technician Program (1)
Western Wisconsin Technical Institute
6th and Vine Streets
LaCrosse, Wisconsin 54601

Respiratory Therapy Technician Program (1)
Milwaukee Area Technical College
1015 North Sixth Street
Milwaukee, Wisconsin 53203

WYOMING

Respiratory Therapy Technician Program (1)
Western Wyoming College
P.O. Box 428
Rock Spring, Wyoming 82901

Respiratory Therapy Aide

Supervised by respiratory therapists and respiratory therapy technicians and having little direct contact with patients, the respiratory therapy aide is mostly concerned with cleaning, disinfecting, sterilizing, and maintaining equipment. She or he may also be responsible for the majority of the clerical duties.

A high school education is the usual prerequisite for admittance into on-the-job hospital training available in some areas. Persons interested in becoming respiratory therapy aides should contact the Chief Respiratory Therapist or the Personnel Director of their local hospital.

According to a 1987 salary survey compiled by the American Association for Respiratory Care, staff respiratory therapy aides in non-supervisory positions earned salaries ranging from $7,000 to $27,000 a year, with average salaries equalling $13,500.

SOURCE:

Dictionary of Occupational Titles

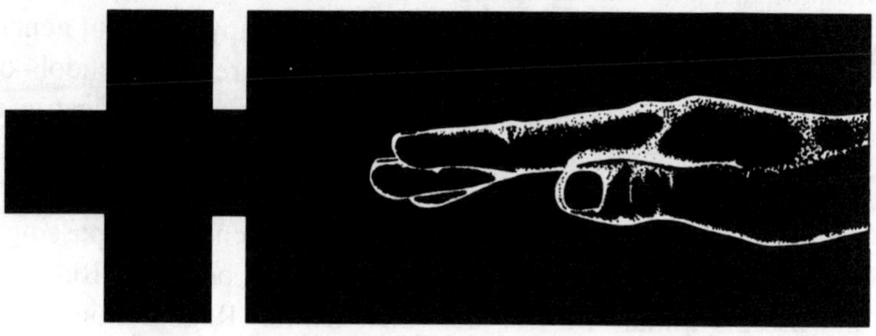

SCIENTIFIC MASSAGE THERAPY

Scientific massage is a systematic manual manipulation of bodily tissues for the purpose of affecting the muscular and nervous systems and the general circulation of the body. It is a method of natural treatment that can be recommended by a physician as a means for restoring the function of muscles and joints, as well as relieving mental and physical fatigue. The qualified practitioner of scientific massage is known as a *massage therapist.*

Massage Therapist

Applying the principles and techniques of scientific massage, the *massage therapist* may be capable of relieving many health disorders and disturbances. The techniques the massage therapist uses may assist in the rehabilitation of sprains, strains, fractures, and dislocations, as well as help eliminate pain from neuritic, arthritic, and rheumatic conditions. The therapist may also be able to apply massage to relieve various forms of paralysis, insomnia, migraine headaches, and other conditions caused by poor functioning of the nervous system. By stimulating the circulatory system, the massage therapist may reduce convalescent periods and improve many conditions after surgery. Shortened recovery time for injured athletes may also be achieved with massage therapy. In addition, massage therapy can also provide relief of muscle tightness caused by stress.

The therapist works with various agents to complement massage, including application of heat and light, hydrotherapy (water treatment), and exercise.

Some massage therapists work in hospitals, clinics, physicians' offices, private practices, sanitariums, and nursing homes while others work in health clubs, spas, and Y.M.C.A.'s.

Length of training programs in massage therapy vary, but generally last one year. The American Massage Therapy Association, Inc., reviews schools of massage therapy and approves them, based on specific curriculum criteria. Certification is available to graduates of curriculum approved schools through membership in the American Massage Therapy Association, Inc. Massage therapists may also become certified in sports massage therapy after graduating from a curriculum approved school and passing a written examination. Massage therapists may also apply to take a test, become a Registered Massage Therapist, and use the initials R.M.T. after their name. Registration requires graduation from a curriculum approved school, successfully passing a written examination, and three years of active membership in the American Massage Therapy Association, Inc. Some states require massage therapists to be licensed. The state's licensing agency (usually located in the state capital) can provide more information.

Specific salary information for massage therapists is not available due to differences in geographic location, experience, and varied places of employment. Many massage therapists do, however, charge fees based on hourly or half-hourly time periods.

The following is a list of schools approved by the National Education Committee of the American Massage Therapy Association, Inc. Currently the American Massage Therapy Association, Inc., approves programs that comprise five hundred (500) hours of classroom instruction with at least six months duration.

For more information about a career as a massage therapist, contact the American Massage Therapy Association, Inc., 1130 W. North Shore Avenue, Chicago, Illinois 60626.

SOURCE:

American Massage Therapy Association, Inc.

Massage Therapist Programs

ARIZONA

Massage Therapist Program
Desert Institute of the Healing Arts
639 North 6th Avenue
Tucson, Arizona 85705

Massage Therapist Program
Phoenix Therapeutic Massage College, Inc.
2545 East Thomas Road
Phoenix, Arizona 85016

CALIFORNIA

Massage Therapist Program
American Institute of Massage Therapy, Inc.
120 East 18th Street
Costa Mesa, California 92627

Massage Therapist Program
Heartwood Healing Arts Institute of California
220 Harmony Lane
Garberville, California 95440

Massage Therapist Program
Institute of Psycho-Structural Balancing
4502 Cass Street
San Diego, California 92109

Massage Therapist Program
Integrative Therapy School
1816 Tribute Road
Sacramento, California 95815

Massage Therapist Program
Mueller College of Massage
4607 Park Boulevard
San Diego, California 92116

Massage Therapist Program
National Holistic Institute
5299 College Avenue
Oakland, California 94618

CANADA

Massage Therapist Program
Canadian College of Massage & Hydrotherapy
85 Church Street, Box 983
Sutton West, Ontario, Canada L0E 1R0

Massage Therapist Program
Sutherland-Chan School & Teaching Clinic
732 Spadina Avenue
Toronto, Ontario, Canada M5S 2J2

COLORADO

Massage Therapist Program
Boulder School of Massage Therapy
1255 Portland Place
Boulder, Colorado 80302

Massage Therapist Program
Stress Massage Institute
Manitou Spa, P.O. Box 1304
Manitou Springs, Colorado 80829

CONNECTICUT

Massage Therapist Program
Connecticut Center for Massage Therapy, Inc.
75 Kitts Lane
Newington, Connecticut 06111

DISTRICT OF COLUMBIA

Massage Therapist Program
Potomac Myotherapy Institute
7826 Eastern Avenue, N.W. Suite LL1
Washington, D.C. 20012

FLORIDA

Massage Therapist Program
Florida School of Massage
5408 S.W. 13th Street
Gainesville, Florida 32608

Massage THerapist Program
Institute of Traditional Healing Arts
3501 S.W. 2nd Avenue, Suite 2500
Gainesville, Florida 32606

Massage Therapist Program
Educating Hands School of Massage
261 S.W. 8th Street
Miami, Florida 33130

Massage Therapist Program
The Humanities Center Schools of Massage
3565 Cypress Terrace
Pinellas Park, Florida 33565

Massage Therapist Program
The Humanities Center Schools of Massage
3805 South Westshore Boulevard
Tampa, Florida 33611

Massage Therapist Program
Institute of Traditional Healing Arts
3501 S.W. 2nd Avenue, Suite 2500
Gainesville, Florida 32606

Massage Therapist Program
Suncoast School of Massage Therapy
4910 West Cypress Street
Tampa, Florida 33607

GEORGIA

Massage Therapist Program
Atlanta School of Massage
Peachwood Park
2300 Peachford Road
Atlanta, Georgia 30338

HAWAII

Massage Therapist Program
Honolulu School of Massage, Inc.
1750 Kalakaua Avenue, Suite 2401
Honolulu, Hawaii 96826

ILLINOIS

Massage Therapist Program
The Chicago School of Massage Therapy
2918 North Lincoln Avenue
Chicago, Illinois 60657

INDIANA

Massage Therapist Program
Alexandria School of Scientific Therapeutics
120 West Church Street
Alexandria, Indiana 46001

Massage Therapist Program
Graham-McClain School of Massage and Multi-Therapy
504 West Third Street
Marion, Indiana 46952

Massage Therapist Program
Lewis School of Massage Therapy
3101 Old Hobart Road
Lake Station, Indiana 46405

IOWA

Massage THerapist Program
Carlson College of Massage Therapy
1756 First Avenue N.E.
Cedar Rapids, IA 52402

MAINE

Massage Therapist Program
Downeast School of Massage
Box 24, Route 220 North
Waldoboro, Maine 04572

MARYLAND

Baltimore Holistic Health Center
School of Therapeutic Massage
6 North Broadway
Baltimore, Maryland 21231

MASSACHUSETTS

Massage Therapist Program
Bancroft School of Massage Therapy
50 Franklin St., Suites 305-370
Worcester, Massachusetts 01608

Massage Therapist Program
Muscular Therapy Institute
222 Third Street
Cambridge, Massachusetts 02142

Massage Therapist Program
New England Institute of Massage
105 Allston Street
Allston, Massachusetts 02134

Massage Therapist Program
Stillpoint Center School of Massage, Inc.
P.O. Box 164
Amherst, Massachusetts 01004

MICHIGAN

Massage Therapist Program
Health Enrichment Massage Therapy
408 Davis Lake Road
Lapeer, Michigan 48446

MINNESOTA

Massage Therapist Program
Northern Lights Institute
P.O. Box 7556
1854 East 38th Street
Minneapolis, Minnesota 55407

NEW HAMPSHIRE

Massage Therapist Program
New Hampshire Institute for Therapeutic Arts-School of Massage Therapy
153 Lowell Road
Hudson, New Hampshire 03051

NEW MEXICO

Massage Therapist Program
New Mexico School of Natural Therapeutics
106 Girard S.E., Suite 107-A
Albuquerque, New Mexico 87106

Massage Therapist Program
The New Mexico Academy of Massage and Advanced Healing Arts
P.O. Box 932
Santa Fe, New Mexico 87504

Massage Therapist Program
Dr. Jay Scherer's Academy of Natural Healing, Inc.
Route 14, Box 314
Santa Fe, New Mexico 87505

NEW YORK

Massage Therapist Program
Swedish Institute, Inc.
875 Avenue of the Americas
New York, New York 10001

OHIO

Massage Therapist Program
Central Ohio School of Massage
35 East Gay Street, Suite 110
Columbus, Ohio 43215

Massage Therapist Program
Self-Health Institutes, Inc.
School of Medical Massage
138 South Main Street
Centerville, Ohio 45459

OREGON

Massage Therapist Program
East-West College of Massage Therapy
2926 N.E. Flanders
Portland, Oregon 97232

PENNSYLVANIA

Massage Therapist Program
Pennsylvania School of Muscle Therapy
651 South Gulph Road
King of Prussia, Pennsylvania 19406

TEXAS

Massage Therapist Program
Asten Center of Natural Therapeutics
200 East Spring Valley, Suite D
Richardson, Texas 75081

Massage Therapist Program
Texas School of Massage Studies
1910 Justin Lane
Austin, Texas 78757

WASHINGTON

Massage Therapist Program
Olympic School of Natural Therapeutics
511 East First Street
Port Angeles, Washington 98362

Massage Therapist Program
Tri-City School of Massage
26 East Third Avenue
Kennewick, Washington 99336

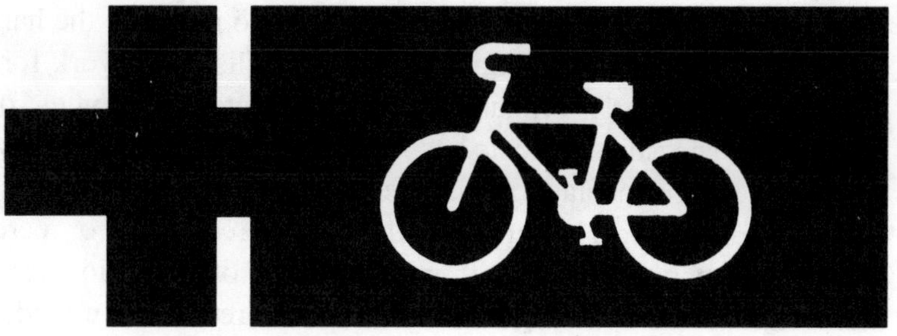

THERAPEUTIC RECREATION

Therapeutic recreation is a specialized allied health field within the recreation profession. Associated with the leisure aspects of medical treatment, therapeutic recreation attempts to physically and socially rehabilitate patients who have chronic physical, psychological, and social handicaps. It involves recreation services that give the patient an opportunity to participate in recreational, leisure and group activities specifically designed to aid in recovery from or adjustment to illness, disability, or a specific social problem. There are two career opportunities in therapeutic recreation: the *therapeutic recreation specialist* and the *therapeutic recreation assistant.*

Therapeutic Recreation Specialist

Also known as a *recreational therapist,* the therapeutic recreation specialist plans, organizes, directs, and counsels medically approved recreation programs. The specialist encourages patients to develop recreational interests and skills and to participate in physical and social activities so that they may better cope with or recover from their illnesses or disabilities. Activities include sports, trips, dramatics, arts and crafts,discussion groups, nature study, and hobbies, and they are administered in accordance with patients' needs, capabilities, and interests. As part of a rehabilitation treatment team, the therapeutic recreation specialist observes and reports on patients' physical, mental, and social progress. This information is then incorporated into the planning of future therapies.

The specialist works in nonmedical as well as medical settings. In the former he or she may work for community recreation agencies to integrate the handicapped into the total community recreation program. Or the specialist may work for schools for the blind, homes for the elderly, orphanages, juvenile detention homes, or prisons. In medical facilities the specialist works in hospitals and rehabilitation centers and is concerned with, among others, the mentally ill, the mentally retarded, and the physically handicapped.

A bachelor's degree, preferably in therapeutic recreation, or recreation with an option in therapeutic recreation, is the minimum level of education for professional status in therapeutic recreation. Programs in therapeutic recreation include classroom as well as a supervised clinical field experience. For executive positions in administration, research, and teaching or in the conducting of training programs a graduate degree is required.

High school students who are interested in a career in therapeutic recreation should become involved with physical education, public speaking, sports, dramatics, music, clubs, and other activities, all of which will help develop skills in basic recreational leadership. Interested students might work as volunteers or paid employees in playgrounds, camps, hospitals, or public and community facilities to gain experience in working with people.

Credentials for the therapeutic recreation specialist are available from the National Council for Therapeutic Recreation Certification for applicants who meet the academic and experience requirements. Prerequisites for certification include 1) minimum of a bachelor's degree in therapeutic recreation or recreation with an option in therapeutic recreation, or 2) minimum of a bachelor's degree in rehabilitation, psychology, sociology, art or music education, dance, drama, early childhood education or related fields plus five-years full time paid experience in a therapeutic recreation program plus 18 semester hours of approved upper division or graduate level therapeutic recreation courses.

A few states currently require therapeutic recreation specialists to meet either certification or licensure criteria. As of 1988, three states, Georgia, North Carolina, and Utah plus the District of Columbia, have enacted licensure legislation. For additional information on state requirements write to the state licensing division, located in the state capital.

Salaries for therapeutic recreation specialists are affected by many factors such as geographic location, type and size of facility, years of experience, and current certification status. Generally average starting salaries for therapeutic recreation specialists equal $18,600 a year according to 1987 figures compiled by the University of Texas Medical Branch. Experienced therapeutic recreation specialists may expect to earn average annual salaries of $24,400.

For further information on career opportunities and certification requirements contact the National Therapeutic Recreation Society, c/o National Recreation and Park Association, 3101 Park Center Drive, Alexandria, Virginia 22302 and the National Council for Therapeutic Recreation Certification, 49 South Main Street, Suite #005, Spring Valley, New York 10977, respectively.

Below is a list, supplied by the National Therapeutic Recreation Society of approved bachelor's degree programs in therapeutic recreation.

SOURCES:

National Therapeutic Recreation Society
Occupational Outlook Handbook

Therapeutic Recreation Specialist Programs

CALIFORNIA

Therapeutic Recreation Program
Department of Recreation Administration
California State University
Chico, California 95429

Therapeutic Recreation Program
Department of Recreation Administration
California State University
Fresno, California 93740

Therapeutic Recreation Program
Department of Recreation and Leisure Studies
California State University
Long Beach, California 90840

Therapeutic Recreation Program
Department of Recreation and Leisure Studies
California State University
Northridge, California 91330

Therapeutic Recreation Program
Department of Recreation and Park Administration
California State University
Sacramento, California 95819

Therapeutic Recreation Program
Department of Recreation and Administration
California Polytechnic State University
San Luis Obispo, California 93407

Therapeutic Recreation Program
Department of Recreation
San Diego State University
San Diego, California 92182

COLORADO

Therapeutic Recreation Program
Department of Recreation Resources
Colorado State University
Fort Collins, Colorado 80523

FLORIDA

Therapeutic Recreation Program
Department of Recreation
University of Florida
Gainesville, Florida 32611

Therapeutic Recreation Program
Department of Leisure Services and Studies
Florida State University
Tallahassee, Florida 32306

GEORGIA

Therapeutic Recreation Program
Department of Recreation and Leisure Studies
University of Georgia
Athens, Georgia 30602

Therapeutic Recreation Program
Department of Therapeutic Recreation
Georgia Southern College
Statesboro, Georgia 30460

ILLINOIS

Therapeutic Recreation Program
Department of Leisure and Environmental
Resources Administration
Aurora University
Aurora, Illinois 60506

Therapeutic Recreation Program
Department of Recreation
Southern Illinois University
Carbondale, Illinois 62901

Therapeutic Recreation Program
Department of Recreation and Leisure Studies
Eastern Illinois University
Charleston, Illinois 61920

Therapeutic Recreation Program
Department of Leisure Studies
College of St. Francis
Joliet, Illinois 60435

Therapeutic Recreation Program
Department of Recreation and Park Administration
Western Illinois University
Macomb, Illinois 61455

Therapeutic Recreation Program
Department of Recreation and Park Administration
Illinois State University
Normal, Illinois 61761

Therapeutic Recreation Program
Department of Leisure Studies
University of Illinois
Urbana, Illinois 61801

INDIANA

Therapeutic Recreation Program
Department of Recreation and Park Administration
Indiana University
Bloomington, Indiana 47401

Therapeutic Recreation Program
Department of Recreation
Indiana State University
Terre Haute, Indiana 47809

IOWA

Therapeutic Recreation Program
Department of Leisure Studies
Iowa State University
Ames, Iowa 50011

Therapeutic Recreation Program
Division of Recreation
University of Northern Iowa
Cedar Falls, Iowa 50614

KENTUCKY

Therapeutic Recreation Program
Department of Recreation and Park Administration
Western Kentucky University
Bowling Green, Kentucky 42101

Therapeutic Recreation Program
Department of Recreation and Park Administration
Eastern Kentucky University
Richmond, Kentucky 40475

LOUISIANA

Therapeutic Recreation Program
Department of Recreation
Grambling State University
Granbling, Louisiana 71245

MARYLAND

Therapeutic Recreation Program
Department of Recreation
University of Maryland
College Park, Maryland 20742

MASSACHUSETTS

Therapeutic Recreation Program
Department of Leisure Studies
University of Massachusetts
Amherst, Massachusetts 01003

Therapeutic Recreation Program
Department of Recreation and Leisure Studies
Springfield College
Springfield, Massachusetts 01109

MICHIGAN

Therapeutic Recreation Program
Department of Recreation and Park Administration
Central Michigan University
Mount Pleasant, Michigan 48859

MINNESOTA

Therapeutic Recreation Program
Division of Recreation, Parks, and Leisure Studies
University of Minnesota
Minneapolis, Minnesota 55455

Therapeutic Recreation Program
Department of Recreation, Parks, and Leisure Services
Mankato State University
Mankato, Minnesota 56001

MISSISSIPPI

Therapeutic Recreation Program
Recreation Department
University of Southern Mississippi
Hattiesburg, Mississippi 39406

MISSOURI

Therapeutic Recreation Program
Department of Recreation and Park Administration
University of Missouri
Columbia, Missouri 65201

NEBRASKA

Therapeutic Recreation Program
Department of Recreation
University of Nebraska
Lincoln, Nebraska 68588

NEW HAMPSHIRE

Therapeutic Recreation Program
Department of Leisure Management and Tourism
University of New Hampshire
Durham, New Hampshire 03824

NEW YORK

Therapeutic Recreation Program
Department of Recreation
Ithaca College
Ithaca, New York 14850

Therapeutic Recreation Program
Department of Recreation and Leisure Studies
New York University
New York, New York 10003

NORTH CAROLINA

Therapeutic Recreation Program
Department of Recreation Administration
University of North Carolina
Chapel Hill, North Carolina 27514

Therapeutic Recreation Program
Division of Recreation and Leisure Studies
University of North Carolina
Greensboro, North Carolina 27412

Therapeutic Recreation Program
Leisure System Studies
East Carolina University
Greenville, North Carolina 27834

Therapeutic Recreation Program
Department of Recreation and Resources Administration
North Carolina State University
Raleigh, North Carolina 27695

Therapeutic Recreation Program
Department of Parks and Recreation Management
University of North Carolina
Wilmington, North Carolina 28403

OKLAHOMA

Therapeutic Recreation Program
Department of Leisure Sciences
Oklahoma State University
Stillwater, Oklahoma 74078

OREGON

Therapeutic Recreation Program
Department of Leisure Studies
University of Oregon
Eugene, Oregon 97403

PENNSYLVANIA

Therapeutic Recreation Program
Department of Recreation and Leisure Services Management
East Stroudsburg State University
East Stroudsburg, Pennsylvania 18301

Therapeutic Recreation Program
Department of Recreation
Lincoln University
Lincoln University, Pennsylvania 19352

Therapeutic Recreation Program
Department of Recreation and Leisure Studies
Temple University
Philadelphia, Pennsylvania 19122

Therapeutic Recreation Program
Department of Parks, Recreation and Environmental Education
Slippery Rock State University
Slippery Rock, Pennsylvania 16057

Therapeutic Recreation Program
Department of Recreation
Pennsylvania State University
University Park, Pennsylvania 16802

Therapeutic Recreation Program
Department of Recreation and Leisure Administration
York College
York, Pennsylvania 17405

SOUTH CAROLINA

Therapeutic Recreation Program
Department of Parks, Recreation and Tourism Management
Clemson University
Clemson, South Carolina 29634

TENNESSEE

Therapeutic Recreation Program
Division of Recreation
University of Tennessee
Knoxville, Tennessee 37996

UTAH

Therapeutic Recreation Program
Department of Recreation Management
Brigham Young University
Provo, Utah 84602

Therapeutic Recreation Program
Department of Recreation and Leisure
University of Utah
Salt Lake City, Utah 84112

VERMONT

Therapeutic Recreation Program
Department of Recreation and Leisure Studies
Lyndon State College
Lyndonville, Vermont 05851

VIRGINIA

Therapeutic Recreation Program
Department of Therapeutic Recreation
Longwood College
Farmville, Virginia 23901

Therapeutic Recreation Program
Department of Leisure Services
Ferrum College
Ferrum, Virginia 24088

Therapeutic Recreation Program
Department of Leisure Studies
Old Dominion University
Norfolk, Virginia 23508

Therapeutic Recreation Program
Department of Recreation and Leisure Studies
Virginia Wesleyan College
Norfolk, Virginia 23502

Therapeutic Recreation Program
Department of Recreation and Leisure Studies
Radford University
Radford, Virginia 24142

Therapeutic Recreation Program
Department of Recreation, Parks, and Tourism
Virginia Commonwealth University
Richmond, Virginia 23284

WASHINGTON

Therapeutic Recreation Program
Department of Recreation
Western Washington University
Bellingham, Washington 98225

Therapeutic Recreation Program
Department of Recreation and Leisure Studies
Eastern Washington University
Cheney, Washington 99004

Therapeutic Recreation Assistant

The *therapeutic recreation assistant* assists the therapeutic recreation specialist in carrying out recreation rehabilitation programs in hospitals and communities. The assistant usually has limited responsibilities in organizing and directing programs and more often specializes in particular activities such as athletics, dramatics, music or arts and crafts.

For training the assistant must graduate from an associate degree program in therapeutic recreation or recreation with an option in therapeutic recreation from a community college or university.

Credentials are available to those individuals who meet the National Council for Therapeutic Recreation Certification's prerequisites. Applicants should have either 1) an associates degree in therapeutic recreation or recreation with an option in therapeutic recreation, or 2) an associates degree in recreation plus one year full-time paid experience in a therapeutic recreation setting, or 3) a major in a related career such as allied health, art, education, dance, drama, gerontology, human services, mental health, music education or physical education, and one year full-time paid experience in a therapeutic recreation setting, or 4) completion of a National Therapeutic Recreation Society approved 750-hour training program for therapeutic recreation paraprofessionals, or 5) four years full-time paid experience in a therapeutic recreation setting.

Salaries for therapeutic recreation assistants vary by geographic location and size and type of facility. According to information provided by the National Therapeutic Recreation Society, salaries range from $9,000 a year for entry level positions, up to $17,000 a year for experienced assistants.

For more information on careers, or National Therapeutic Recreation Society approved training programs for therapeutic recreation paraprofessionals, write the National Therapeutic Recreation Society, c/o National Recreation and Park Association, 3101 Park Center Drive, Arlington, Virginia 22302.

Information on certification requirements can be obtained through the National Council for Therapeutic Recreation Certification, 49 South Main Street, Suite #005, Spring Valley, New York 10977.

For training programs contact community colleges and universities in your area or write to the National Therapeutic Recreation Society at the above address.

SOURCES:

National Therapeutic Recreation Society
Occupational Outlook Handbook

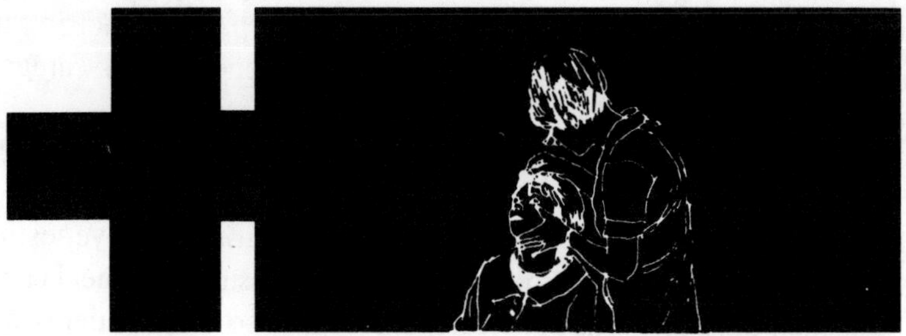

VISION CARE

There are many specialized fields in the medical practice of vision care, including optometry, ophthalmology, orthoptics, and opticianry. The optometrist is a doctor of optometry who examines eyes and related structures, detects visual abnormalities, and prescribes either corrective lenses or orthoptic procedures to preserve or restore maximum vision, or refers the patient to an ophthalmologist. The ophthalmologist is a medical physician who specializes in the diagnosis and treatment of all eye diseases and abnormal eye conditions. The ophthalmologist also prescribes drugs, corrective lenses, and other treatments. Both the optometrist and the ophthalmologist are professionally licensed medical practitioners and have graduated from schools of optometry and medicine, respectively.

Orthoptics is the clinical science of ocular motility, and orthoptists use visual training aids in the treatment of crossed eyes and other eye disorders. Opticianry is the science of optics; and opticians translate, fill, and adjust ophthalmic and optometric prescriptions, products, and accessories. The optician may be employed either as a dispensing optician, an ophthalmic laboratory technician, or as both.

Discussed below are the allied health careers in vision care of the *paraoptometric, (optometric assistant, optometric technician),* the *ophthalmic medical assistant,* the *orthoptist,* the *dispensing optician,* and the *ophthalmic laboratory technician.*

Paraoptometric: Optometric Assistant, Optometric Technician

The paraoptometric serves as a technical aide, under the direct supervision of an optometrist, and may be classified as either an *optometric assistant* or as a more highly trained *optometric technician*. The functions of a paraoptometric vary, but usually include several responsibilities in one or more of three general work categories: office, technical, and ophthalmic duties.

Office duties include scheduling appointments, record keeping, recording patients' case histories, preparing patients for examinations, and recording examination results. Technical duties consist of assisting the optometrist with eye testing procedures such as determining angle and width of visual field, measuring corneal curvature, and measuring intraocular pressure. The paraoptometric may also assist patients with vision training and eye coordination exercises if they suffer from focusing defects. If the optometrist dispenses corrective lenses, then the paraoptometric may also assist in facial measurement and frame selection, or in the fitting of contact lenses. The paraoptometric often provides instruction to patients on lens care procedures.

In some circumstances the paraoptometric, if sufficiently trained, may be engaged in ophthalmic duties in a laboratory, where she or he modifies conventional glasses or contact lenses, keeps an inventory of ophthalmic materials, and cleans and cares for the laboratory instruments.

In a small optometrist's practice, the paraoptometric may perform all of the above duties, whereas in a larger practice there may be specialization in either vision training, chairside assistance, office management, or laboratory or contact lens work. Most paraoptometrics are employed by optometrists in their private practices, while the remainder work in health clinics and vision care centers.

The paraoptometric may work with patients of all ages, from young children with vision or reading problems to the elderly who may require special therapeutic devices to improve declining vision.

Although most are trained on-the-job in an optometrist's office, the optometric assistant may, as an alternative, receive formal training in a one-year certificate program offered by a community college or vocational-technical school. The optometric technician, on the other hand, must complete a two-year associate degree program to gain more comprehensive training in the technical aspects of optometry. Optometric technician programs are offered at community and junior colleges, vocational-technical institutes, and through several schools of optometry.

High school graduation or its equivalent is required for acceptance into an academic or an on-the-job training program, and recommended high school subjects include courses in English, mathematics and office procedures.

Registration as a paraoptometric assistant and technician is available to those individuals who meet specific educational and/or experience requirements and successfully pass the American Optometric Association's registration examination.

Depending upon the size and the type of optometrist's practice, geographic location, and level of education, starting salaries generally range from $7,500 to $9,500 a year for the optometric assistant, and $8,500 to $15,000 for the optometric technician.

Below is a list, supplied by the American Optometric Association, of schools that offer certificate and associate degree programs in paraoptometrics. Those interested in on-the-job training as an optometric assistant, should contact their local or state optometric society or refer to the yellow pages of the telephone directory for potential employers who may have entry-level positions.

For additional information on registration or career opportunities as a paraoptometric, contact the American Optometric Association, 243 North Lindbergh Avenue, St. Louis, Missouri 63141.

KEY:

(1) One-year program awarding certificate

(2) Two-year program awarding associate degree

SOURCES:

American Optometric Association
Occupational Outlook Handbook

Paraoptometric Programs

FLORIDA

Optometric Assistant Program (1)
McFatter Vocational Technical Center
6500 Nova Drive
Davie, Florida 33310

Optometric Technology Program (2)
Miami-Dade Community College
Medical Center Campus
950 N.W. 20th Street
Miami, Florida 33127

Optometric Technology Program (2)
St. Petersburg Community College
P.O. Box 13489
St. Petersburg, Florida 33733

Optometric Assistant Program (1)
Erwin Vocational Technical Area Center
2010 E. Hillsborough Avenue
Tampa, Florida 33610

INDIANA

Optometric Technology Program (2)
Indiana University
School of Optometry
800 E. Atwater Avenue
Bloomington, Indiana 47405

IOWA

Optometric Assistant Program (1)
North Iowa Area Community College
Health Programs Department
Mason City, Iowa 50401

MARYLAND

Optometric Assistant Program (1)
Howard Community College
Little Patuxent Parkway
Columbia, Maryland 21044

MASSACHUSETTS

Optometric Technology Program (2)
NEWENCO
424 Beacon Street
Boston, Massachusetts 02116

MICHIGAN

Optometric Technology Program (2)
Ferris State College
School of Allied Health
Big Rapids, Michigan 49307

Optometric Technology Program (2)
Macomb County Community College
44575 Garfield
Mt. Clemens, Michigan 48044

MINNESOTA

Optometric Assistant Program (1)
Granite Falls Area Vocational Technical Institute
Granite Falls, Minnesota 56241

Optometric Assistant Program (1)
St. Cloud Area Vocational Technical Institute
1540 Northway Drive
St. Cloud, Minnesota 56301

NEBRASKA

Optometric Assistant Program (1)
Mid-Plains Community College
Interstate 80 at Highway 83
North Platte, Nebraska 69101

OHIO

Optometric Technology Program (2)
Columbus Technical Institute
550 East Spring
Columbus, Ohio 43215

Optometric Technology Program (2)
Owens Technical College
Oregon Road
Toledo, Ohio 43699

PENNSYLVANIA

Optometric Technology Program (2)
Manor Junior College
Fox Chase and Forrest Avenue
Jenkintown, Pennsylvania 19046

SOUTH CAROLINA

Optometric Technology Program (2)
Greenville Technical
P.O. Box 5616 Station B
Greenville, South Carolina 29606

WASHINGTON

Optometric Technology Program (2)
Spokane Community College
N. 1810 Greene Street
Health Science Building
Spokane, Washington 99207

WISCONSIN

Optometric Assistant Program (1)
Lakeshore Technical Institute
1290 North Avenue
Cleveland, Wisconsin 53015

Optometric Technology Program (2)
Madison Area Technical College
211 North Carroll Street
Madison, Wisconsin 53703

Ophthalmic Medical Assistant

The *ophthalmic medical assistant* aids and is supervised by the ophthalmologist in the diagnosis and treatment of medical and surgical eye problems. The ophthalmic medical assistant collects data necessary for the ophthalmologist to make diagnoses, and assists him or her in the care of patients.

The ophthalmic assistant performs a large number of routine technical procedures involving vision measurement tests and direct patient care. The assistant records medical histories, measures patients' visual acuity, eye movement, field of vision, color vision, intraocular pressure, corneal curvature, and also measures the power of corrective lenses. In direct patient care, the ophthalmic assistant changes eye dressings and administers eye drops. The assistant may also make adjustments and minor repairs to ophthalmic instruments and corrective lenses.

Ophthalmic medical assistants work primarily for ophthalmologists in their private practices, but they are also employed by hospitals, clinics, and university research and training centers.

Certification by the Joint Commission on Allied Health Personnel in Ophthalmology is awarded at one of three proficiency levels: assistant, technician, and technologist. Certification at each level is granted after meeting specific educational and experience requirements, sponsorship by an ophthalmologist, a current CPR (cardiopulmonary resuscitation) certificate and successful passing of a certification examination. As an example; candidates for the assistant (beginning) level, must have one year of work experience and successfully complete an approved training program or an approved home study course. Different educational guidelines and amount of work experience apply with higher levels of certification.

Training to become an ophthalmic medical assistant varies with the respective occupational title. Programs are affiliated with colleges and universities and offer courses lasting from a few weeks (assistant level), to four year bachelor degree programs (technologist level). Information on the American Academy of Ophthalmology's home study course can be obtained by writing to them at P.O. Box 7424, San Francisco, California 94120-7424.

Salaries for ophthalmic medical assistants vary because of geographic location, type of employee, level of certification, and amount of work experience. Recent annual average salaries for ophthalmic assistants, ranged from $9,300 in the Northeast, to $10,700 in the South, $11,300 in the Midwest and $12,300 in the West, according to a recent survey conducted for *20/20 Magazine*.

For further information on education, training, or certification as an ophthalmic medical assistant, interested persons should write to and ask for specific information from the Joint Commission on Allied Health Personnel in Ophthalmology, 1812 North Street, Paul Road, St. Paul, Minnesota 55109. Information on specific program requirements, length of programs, and fees should be directed to the Program Director at the schools in question.

Below are three lists of training programs provided by the Joint Commission on Allied Health Personnel in Ophthalmology, the first being accredited by the Committee on Allied Health Education and Accreditation of the American Medical Association, and the second, by the Joint Commission on Allied Health Personnel in Ophthalmology, and the third, by the Canadian Medical Association. The Home Study Course for Ophthalmic Medical Assistants offered by the American Academy of Ophthalmology, is approved by the Joint Commission on Allied Health Personnel in Ophthalmology and is also listed below.

KEY:

(1) Programs accredited by the AMA's Committee on Allied Health Education and Accreditation

(2) Programs approved by the Joint Commission on Allied Health Personnel in Ophthalmology

(3) Programs approved by the Canadian Medical Association
(a) Programs for the ophthalmic medical assistant

(b) Programs for the ophthalmic medical technician or technologist
(c) Home Study Course

SOURCES:

Joint Commission on Allied Health Personnel in Ophthalmology
American Academy of Ophthalmology
20/20 Magazine

Ophthalmic Medical Assistant Programs

CALIFORNIA

Ophthalmic Assistant Program (2,a)
Ocular Technician School
Naval School of Health Sciences
San Diego, California 92134-5000

Ophthalmic Assistant Program (2,a)
Jules Stein Eye Program
800 Westwood Plaza
Los Angeles, California 90027

Home Study Course for Ophthalmic Medical Assistants (2,a,c)
American Academy of Ophthalmology
P.O. Box 7424
San Francisco, California 94120-7424

DISTRICT OF COLUMBIA

Ophthalmic Technology Assistant Program (1,b,2,b)
Department of Ophthalmology
Georgetown University Medical Center
3800 Reservoir Road, N.W.
Washington, DC 20007

FLORIDA

Ophthalmic Technology Program (1,b)
Department of Ophthalmology, College of Medicine
University of Florida
Gainesville, Florida 32610

GEORGIA

Ophthalmic Technology Program (1,b)
Orthoptic/Ophthalmic School
Emory University School of Medicine
1327 Clifton Road, N.E.
Atlanta, Georgia 30322

ILLINOIS

Ophthalmic Technician Program (1,b)
Triton College
2000 N. Fifth Avenue
River Grove, Illinois 60171

LOUISIANA

Ophthalmic Assistant Program (2,a)
Department of Ophthalmology
Tulane Medical Center
1430 Tulane Avenue
New Orleans, Louisiana 70112

MASSACHUSETTS

Ophthalmic Technology Assistant Program (1,b,2,a)
Department of Ophthalmology
Boston University Medical Center
80 East Concord Street
Boston, Massachusetts 02118

MICHIGAN

Ophthalmic Medical Assistant Program (1,b)
Detroit Institute of Ophthalmology
15415 E. Jefferson Avenue
Grosse Point Park, Michigan 48230

MINNESOTA

Ophthalmic Technician Program (1,b)
St. Paul Ramsey Medical Center
640 Jackson Street
St. Paul, Minnesota 55101

NEW JERSEY

Ophthalmic Technician Program (2,b)
Department of Ophthalmology
Eye Institute of New Jersey
15 South 9th Street
Newark, New Jersey 07107

NEW YORK

Ophthalmic Assistant Program (1,b)
New York Eye and Ear Infirmary
310 East 14th Street
New York, New York 10003

OHIO

Ophthalmic Assistant Program (2,a)
Mt. Sinai Medical Center
One Mt. Sinai Drive
Cleveland, Ohio 44106

PENNSYLVANIA

Ophthalmic Technology Program (1,b)
Scheie Eye Institute
University of Pennsylvania
51 North 39th Street
Philadelphia, Pennsylvania 19104

SOUTH CAROINA

Ophthalmic Technician Program (1,b)
Medical University of South Carolina
171 Ashley Avenue
Charleston, South Carolina 29425

TEXAS

Eye Specialist Program (2,a)
Academy of Health Sciences
Department of the Army
Ft. Sam Houston, Texas 78234

CANADA

Ophthalmic Technician Program (3,b)
Canadian Forces Medical Service
National Defense Medical Centre
Ottawa, Ontario, Canada K1A 0K6

Ophthalmic Assistant Program (3,b)
Centennial College
Box 631, Station A
Scarborough, Ontario, Canada M1K 5E9

Ophthalmic Medical Assistant Program (2,a)
Department of Ophthalmology
Stanton Yellowknife Hospital
Box 10
Yellowknife, NWT, Canada X1A, 2N1

Orthoptist

Under the supervision of an ophthalmologist the *orthoptist* is an eye muscle specialist who diagnoses and treats defects in eye coordination. The orthoptist performs diagnostic tests for visual acuity, binocular cooperation, and focusing ability, in both children and adults, and then instructs patients in the proper use of their eyes in corrective eye exercises. With appropriate training the orthoptist may also assist the ophthalmologist with visual field determination and glaucoma testing of patients, or with visual devices such as developmental glasses or prisms.

Most orthoptists work for one or more ophthalmologists in their private practice, or they are employed by clinics, hospitals, or medical schools. Some orthoptists do research, while others teach.

The prerequisite for entrance into most training programs in orthoptics is completion of two years in an accredited college or university. Some programs have additional requirements, and interested persons should contact the program directly. Training programs are 24 months in length. Some programs are shorter for those individuals certified as an ophthalmic medical technician or ophthalmic medical technologist, and wish to receive specialized training in orthoptics. Certification is awarded for those individuals who complete an accredited training program and who successfully pass the American Orthoptic Council examinations.

Depending upon geographic location and type of employer, certified orthoptists can earn starting salaries ranging from $17,500 to $23,000 a year. Certified orthoptists with several years experience may earn up to $40,000.

Below is a list of accredited training centers supplied by the American Orthoptic Council. For more information on career opportunities, training prerequisites, and certification requirements in orthoptics, interested persons should contact the American Orthoptic Council, 3914 Nakoma Road, Madison, Wisconsin 53711.

SOURCE:

American Orthoptic Council

Orthoptist Programs

CALIFORNIA

Orthoptist Program
Division of Ophthalmology Children's Hospital of Los Angeles
4650 Sunset Boulevard
Los Angeles, California 90027

FLORIDA

Orthoptist Program
Department of Ophthalmology
University of Florida
College of Medicine
Gainesville, Florida 32610

Orthoptist Program
Bascom Palmer Eye Institute
University of Miami School of Medicine
P.O. Box 016880
Miami, Florida 33101

GEORGIA

Orthoptist Program
Emory University Orthoptic Training School
School of Medicine
Atlanta, Georgia 30322

ILLINOIS

Orthoptist Program
Illinois Eye and Ear Infirmary
University of Illinois at Chicago
1855 West Taylor Street
Chicago, Illinois 60612

Orthoptist Program
Department of Ophthalmology and Visual Science
University of Chicago
939 East 57th Street
Chicago, Illinois 60637

IOWA

Orthoptist Program
Department of Ophthalmology
The University of Iowa Hospitals
Iowa City, Iowa 52242

LOUISIANA

Orthoptist Program
Children's Hospital of New Orleans
136 South Roman
New Orleans, Louisiana 70112

MARYLAND

Orthoptist Program
The Wilmer Institute
John Hopkins Hospital
Baltimore, Maryland 21205

MASSACHUSETTS

Orthoptist Program
Department of Ophthalmology
Tufts New England Medical Center
171 Harrison Avenue
Boston, Massachusetts 02111

MICHIGAN

Orthoptist Program
W.K. Kellogg Eye Center
University of Michigan
990 Wall Street
Ann Arbor, Michigan 48105-1910

Orthoptist Program
Kresge Eye Institute of Wayne State University
3994 John Road
Detroit, Michigan 48201

NEW YORK

Orthoptist Program
School of Orthoptics
New York Eye and Ear Infirmary
310 East 14th Street
New York, New York 10003

Orthoptist Program
School of Orthoptics
Presbyterian Hospital
New York, New York 10032

SOUTH CAROLINA

Orthoptist Program
Department of Ophthalmology
Medical University of South Carolina
171 Ashley Avenue
Charleston, South Carolina 29401

TEXAS

Orthoptist Program
Hermann Eye Center
University of Texas Medical School
6411 Fannin
Houston, Texas 77030-1697

Orthoptist Program
Baylor College of Medicine
Department of Ophthalmology
P.O. Box 20269
Houston, Texas 77025

WISCONSIN

Orthoptist Program
University of Wisconsin Hospital
Pediatric Eye Clinic
600 Highland Avenue
Madison, Wisconsin 53792

CANADA

Orthoptist Program
Health Centre for Children
715 West 12th Avenue
Vancouver, British Columbia, Canada V52 1M9

Orthoptist Program
Izaak Walton Killam Hospital for Children
5850 University Avenue
Box 3070
Halifax, Nova Scotia, Canada B3J 3G9

Orthoptist Program
Hospital for Sick Children
555 University Avenue
Toronto, Ontario, Canada M5G 1X8

Orthoptist Program
University Hospital
Department of Ophthalmology
Orthoptic Clinic
Saskatoon, SK, Canada S7N 0X0

Dispensing Optician

Also known as an *ophthalmic dispenser,* the dispensing optician supplies, adapts, and fits eyeglasses and/or contact lenses prescribed by ophthalmologists and optometrists. The dispensing optician does not examine eyes or prescribe corrective lenses.

Upon receipt of the prescription for eyeglasses, the dispensing optician measures the client's facial contours and assists the client in lens and frame selection. The dispenser then either writes a work order for an ophthalmic laboratory to grind the lenses, or does the grinding himself. After the lenses are ground and inserted into the frames, the dispensing optician adjusts the frames and fits them properly and comfortably onto the client's face. The dispensing optician also provides follow up care, in the event eyeglass frame readjustment or repair is needed.

In the fitting of contact lenses, which requires considerably more expertise, the dispensing optician measures the curvature of the client's corneas (the front transparent part of the eye over which the contact lenses will fit) with a special instrument, and then prepares the appropriate specifications for the contact lens manufacturer. The optician instructs the client on how to insert, remove, and care for the contact lenses.

Most dispensing opticians are employed in retail optical shops, while the remainder may own their own shops, own a franchise from a large optical chain, work for ophthalmologists or optometrists, or are employed by ophthalmic goods manufacturers or wholesalers. A dispensing optician may be employed to only supply corrective lenses, or may be trained as an ophthalmic laboratory technician, a contact lens fitter, or ocularist, (one who makes and fits artificial eyes).

The two methods of becoming trained as a dispensing optician are on-the-job training apprenticeships and formal optician educational programs. These are offered by community colleges, vocational-technical schools, and the Armed Forces. Apprenticeships last three to four years, and include training in optical mathematics and physics, laboratory equipment, and office management and sales. Formal dispensing programs offered by schools are twenty-four months in length and award associate degrees upon graduation. The National Academy of Opticianry, at 10111 Martin Luther King Highway, Suite 112, Bowie, Maryland 20715-4299, offers a home-study course with an award of a Certificate of Completion.

Currently, twenty-six states require that their practicing dispensing opticians be licensed. Licensure information is available from the state's licensing division, located in the state capitol. Certification examinations are available in dispensing opticianry and contact lens-fitting, from the American Board of Opticianry/National Contact Lens Examiners, 10341 Democracy Lane, P.O. Box 10110, Fairfax, Virginia 22030.

Recommended high school courses for those students interested in a career in opticianry include physics, algebra, geometry, and mechanical drawing.

According to an annual survey report conducted for *20/20 Magazine*, average regional salaries for opticians ranged from $18,400 in the West, to $19,200 in the South, $23,000 in the Midwest and $24,300 in the Northeast. According to the *Occupational Outlook Handbook,* salaries for apprentices usually start at about 60 percent of those skilled apprentices. By the end of the apprenticeship, however, their salaries are at par with beginning salaries of experienced workers.

A list of educational programs for dispensing opticians is listed following the section for ophthalmic laboratory technicians. Persons interested in further information on career opportunities in opticianry should contact the Optician's Association of America, 10341 Democracy Lane, P.O. Box 10110, Fairfax, Virginia 22030. Persons interested in potential dispensing opticianry apprenticeships in their area should contact either the state licensing board; the National Academy of Opticianry, 10111 Martin Luther King Highway, Suite 112, Bowie, Maryland 20715; their state opticianry association; or employer, if currently employed in the opticianry field.

SOURCES:

Optician's Association of America
American Board of Opticianry/National Contact Lens Examiners
National Academy of Opticianry
Commission on Opticianry Accreditation
20/20 Magazine
Occupational Outlook Handbook

Ophthalmic Laboratory Technician

Also called an *optical mechanic*, the ophthalmic laboratory technician grinds and polishes eyeglass lenses according to the specifications of a prescription, and then inserts the lenses into frames. In a large laboratory the technician may specialize in either grinding and polishing of stock-size lens blanks, or in the cutting, edging, and smoothing and assembling the lenses and the frames. Many ophthalmic laboratory technicians are also trained to become contact lens fitters and/or dispensing opticians.

Formal training programs for the ophthalmic laboratory technician, one year in length, are offered by community colleges and vocational technical schools. Additional training is required to grind contact lenses. Further information on training in the ophthalmic laboratory may be obtained from the Optician's Association of America, 10341 Democracy Lane, P.O. Box 10110, Fairfax, Virginia 22030.

According to an annual salary report conducted for *20/20 Magazine*, average regional salaries for laboratory technicians ranged from the lowest, $8,600 in the West, to the highest, $12,000 in the Midwest.

Below is a list of formal educational programs in opticianry, accredited by the Commission on Opticianry Accreditation, for dispensing opticians and for ophthalmic laboratory technicians.

KEY:

(1) Dispensing optician program

(2) Ophthalmic laboratory technician program

SOURCES:

Optician's Association of American
Commission on Opticianry Accreditation
20/20 Magazine

Dispensing Optician and Ophthalmic Laboratory Technician Programs

ARIZONA

Dispensing Optician Program (1)
Pima Community College
2202 W. Anklam Road
Tucson, Arizona 85709-0001

CALIFORNIA

Dispensing Optician Program (1)
Canada College
4200 Farm Hill Boulevard
Redwood City, California 94061

FLORIDA

Dispensing Optician Program (1)
Miami-Dade Community College
950 N.W. 20th Street
Miami, Florida 33127

Ophthalmic Laboratory Technician Program (2)
St. Petersburg Vocational Technical Institute
901 34th Street, South
St. Petersburg, Florida 33711

Dispensing Optician Program (1)
Hillsborough Community College
P.O. Box 30030
Tampa, Florida 33630

MINNESOTA

Ophthalmic Laboratory Technician Program (2)
Anoka Area Vocational Technical Institute
1355 West Main
Anoka, Minnesota 55303

Ophthalmic Laboratory Technician Program (2)
Eveleth Area Vocational Technical Institute
Eveleth, Minnesota 55734

NEW JERSEY

Dispensing Optician Program (1)
Camden County College
P.O. Box 200
Blackwood, New Jersey 08012

Dispensing Optician Program (1)
Essex County College
303 University Avenue
Newark, New Jersey 07102

NEW YORK

Dispensing Optician Program (1)
New York City Technical College
300 Jay Street
Brooklyn, New York 11201

Dispensing Optician Program (1)
Erie Community College
North Campus
Main Street and Youngs Road
Buffalo, New York 14221

Dispensing Optician Program (1)
Mater Del College
Riverside Drive
Ogdensburg, New York 13669

NORTH CAROLINA

Dispensing Optician Program (1)
Durham Technical Community College
1637 Lawson Street
Durham, North Carolina 27703

OHIO

Dispensing Optician Program (1)
Cuyahoga Community College
4250 Richmond Road
Warrensville Township, Ohio 44122

TEXAS

Dispensing Optician Program (1)
El Paso Community College
P.O. Box 20500
El Paso, Texas 79998

VIRGINIA

Dispensing Optician Program (1)
J. Sargeant Reynolds Community College
P.O. Box C-32040
Richmond, Virginia 23261-2040

OTHER CAREERS WITHIN THE HEALTHCARE FACILITY

In hospitals and other healthcare facilities there are many clerical and staff positions that do not require specific health-related education or training. For example, in many hospital administrative, and physical plant departments there are jobs and careers at all levels - from clerk and secretary, to technican and engineer, to administrative assistant and unit manager that require no formal medical or health education. Thus in *finance, business, communications, information management, human resources, public relations, patient admissions, purchasing, housekeeping, volunteer services, central services,* and *security* and *maintenance,* a general educational background ranging from a high school education to vocational training to a bachelor's degree in social sciences or business may very well be sufficient training for certain job responsibilities.

For information on career opportunities in these fields, interested students should talk with Directors of Human Resources at area healthcare facilities, instructors at postsecondary institutions and with individuals currently employed in the healthcare field.

One other way to learn more about careers in healthcare administration is through membership in professional organizations. Members, through newsletters and other publications, are kept abreast of healthcare issues and can share ideas and expertise with other professionals in their field. Often these organizations offer student and affiliate memberships. The American Hospital Association offers several personal membership groups to professionals in the health fields of volunteer services, healthcare education and training, social work, hospital engineering, hospital risk management, marketing, personnel administration, information management, patient representation, ambulatory care, central service and materials management. For information on the Personal Membership Groups, write to The American Hospital Association, 840 North Lake Shore Drive, Chicago, Illinois 60611.

Central Service Technician

Working in a hospital's Central Service Department the *central service technician's* primary responsibility is the cleaning and sterilizing of medical supplies, instruments, and equipment, according to prescribed procedures and techniques. Usually working under minimal supervision of the director of central service, who is usually a registered nurse, the technician receives or collects contaminated surgical instruments, gloves, containers, treatment trays, syringes, and other supplies and equipment from operating rooms, patient wards, emergency units, outpatient departments, and laboratories, and either disinfects these items with antiseptic solutions or gases, or sterilizes them in steam autoclaves or in similar equipment. The technician then stores the items or distributes them to their appropriate hospital unit or department.

The central service technician also assembles, labels, and seals sterile and nonsterile treatment and dressing trays or packs including blood transfusion sets, surgical trays, intravenous infusion sets, and obstetrical packs. The technician is also responsible for being able to operate and sometimes repair or adjust equipment such as resuscitators, ambulance equipment, orthopedic equipment, oxygen tents and masks, and some monitoring equipment.

Although some employers prefer their central service technicians to be licensed practical nurses, most require only high school education as the entrance requirements for their three-to-six months on-the-job training programs. Courses in central service technology have been recently introduced into vocational-technical schools and are expected to increase in number in accordance with the continued rise in demand for more highly trained technicians. With experience, competence, and training the central service technician may advance to senior central service technician or to departmental assistant supervisor.

For additional information on career opportunities in central service technology, interested persons should contact the Personnel Director of their local hospital or the American Society for Healthcare Central Service Personnel of the American Hospital Association, 840 North Lake Shore Drive, Chicago, Illinois 60611.

SOURCE:

American Society for Healthcare Service Personnel of the American Hospital Association

---

Hospital Admitting Officer

In a hospital the *admitting officer* arranges the admission and discharge of patients in accordance with physicians' requests, hospital policies, and the availability of facilities in the hospital. As the first person to meet the incoming patient, the admitting officer should be courteous and understanding and not cause the patient any undue anxiety. She or he interviews the patient or the patient's relatives for biographical data and explains hospital services, charges, insurance coverages, and payment procedures. The admitting officer also notifies the appropriate ward and hospital department of the patient's admittance. Other duties may include the supervising and the training of *assistant admitting officers* and *admitting clerks* in a large healthcare facility. Or, in a small healthcare facility, the admitting officer may work alone in the admitting office but also carry out certain duties in the credit department. Whatever the place of employment the admitting officer is responsible to the controller, associate administrator, or business manager.

A bachelor's degree with a major in psychology, sociology, personnel relations, or business administration, plus two-to-three months of on-the-job training is the usual educational requirement for the position of admitting officer. One-or-two years experience working in a healthcare facility or social agency is also required by some hospitals for employment.

Salaries for admitting officers vary depending upon experience and the size and location of the facility.

For additional information on career opportunities and training as an admitting office, an assistant admitting officer, or as an admitting clerk, interested persons should contact the Personnel Director of their local hospital.

Ward Clerk

Also known as nursing units, pavilions, or floors, hospital wards are areas in a hospital where nursing care is provided to a group of patients. The *ward clerk* assists the unit's nursing staff by performing a variety of clerical tasks that ensure the efficient operation of the nursing unit. The ward clerk provides services both for the patients and also for the management of the hospital. These services can be divided into four categories: reception, communication, clerical, and safety.

Receptionist duties include receiving new patients, directing visitors, and providing patient information to physicians, nurses, and other medical staff upon request. Communication duties include answering the phone, answering patient requests on the intercom system, and delivering mail and messages for patients. With a certain degree of knowledge of medical terminology the ward clerk also can operate hospital communication systems and help to coordinate the activities of medical personnel on the ward. The ward clerk's clerical duties include transcribing physicians' orders, copying and compiling data on patients' charts, and scheduling tests and other appointments for patients. She or he also maintains essential records for the operation of the nursing unit such as recording hours worked and absenteeism of unit personnel, filing records and reports, verifying stock inventory, and requesting additional supplies and equipment when shortages occur. Finally, the clerk's responsibilities for ward safety include helping keep work areas clean, eliminating potential accident hazards, and making emergency code calls when required.

Most training of ward clerks has previously occurred on-the-job, but more and more hospitals today are tending to employ candidates who have graduated from a formal educational course in ward clerk skills. These courses are offered by secondary schools, community colleges, vocational schools, and adult educational centers and usually last from a period of six weeks to one year.

Recommended high school courses for students who are looking into a career as a ward clerk include English, secretarial skills, and mathematics.

Persons interested in career opportunities and training as a ward clerk should contact the Personnel Director of their local hospital.

Appendix A: State Departments of Public Health

ALABAMA

Department of Public Health
Montgomery, Alabama 36130

ALASKA

Department of Health and Social Services
Division of Public Health
P.O. Box H
Juneau, Alaska 99811

ARIZONA

Department of Health Services
1740 West Adams Street
Phoenix, Arizona 85007

ARKANSAS

State Department of Health
4815 West Markham Street
Little Rock, Arkansas 72205

CALIFORNIA

Department of Health Services
714 P Street
Sacramento, California 95814

COLORADO

State Department of Health
4210 East Eleventh Avenue
Denver, Colorado 80220

CONNECTICUT

Department of Health Services
150 Washington Street
Hartford, Connecticut 06106

DELAWARE

Department of Health and Social Services
Division of Public Health
P.O. Box 637
Dover, Delaware 19903

DISTRICT OF COLUMBIA

Department of Human Services
1875 Connecticut Avenue, N.W., Room 825
Washington, D.C. 20009

FLORIDA

Department of Health and Rehabilitative Services
State Health Office
1323 Winewood Boulevard
Tallahassee, Florida 32399

GEORGIA

Department of Human Resources
Division of Public Health
878 Peachtree Street, N.E.
Atlanta, Georgia 30309

HAWAII

Department of Health
P.O. Box 3378
Honolulu, Hawaii 96801

IDAHO

Department of Health and Welfare
Statehouse
Boise, Idaho 83720

ILLINOIS

Department of Public Health
535 West Jefferson Street
Springfield, Illinois 62761

INDIANA

Indiana State Board of Health
1330 West Michigan Street
Indianapolis, Indiana 46206

IOWA

Department of Health
Lucas State Office Building
Des Moines, Iowa 50319

KANSAS

Department of Health and Environment
Forbes Air Force Base
Topeka, Kansas 66620

KENTUCKY

Department for Health Services
275 East Main Street
Frankfort, Kentucky 40601

LOUISIANA

Department of Health and Human Resources
P.O. Box 3776
Baton Rouge, Louisiana 70821

MAINE

Department of Human Services
State House
Augusta, Maine 04330

MARYLAND

Department of Health and Mental Hygiene
201 West Preston Street
Baltimore, Maryland 21201

MASSACHUSETTS

Department of Public Health
150 Tremont Street
Boston, Massachusetts 02111

MICHIGAN

Department of Public Health
3423 North Logan Street
Lansing, Michigan 48909

MINNESOTA

Department of Health
717 Delaware Street, S.E.
Minneapolis, Minnesota 55440

MISSISSIPPI

Board of Health
P.O. Box 1700
Jackson, Mississippi 39215

MISSOURI

Department of Social Services
Division of Health
Jefferson City, Missouri 65102

MONTANA

Department of Health and Environmental Sciences
Cogswell Building
Helena, Montana 59620

NEBRASKA

Department of Health
301 Centennial Mall S.
Lincoln, Nebraska 68509

NEVADA

Department of Human Resources
Capitol Complex
Carson City, Nevada 89710

NEW HAMPSHIRE

Department of Health and Welfare
Division of Public Health Services
6 Hazen Drive
Concord, New Hampshire 03301

NEW JERSEY

Department of Health
CN 360
Trenton, New Jersey 08625

NEW MEXICO

Department of Health and Environment
435 Michaels Drive
Santa Fe, New Mexico 87501

NEW YORK

Department of Health
Empire State Plaza, Tower Building
Albany, New York 12237

NORTH CAROLINA

Department of Human Resources
Division of Health Services
225 North McDowell Street
Raleigh, North Carolina 27602

NORTH DAKOTA

Department of Health
State Capitol
Bismarck, North Dakota 58505

OHIO

Department of Health
246 North High Street
Columbus, Ohio 43215

OKLAHOMA

Department of Health
P.O. Box 53551
Oklahoma City, Oklahoma 73152

OREGON

Department of Human Resources
Health Division
1400 Southwest Fifth Avenue
Portland, Oregon 97201

PENNSYLVANIA

Department of Health
P.O. Box 90
Harrisburg, Pennsylvania 17120

RHODE ISLAND

Department of Health
75 Davis Street
Providence, Rhode Island 02908

SOUTH CAROLINA

Department of Health and Environmental Control
2600 Bull Street
Columbia, South Carolina 29201

SOUTH DAKOTA

Department of Health
State Capitol Building
Pierre, South Dakota 57501

TENNESSEE

Department of Public Health
344 Cordell Hull Building
Nashville, Tennessee 37219

TEXAS

Department of Health
1100 West Forty-Ninth Street
Austin, Texas 78756

UTAH

Department of Health
P.O. Box 2500
Salt Lake City, Utah 84110

VERMONT

Health Department
60 Main Street
Burlington, Vermont 05401

VIRGINIA

Department of Health
400 Madison Building
Richmond, Virginia 23219

WASHINGTON

Department of Social and Health Services
Health Services Division
Mail Stop OB-44
Olympia, Washington 98504

WEST VIRGINIA

Department of Health
1800 Washington Street, East
Charleston, West Virginia 25305

WISCONSIN

Department of Health and Social Services
Division of Health
1 West Wilson Street
Madison, Wisconsin 53707

WYOMING

Division of Health and Medical Services
Hathaway Building
Cheyenne, Wyoming 82002

Appendix B: List of Associations

American Academy of Ophthalmology
P.O. Box 7424
San Francisco, California 94120-7424

American Academy of Physician Assistants
950 North Washington Street
Alexandria, Virginia 22314

American Art Therapy Association, Inc.
505 East Hawley Street
Mundelein, Illinois 60060

American Association for Counseling and Development
5999 Stevenson Avenue
Alexandria, Virginia 22304

American Association for Laboratory Animal Science
70 Timber Creek Drive, Suite 5
Cordova, Tennessee 38018

American Association for Medical Transcription
P.O. Box 6187
Modesto, California 95355

American Association for Music Therapy
66 Morris Avenue, P.O. Box 359
Springfield, New Jersey 07081

American Association for Respiratory Care
1720 Regal Row
Dallas, Texas 75235

American Association of Blood Banks
1117 North 19th Street
Arlington, Virginia 22209

American Association of Dental Examiners
211 East Chicago Avenue
Chicago, Illinois 60611

American Association of Medical Assistants
20 North Wacker Drive, Suite 1575
Chicago, Illinois 60606

American Association of Nurse Anesthetists
216 Higgins Road
Chicago, Illinois 60068

American Association of Occupational Health Nurses
3500 Piedmont Road, N.E.
Atlanta, Georgia 30305

American Board of Opticianry/National Contact Lens Examiners
10341 Democracy Lane, P.O. Box 10110
Fairfax, Virginia 22030

American Board of Registration of Electroencephalographic Technologist's Examination
Psychological Corporation
555 Academic Street
San Antonio, Texas 78204

American Cardiology Technologists Association
1980 Issac Newton Square South
Reston, Virginia 22090

American College of Health Care Administrators
325 S. Patrick Street
Alexandria, Virginia 22314

American College of Hospital Administrators
840 N. Lake Shore Drive
Chicago, Illinois 60611

American College of Nurse-Midwives
1522 "K" Street, N.W.
Washington, D.C. 20005

American Dance Therapy Association
2000 Century Plaza, Suite 108
Columbia, Maryland 21044

American Dental Assistants Association
666 N. Lake Shore Drive
Chicago, Illinois 60611

American Dental Association
Division of Educational Measurements
211 East Chicago Avenue
Chicago, Illinois 60611

American Dental Hygienists' Association
444 N. Michigan Avenue, Suite 3400
Chicago, Illinois 60611

American Dietetic Association
216 West Jackson
Chicago, Illinois 60606

American Fund for Dental Health
211 East Chicago Avenue
Chicago, Illinois 60611

American Healthcare Association
1201 "L" Street, N.W.
Washington, D.C. 20005

American Heart Association
7320 Greenville Avenue
Dallas, Texas 75231

American Home Economic Foundation
2010 Massachusetts Ave., NW
Washington, D.C. 20036-1028

American Hospital Association
840 North Lake Shore Drive
Chicago, Illinois 60611

American Industrial Hygiene Association
475 Wolf Ledges Parkway
Akron, Ohio 44311-1087

American Kinesiotherapy Association, Inc.
259-08 148th Road
Rosedale, New York 11422

American Library Association
50 E. Huron Street
Chicago, Illinois 60611

American Massage Therapy Association, Inc.
1130 W. North Shore Avenue
Chicago, Illinois 60626

American Medical Record Association
875 N. Michigcan Avenue, Suite 1850
Chicago, Illinois 60611

American Medical Technologists
710 Higgins Road
Park Ridge, Illinois 60068

American Medical Writer's Association
9650 Rockville Pike
Bethesda, Maryland 20814

American National Red Cross
431 18th Street, N.W.
Washington, D.C. 20006

American Nephrology Nurses Association
4903 Glenmeadow Drive
Houston, Texas 77096

American Nurses Association
2420 Pershing Road
Kansas City, Missouri 64108

American Occupational Therapy Association, Inc.
1383 Piccard Drive
Rockville, Maryland 20850

American Optometric Association
243 North Lindbergh Avenue
St. Louis, Missouri 63141

American Orthoptic Council
3914 Nakoma Road
Madison, Wisconsin 53711

American Physical Therapy Association
1111 North Fairfax Street
Alexandria, Virginia 22314

American Psychiatric Association
1400 "K" Street, N.W.
Washington, D.C. 20005

American Psychological Association
1200 17th Street, N.W.
Washington, D.C. 20036

American Registry for Diagnostic Medical Sonographers
32 E. Hollister Street
Cincinnati, Ohio 45219

American Registry of Radiologic Technologists
2600 Wayzata Boulevard
Minneapolis, Minnesota 55405

American Society for Healthcare Central Service Personnel
840 North Lake Shore Drive
Chicago, Illinois 60611

American Society of Clinical Pathologists
2100 W. Harrison Street
Chicago, Illinois 60612

American Society of Cytology
130 South 9th Street
Philadelphia, Pennsylvania 19107

American Society of Directors of Volunteer Services
840 North Lake Shore Drive
Chicago, Illinois 60611

American Society of Electroneurodiagnostic Technologists
Sixth at Quint
Carroll, Iowa 51401

American Society of Radiologic Technologists
15000 Central Avenue, S.E.
Albuquerque, New Mexico 87123

American Society of Safety Engineers
1800 E. Oakton Street
Des Plaines, Illinois 60018-2187

American Veterinary Medical Association
930 North Meacham Road
Schaumburg, Illinois 60196

Association for Medical Illustrators
2692 Huguenot Springs Road
Midlothian, Virginia 23113

Association for the Advancement of Health Education
1900 Association Drive
Reston, Virginia 22091

Association for the Advancement of Medical Instrumentation
3330 Washington Boulevard
Arlington, Virginia 22201

Association of Operating Room Nurses
10170 E. Mississippi Avenue
Denver, Colorado 80231

Association of Physician Assistant Programs
950 North Washington Street
Alexandria, Virginia 22314

Association of Schools of Public Health
1015 15th Street, N.W., Suite 404
Washington, D.C. 20005

Association of Surgical Technologists, Inc.
8307 Shaffer Parkway
Littleton, Colorado 80127

Association of University Programs in Health Administration
1911 N. Fort Myer Drive, Suite 503
Arlington, Virginia 22209

Biological Photographic Association
115 Stoneridge Drive
Chapel Hill, North Carolina 27514

Biomedical Engineering Society
P.O. Box 2399
Culver City, California 90231

Board for Certification in Orthotics and Prosthetics
717 Pendleton Street
Alexandria, Virginia 22314

Broadcast Education Association
1771 "N" Street, N.W.
Washington, D.C. 20036

Canadian Nurses Association
50 The Driveway
Ontario, Canada K2P 1E2

Cardiovascular Credentialing International
2801 Farhills
Dayton, Ohio 45419

Certification Board for Music Therapists
c/o ASI Processing Center
718 Arch Street
Philadelphia, Pennsylvania 19106

Dental Assisting National Board, Inc.
216 East Ontario Street
Chicago, Illinois 60611

Dietary Managers Association
400 East 22nd Street
Lombard, Illinois 60148

Emergency Nurses Association
230 E. Ohio Street
Chicago, Illinois 60611

Health Occupations Students of America
4108 Amon Carter Boulevard
Fort Worth, Texas 76155

Health Sciences Communications Association
6105 Lindell Boulevard
St. Louis, Missouri 63112

Institute of Food Technologists
221 North LaSalle Street
Chicago, Illinois 60601

International Society for Clinical Laboratory Technology
818 Olive Street
St. Louis, Missouri 63101

Joint Commission on Allied Health Personnel in Ophthalmology
1812 North Street, Pave Road
St. Paul, Minnesota 55109

Joint Review Committee for Respiratory Therapy Education
1701 W. Euless Blvd., Suite 200
Euless, Texas 76040

Medical Library Association
6 North Michigan Avenue, Suite 300
Chicago, Illinois 60602

National Academy of Opticianry
10111 Martin Luther King Hwy., Suite 112
Bowie, Maryland 20715-4299

National Association for Drama Therapy
19 Edwards Street
New Haven, Connecticut 06511

National Association for Music Therapy
505 Eleventh Street, S.E.
Washington, D.C. 20003

National Association for Poetry Therapy
225 Williams Street
Huron, Ohio 44839

National Association of Dental Laboratories
3801 Mt. Vernon Avenue
Alexandria, Virginia 22305

National Association of Emergency Medical Technicians
9140 Ward Parkway
Kansas City, Missouri 64114

National Association of Pediatric Nurse Associates and Practitioners
1101 Kings Highway North
Cherry Hill, New Jersey 08034

National Association of Social Workers
7981 Eastern Avenue
Silver Spring, Maryland 20910

National Athletic Trainers Association
P.O. Box Drawer 1865
Greenville, North Carolina 27834

National Board for Respiratory Care
11015 West 75th Terrace
Shawnee Mission, Kansas 66214

National Certification Agency for Medical Laboratory Personnel
P.O. Box 705, Ben Franklin Station
Washington, D.C. 20044

National Committee on Certification of Physician's Assistants
2845 Henderson Mill Road, N.E.
Atlanta, Georgia 30341

National Council for Therapeutic Recreation Certification
49 South Main Street, Suite #005
Spring Valley, New York 10977

National Environmental Health Association
720 S. Colorado Boulevard, Suite 970
South Tower
Denver, Colorado 80222

National Executive Housekeepers Association
1001 Eastwind Dr., Suite 301
Westerville, Ohio 43081

National Federation of Licensed Practical Nurses
P.O. Box 11038
Durham, North Carolina 27703

National Home Caring Council
A Division of the Foundation for Hospice and Home Care
591 "C" Street, N.E., Stanton Park
Washington, D.C. 20002

National Institute for Occupational Safety and Health
Robert A. Taft Laboratories
4676 Columbia Parkway
Cincinnati, Ohio 46226

National League for Nursing
10 Columbus Circle
New York, New York 10019

National Mental Health Association
1021 Prince Street
Alexandria, Virginia 22314

National Registry of Emergency Medical Technicians
P.O. Box 29233
Columbus, Ohio 43229

National Rehabilitation Counseling Association
633 South Washington Street
Alexandria, Virginia 22314

National Therapeutic Recreation Society
c/o National Recreation and Park Association
3101 Park Center Drive
Alexandria, Virginia 22302

Nuclear Medicine Technology Certification Board
136 Madison Avenue
New York, New York 10016

Nurses Association of the American College of
Obstetricians and Gynecologists
600 Maryland Avenue, S.W.
Washington, D.C. 20024

Oncology Nursing Society
1016 Greentree Road
Pittsburgh, Pennsylvania 15220

Optician's Association of America
10341 Democracy Lane, P.O. Box 10110
Fairfax, Virginia 22030

Society for Public Health Education, Inc.
2001 Addison Street, Suite 220
Berkeley, California 94704

Society of Biomedical Equipment Technicians
3330 Washington Boulevard
Arlington, Virginia 22201

Society of Diagnostic Medical Sonographers
12225 Greenville Avenue, Suite 434
Dallas, Texas 75243

Society of Nuclear Medicine
136 Madison Avenue
New York, New York 10016